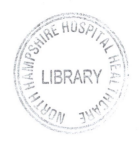

Essential Coloproctology for Nurses

This publication has been made available to you by:

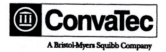

A Bristol-Myers Squibb Company

as part of their commitment to
continuing professional development in stoma care

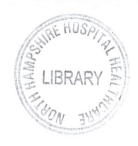

Essential Coloproctology for Nurses

Theresa Porrett RGN

*Nurse Practitioner in Coloproctology, Homerton Hospital,
London, UK*

Norma Daniel RN, MS, CNOR, RNFA

*Surgical Nurse Clinician, Colorectal Department,
Cleveland Clinic Florida, Florida, USA*

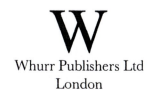

Whurr Publishers Ltd
London

© 1999 Whurr Publishers Ltd
First published 1999 by
Whurr Publishers Ltd
19b Compton Terrace, London N1 2UN, England

Reprinted 1999

British Library Cataloguing in Publication Data
A catalogue record for this book is available from the British
Library.

ISBN 1 86156 085 0
Printed and bound by CPI Antony Rowe, Eastbourne
Reprinted 2006

Printed and bound in the UK by Athenaeum Press Ltd,
Gateshead, Tyne & Wear

Contents

Acknowledgements   ix
Preface   xi
Foreword   xiii
Introduction   xv

Chapter 1   **1**
Developing and Extended Practice: The UK and US Perspectives
Marion Allison and Chantal Leconte

Chapter 2   **21**
Anatomy and Physiology of the Colon, Rectum and Anus
J. Marcio N. Jorge

Chapter 3   **52**
Investigation and Examination of a Patient with Colorectal Problems
Laurence R. Sands and Norma Daniel

Chapter 4   **76**
Common Anal Conditions
Peter J. Lunniss and Theresa Porrett

Chapter 5   **97**
Colorectal Cancer
Eric G. Weiss and Thelma E. Johnson

Chapter 6   **119**
Inflammatory Bowel Disease: The Nursing Implications
Jacqueline Joels

Chapter 7   **146**
Familial Adenomatous Polyposis
Juan J. Nogueras and Ellen McGannon

Chapter 8   **165**
Faecal Stomas
Siobhan McCahon

Chapter 9   **188**
Diverticular Disease
Marc E. Sher, Leslie Cheney and Julia Ricciardi

Chapter 10   **206**
Constipation
Elinor Teahon

Chapter 11   **222**
Irritable Bowel Syndrome
Paula Taylor

Chapter 12   **256**
Laparoscopic Colorectal Surgery
Mara Rita Salum, Steven D. Wexner, Norma Daniel and Muraleen Gustin

Chapter 13   **292**
The Modern Management of Faecal Incontinence
Barbara Stuchfield and A.J.P. Eccersley

Chapter 14   **318**
Sexually Transmitted Diseases and the Acquired Immune Deficiency
Syndrome
Stephanie L. Schmitt

Chapter 15   **332**
Colorectal Problems in Paediatric Patients
Alberto Peña and Kathleen O'Connor Guardino

Chapter 16   **358**
Infectious Colitis
Margaret J. Gorensek

Chapter 17   379

Rectal Prolapse, Volvulus of the Colon and Intussusception
Luke Meleagros

Chapter 18   401

Drug Considerations in Coloproctology
Stephanie E. Guerriero and Thomas Guerriero

Index   421

Acknowledgements

This book did not write itself but was created out of the efforts of many people who have supported, helped, reviewed and guided us. We would like to thank all the contributors for taking time out of their busy schedules to write chapters for us.

Terri would particularly like to thank Bradley for his patience and understanding, the Homerton Hospital Surgical Nurse Team for their wonderful sense of humour and Mr P.J. Lunniss, Senior Lecturer and Honorary Consultant in Coloproctology for his advice, support and editorial assistance.

Norma would particularly like to mention Dr Steven Wexner for his insightful guidance and encouragement, Elektra McDermott for her editorial assistance, Robert Cravero in the Photography Department at the Cleveland Clinic, Florida for his expertise and her daughters Lauren and Marsha for their support and understanding.

Preface

Coloproctology as a distinct surgical speciality has developed rapidly in the last 15 years. There have been many advances in the surgical options, treatment and management for patients with colorectal disease. This book has been written as a reference for all nurses who work in the speciality of coloproctology. Nurses from all areas of the health care environment come into contact with patients with colorectal problems and therefore this text has been written so that it is appropriate and relevant for nurses working in a variety of health care settings such as the operating room, clinic or acute care setting. The number of specialist nursing roles in coloproctology is increasing and it is hoped that this text will provide a valuable and relevant reference for those wishing to develop their expertise in this field.

We have attempted to deal with all aspects of coloproctology through the contributions of experts in the field, who in each chapter have emphasized the nursing implications of each topic covered. Patients with colorectal problems often feel stigmatized by the nature of their condition and many find the subject embarrassing and difficult to discuss. It is often the sensitive and informed nurse who supports, educates and advises the patient through his/her investigations, treatment and adaptation and therefore the impact that nurses can have on the quality of care outcomes should not be underestimated.

By choosing expert contributors from the UK and USA we hope we have presented the reader with current best practice examples. Although health care systems vary we can all learn from the experiences of our colleagues and the methods and treatment modalities they have developed.

We hope that the reader will find the information contained in this text useful in the management and understanding of patients with colorectal problems and that it will go some way to ensuring that the level of nursing services for patients continues to develop alongside our medical colleagues.

Theresa Porrett
Norma Daniel

Foreword

One of the most important recent developments in clinical practice has been the widening role of the nurse in the management of patients. This has been associated with the introduction of nursing degree courses. The increasing sub-specialization in medicine and surgery has had its counterpart in nursing, with the appearance of specialist nurses even within a sub-speciality such as coloproctology. Stoma care has been established as a discipline for 30 years, but there are now nurse practitioners in proctology, incontinence, nutrition, pouch support, endoscopy, large bowel cancer and other fields.

The contribution these professionals have made to the patient through this multidisciplinary approach has been immense. The expanding role of the nurse has relieved some of the clinical burden due to increasing patient demand, but it has had much more important consequences. The nurse has a different relationship with the patient and can offer skills and support which doctors cannot supply. The opportunity to develop an extended role in nursing must be attractive to young people contemplating a career. The nurse practitioner can contribute to research in collaboration with doctors but can also initiate projects on certain aspects of care that no other group can do.

Coloproctology is a rewarding speciality. The diseases are common, they often affect young people and many can be cured. For example, large bowel cancer is one of the most prevalent tumours in industrial societies. If treated at an early stage it can be cured and high-risk groups are being increasingly recognized by clinical method, epidemiology and gene analysis. The nurse has a vital role to play in all these aspects.

Essential Coloproctology for Nurses is a timely publication. It deals with all aspects of the speciality in a practical and authoritative way. It takes the reader through the basics of anatomy and physiology and leads on to detailed chapters on clinical technique and the various colorectal diseases. The emphasis is practical but based on more than adequate theoretical information. The references are well chosen and will offer the reader a useful source of further information. The authorship reflects the multidisciplinary nature of modern practice with recognized experts in nursing, dietetics and colorectal surgery.

The book will be essential reading for any nurse involved with patients with a colorectal disorder, but in particular it will be a vital resource for those contemplating a closer interest in colorectal disease.

Professor R.J. Nicholls
Postgraduate Dean, St Mark's Hospital
Harrow, Middlesex

Introduction

Essential Coloproctology for Nurses covers key nursing issues in coloproctology. Chapter 1 deals with the implications for nurses wishing to extend their practice in the field of coloproctology, and Chapter 2 reviews the anatomy and physiology of the colon, rectum and anus prior to looking at specific disease management. Chapter 3 identifies the specific examination and investigations patients with colorectal problems may undergo. The following chapters look specifically at issues surrounding colorectal cancer, inflammatory bowel disease, familial adenomatous polyposis, diverticular disease and irritable bowel syndrome, and a general chapter outlines the issues surrounding stoma care. Faecal incontinence and constipation are common problems and the many treatment options are outlined. There are specialist chapters on sexually transmitted diseases and AIDS, laparoscopic surgery, colorectal problems in paediatric patients and infectious colitis, and the final chapter looks at pharmacology as applied to colorectal problems.

Chapter 1
Developing and Extended Practice

THE UK PERSPECTIVE

MARION ALLISON RGN, Lecturer in Stoma Care, City University, St Bartholomew School of Nursing, London

In the United Kingdom, stoma care nursing as a specialism has developed and evolved since the inception of the first post at St Bartholomew's Hospital in London in 1972. The nature of the service now offered is comprehensive, encompassing provision of specialist care before and after surgery in hospital and community settings. The importance of fulfilling the key sub-roles is widely recognized; whilst provision of direct, expert clinical care remains the primary focus (Sparacino and Cooper, 1990), educative, research, consultancy, service management and change agent elements are implemented and integrated in various ways according to patient need and the individual nurse's expertise and interests.

The local working situation inevitably varies due to the needs of patients, the nature of surgery undertaken, and the resources available within the multidisciplinary team. The wider context of reforms in the provision of health care within the National Health Service in the 1990s and publication of guidelines by the nursing profession have additionally served to bring about a reappraisal of the specialist service offered to patients, and of the direction in which this service should develop in the future.

Preparation required for specialist practice and the specific nature of that practice have only recently been defined on a national basis (UKCC, 1994). However, diversity rather than uniformity may be the hallmark of specialist nursing in this field in the future, as new opportunities arising from developments within and outside nursing are analysed and assimilated into practice by individual practitioners. This chapter explores recent significant influences on specialist practice in stoma care nursing in the United Kingdom and considers the associated implications for practitioners.

Role Development in the First 20 Years

In reviewing stoma care nursing practice and the changes that have occurred since it began 25 years ago, it could be argued that role evolution or development is the norm in this field, rather than the exception. There has been a transition from a predominantly acute, hospital-based service, focusing specifically on the needs of people with a stoma, to one which crosses traditional health care boundaries and assists the patient through all stages of rehabilitation and adaptation. The client base has widened and it is unexceptional for the stoma care nurse to include specialist care for people with enterocutaneous fistulae, percutaneous gastrostomy and complicated wounds in his or her everyday practice.

These activities may have been initiated by the specialist nurse identifying areas of unmet patient need and negotiating to include them in his/her practice or through delegated responsibility arising as a consequence of new colorectal surgical developments and techniques. What makes such delegated role development acceptable and appropriate in the latter situation is usually recognition that the unique core skills possessed by the specialist nurse and utilized with the existing client group will also be of benefit to and required by patients undergoing associated surgery.

Developing New Roles: Significant Government Influences

It is mainly in the past decade that the expanded and extended nursing role has been of increased interest (Mitchinson, 1996). However, it was in 1977 that the Department of Health and Social Security first produced guidelines which clearly stated legal and ethical implications of role extension for the professionals involved and the health authorities for which they worked (DHSS, 1977). It was recognized that in both primary and specialist health care, nurses had become increasingly involved in tasks, procedures and decision making which had previously been a medical responsibility. A number of contributory factors were identified; these included increasing complexity of treatment and growth in the specialist expertise of the nurse. The Department welcomed this trend, and provided a framework within which the nurse's role could be extended. The guidelines were intended to facilitate the flexible and efficient provision of patient care, allowing doctors greater freedom in the allocation of their time and increasing the job satisfaction of nurses.

However, in 1989, the Department considered it necessary to issue a further circular to address the difficulties which had become apparent in implementing new role developments (DHSS, 1989). These related, first, to the distance of the health authority from the clinical context in which role developments were taking place, with a resulting lack of clearly stated policies and inconsistency between health authorities. Associated with this deficiency was a lack of parity in the training provided for nurses who were undertaking delegated activities, with the consequences that in some areas this was totally inadequate and that nurses who moved between health authorities were often required to repeat their preparation. Finally, the nursing profession had reached no national consensus as to which activities actually constituted an extended role.

In the circular, the extended nursing role was clearly defined as those 'activities normally undertaken by doctors but which may be delegated in appropriate circumstances, and which may be performed by nurses with appropriate training and competence'. The term 'activities' was chosen carefully – it was intended to discourage a task-orientated approach to role development, and emphasized that the nurse's concern was with the patient as a whole person. Finally, it was stated that role-extension initiatives developed in the clinical settings in which the delegated activities were to be performed should take place only in the context of an approved policy developed by the employing authority.

Training for competence was also considered. It was recognized that approved post-registration courses could not cover all activities that were appropriate for delegation and, in these situations, training courses could either be organized at local level or individual training could be provided within the relevant clinical environment. Assessment of competence would be undertaken by the most appropriate health professional in each specific situation, who might be the clinical nurse to whom the individual practitioner was accountable, a consultant or a general practitioner.

Implementation of the recommendations stated above was intended to ensure that there would be a sound basis for the further development of the nurse's role and that, by approving policies, the employing health authority would accept liability for the nurse's actions.

However, in the intervening years, massive changes in the Health Service were being driven by new political, economic and social forces (Wright, 1995). These included widespread NHS reorganization and the introduction of a market-led service. The reorganization White Paper *Working for Patients* (DoH, 1989) considered that there should be a reappraisal of traditional patterns and working practices within the health professions, including the extended role of nurses to cover specific duties normally undertaken by doctors.

Further debate was inevitable when, within a year, the National Health Service Management Executive report on reducing junior doctors' hours was published (NHSME, 1990). This document claimed that 'doctors in training at present undertake many duties which could be more appropriately carried out by non-medical staff, such as nurses'. The response within the nursing profession was divided; some nurses saw this as an opportunity to further their practice and improve the quality of the service offered to patients. Others were concerned that these recommendations further legitimized the perpetuation of past practices in which tasks that doctors had previously found inconvenient or boring were passed on to nurses (McAlister, 1995).

Developing New Roles: Influence of the Nursing Profession

Concurrent with the major changes occurring in the Health Service and the medical profession in the late 1980s and early 1990s, nurses were also having to address some fundamental questions. Some of these arose as responses to new practice roles, derived from initiatives originally implemented in the United States. Others related to the position and future responsibilities of the nurse in the context of cultural changes in the new NHS and in society at large. Business principles and financial constraints now govern health service provision; health service users are becoming more aware of their health care needs and becoming more involved in decision making. In common with other health professionals, nurses are having to justify their practice, not just in terms of role function and the specific nature of nursing practice, but also in the relative social and economic worth of their practice. In doing so, the most important issues of all – the true nature of professional nursing practice, and the unique contribution that nurses have to offer – inevitably have to be considered.

It is through such questioning and analysis that traditional patterns of thought and practice are challenged, including the subordination of nurses to the medical profession; it is now rightly recognized that nursing is a profession allied to medicine, with a specific knowledge base and scope of practice. However, the impetus to develop the role of the nurse in an effort to raise the professional status of nursing is misguided, and may actually threaten its continued existence. Hunt and Wainwright (1994) most aptly summarize the only legitimate driving forces for the development of future nursing roles:

> If role expansion is about anything, it is about nurses taking their *own* initiative, doing their own thinking and making their own decisions based on their own experience and education, to improve practice for the benefit of patients and clients. (p. xv)

Bearing this definition in mind, it is now possible to explore the nursing roles that have been developed and consider their implications for role development. In the United Kingdom it is recognized that the role activities and scope of responsibility of specialist nurses differ from those of other clinical nurses. This differentiation arises from three clearly defined characteristics of the specialist nurse: the demonstration of expert clinical practice in a specific area, or with a specific client group; further post-registration education to develop an appropriate knowledge base for practice; and practice based on research findings (Humphris, 1994).

However, role enactment varies within and across specialties; this has compounded difficulties in clearly defining the new nursing roles of nurse practitioner and advanced nurse practitioner, and in differentiating them from nurse specialism and from each other. In the United Kingdom, the nurse practitioner has been defined as 'a registered nurse who has been specially prepared to carry out and integrate a more medical model of care into his/her nursing practice, with the purpose of improving health assessment, management and delivery of services at the first level of access' (Castledine, 1995). Concerns have previously been expressed about introducing medical elements into the nurse's activities, yet this has been done successfully, with positive benefits for patients. The key factor for successful implementation would appear to be that aspects of the physician's role are incorporated into an expanded nursing role, thereby enhancing the quality and range of care delivered to patients; the rationale for incorporating medical or technical tasks into practice is to facilitate the provision of more effective, holistic and personal care (Wright, 1995). The end result is a unique nursing role which moves beyond the traditional boundaries of professional nursing practice (Mitchinson, 1996; Porrett, 1996).

The publication of standards for post-registration education and practice (UKCC, 1994) endorsed specialist and advanced clinical roles and defined what was to be expected of such practitioners (Figure 1.1). Both roles require nurses to be expert in their chosen field of practice, with an appropriate depth of knowledge, although the level of preparation for effective practice differs. For the specialist practitioner this is at first-degree level and whilst there is no specific stipulation for the advanced practitioner, it is suggested that this will probably be master's level study. However, such programmes need to be flexible, to ensure that students can determine their own learning objectives which both meet their organizational and personal needs, and reflect the development of advanced practice in the clinical setting (Bowles and Cassidy, 1997). The demonstration of advanced clinical practice, and its formal assessment, is still an issue which needs to be fully resolved in some academic institutions.

There is no national policy relating to the activities, grading, level of responsibility and role boundaries of nurses employed as nurse practitioners, specialist practitioners or advanced practitioners in the

---

Definition of the specialist role

There is therefore a need for some practitioners to be able to exercise higher levels of judgement and discretion in clinical care to function as specialist nursing practitioners. Such practitioners will demonstrate higher levels of clinical decision making, and will be able to monitor and improve standards of care through supervision of practice, clinical nursing audit, developing and leading practice, contributing to research, teaching and supporting professional colleagues. (UKCC, 1994, p. 9)

Definition of the advanced role

Advanced nursing practice is concerned with adjusting the boundaries for the development of future practice, pioneering and developing new roles responsive to changing need and with advancing clinical practice, research and education to enrich professional practice as a whole ... It is concerned with the continuing development of the professions in the interests of patients, clients and the health services. (UKCC, 1994, p. 20)

Figure 1.1: Definition of nursing roles.

United Kingdom. The numbers of these nurses within Health Care Trusts throughout the country are increasing as areas of unmet patient need are identified and plans implemented to rectify this. As it is unlikely that a consensus will ever be achieved, it is probably more constructive to consider them all as examples of advanced nursing roles which have different emphases according to the local situation, and focus attention instead on the principles which should underpin the practice of each nurse who occupies such a post.

The Scope of Professional Practice

The document of this name, published by the UKCC in 1992, was timely, as it both responded to changes already occurring as nurses at the forefront of practice developed innovative new roles, and aimed to shape future thinking about such role advancement. It acknowledged that the context of clinical practice was continually changing, and that nursing should be sensitive, relevant and responsive, with the capacity to adjust to these circumstances. The Code of Professional Conduct was described as the 'firm bedrock' upon which decisions about adjustments to the scope of professional practice should be made.

The term 'extended role' was perceived as limiting the parameters of practice and preventing many practitioners from achieving their full potential in adjusting practice to meet changing health care needs, and it was recommended that it should no longer be used. Instead, six principles were listed which would form the framework for a realistic, effective, flexible and rational approach to any adjustments in the scope of practice (Figure 1.2). Local policies and practices should be underpinned by the six principles and by reference to the Code of Professional Conduct.

The position statement incorporated major changes to the manner in which role development in nursing practice was to take place; from giving guidance on the specific to the general, and from external control to the exercise of professional discretion (Hunt and Wainwright, 1994). Nurses were to be personally accountable for their decisions and actions and attain a greater freedom to exercise professional judgement and discretion in developing nursing practice roles. Many nurses agree that the document offered new opportunities to develop initiatives which had previously remained ideals, and that the fear that it was simply the means by which they would relieve doctors of their inappropriate duties has not been realized (Koefman, 1995; Tolley, 1995). The implications of the principles for future practice are, however, potentially far reaching and require further exploration.

The registered nurse, midwife or health visitor:

9.1   must be satisfied that each aspect of practice is directed to meeting the needs and serving the interests of the patient or client;

9.2   must endeavour always to achieve, maintain and develop knowledge, skill and competence to respond to those needs and interests;

9.3   must honestly acknowledge any limits of personal knowledge and skill and take steps to remedy any relevant deficits in order effectively and appropriately to meet the needs of patients and clients;

9.4   must ensure that any enlargement or adjustment of the scope of personal professional practice must be achieved without compromising or fragmenting existing aspects of professional practice and care and that the requirements of the Council's Code of Professional Conduct are satisfied throughout the whole area of practice;

9.5   must recognise and honour the direct or indirect personal accountability borne for all aspects of professional practice and

9.6   must, in serving the interests of patients and clients and the wider interests of society, avoid any inappropriate delegation to others which compromise those interests.

Source: UKCC (1992).

Figure 1.2: Principles for adjusting the scope of practice.

The Scope of Professional Practice and the Individual Nurse

The Scope document (UKCC, 1992) clearly states that the aim of role development should be to benefit patients and to achieve direct improvements in patient care. This is further explored in a later publication (UKCC, 1997):

> *Scope* recognises that every nurse ... is accountable for their practice and it is their professional judgement that can provide innovative solutions to meeting the needs of patients and clients in a health service that is constantly changing ... This is a revolutionary approach. It means that new services can be set up with nurses ... themselves deciding what skills and knowledge they need ... It

puts the onus on the individual practitioner to define the limits of their practice and to refer to appropriate others when necessary. (p. 4)

The assumption is that nurses will be able to define the boundaries of their own practice; undoubtedly, nurse-led services can extend the range and quality of services available to patients and uniquely fill areas of unmet patient need. Successful examples of such innovatory practices are evident in the United Kingdom with the recent development of the roles of the Nurse Practitioner in Coloproctology (Porrett, 1996) and Colorectal Nurse Specialists.

However, to consider that nurses have complete freedom to develop further areas of practice or implement new roles is a simplistic view that ignores the complex situation within which they work and which directly affects the degree of autonomy and independence which can be exercised. Nurses are part of a multidisciplinary team; the success of new initiatives is dependent on the support and cooperation of other team members, particularly medical colleagues, whose expertise and assessment will inevitably be required in preparing the nurse whose role development includes learning such skills as rectal examination and flexible sigmoidoscopy.

Business managers in healthcare trusts have a primary responsibility to ensure that services provided are both cost effective and of a high quality. As the health service is now finance dominated, the extent to which nursing-led services can be developed is dependent on the nurse presenting a convincing case, not simply in terms of benefit to patients, but also at a competitive cost.

It is also essential that a strong case for role development can be presented to the Director of Nursing, Directorate Managers and Trust Chief Executives as these Executive Board members are responsible for the implementation of an overall strategy for the planning and delivery of patient services within each Trust, and any new initiatives have to be consistent with the strategic plan. The employing authority is vicariously liable for the actions of the nurse, so it is at Trust level that approval should be given to new protocols and policies for practice if nurses are intending to move beyond the boundaries of their former job description. Approaches to management at this level have an added benefit in raising the profile of the nursing contribution to patient care and ensuring that its value is recognized.

Nurses are therefore not totally free to determine their own role and the parameters of their practice, because of the hierarchical relationship that exists between health service managers, nurse managers and nurses in clinical practice (Mitchinson, 1996), and because their work is interdependent with that of others in the multidisciplinary team. Any proposed new developments in practice have to be planned with these considerations in mind. As Wainwright (1994) points out, it may not be possible to achieve nursing's full potential as suggested by the *Scope of Professional Practice* paper, until nurses have the requisite authority to permit them greater autonomy and independence in their professional practice.

Individual accountability of the nurse is emphasized in all decision making and implementation related to the principles for developing the scope of practice. This includes ensuring that the nurse is competent to fulfil all aspects of her/his role. With innovative practices, there will not be a prescribed course of preparation and individual plans will need to be made at local level. To determine that the nurse has acquired the prerequisite knowledge and skills, these should also be assessed. This involves fundamental questions of who is most appropriate to undertake this, and what standards will be used to make the judgement. Clear specification of assessment is of vital importance, although Ashwell and Saxton (1992) point out that some competencies concerned with personal or social skills may be relatively intangible, and therefore problematic to assess. The standards used to ascertain whether the nurse is competent are clear:

> The patient is entitled to the standard of care which would be expected of the skilled practitioner exercising and professing to have that special skill ... whether the task is undertaken by a doctor or by a nurse. (Dimond, 1994, p.65)

The position of the Royal College of Nursing in relation to support of its members undertaking new role development is outlined by Porrett (1996); provided that formal preparation and assessment of competence to carry out technical procedures is undertaken the nurse has indemnity cover to incorporate them into his or her new role.

There is no doubt that the opportunities for nurses to shape the future of their professional practice are greater now than ever before. In the specialist practice areas of coloproctological and stoma care nursing, nurses are demonstrating their unique contribution in providing nurse-led services which enhance the quality and range of health care provision for patients. There are many issues still to be considered, not least the way in which nursing and medicine can develop together as complementary disciplines. The boundaries between these two professions are becoming less distinct and more mutually interdependent with increased multidisciplinary teamwork. Nurses have a responsibility to ensure that the uniquely caring function, core skills and values of nursing underpin all new role developments intended to improve patient care, in order to survive in a changing climate of health care provision.

The debate is not over, but as Koefman (1995) asserts, this should no longer be about 'what is a doctor's role and what is a nurse's?' The proper question to ask is 'who is the right person in the right place at the right time to provide the most appropriate and effective service to meet the patient's needs?'

THE US PERSPECTIVE

CHANTAL LECONTE RN BSH MBA, Administrator, Cleveland
    Clinic Hospital, Florida, USA

Factors that Have Influenced the Evolution of Extended Nursing Practice in the United States

In order to understand the evolution of nursing in the United States, one must identify and consider some of the different factors that influenced the development of this discipline as a profession. Those factors, which include the traditional role of women, apprenticeship, humanitarian aims, religious ideals, intuition, common sense, trial and error, theories and research, as well as the influences of medicine, technology, politics, war, economics and feminism, served as catalysts to facilitate the progression of nursing from a submissive role toward a collaborative role (Shaw, 1993).

Prior to the 1860s, a formal education was not a prerequisite to the practice of nursing. Nurses who provided care based on intuition and trial and error were generally uneducated women caregivers or minimally trained individuals from religious or military groups whose primary function was not nursing (Shaw, 1993). The lack of supporting scientific principles and theories resulted in a projected craft or folk image of the practice. As nurses started to interact with physicians, the folk image was gradually replaced by the servant image. For years, the nurse–physician relationship endured a pattern of physician superiority and nurse deference, paralleling the male–female societal relationships. Consequently, nurses were viewed by society as occupying a position of lower status and as subordinate to the medical profession.

The 1860s witnessed the emergence of the first nursing theorist, Florence Nightingale. Nightingale viewed nursing as a discipline with organized concepts and social relevance distinct from medicine (Shaw, 1993). She initiated the requirement for formal nursing education and opened the first school of nursing dedicated to the training of qualified nurses. Although her contribution is one of the most important hallmarks in the history of nursing, it did not at that time address the nurse–physician relationship, which remained a unilateral one, with most of the authority and decision making assumed by the physician. According to Seifert (1993), nurses remained inactive in the planning of patient care, were expected to follow physicians' orders, and were forbidden to provide patients with explanations.

In 1903, the Nurse Practice Act was implemented by North Carolina, with other states following shortly thereafter. The general purpose of the Practice Act, which included the major rights and requirements of nursing practice that remain relevant today, was to protect the patient by limiting the practice of nursing to qualified licensees, and by preventing impostors from delivering substandard care.

The decades to follow witnessed a progressive revolution in nursing throughout America. This professional revolution paralleled the massive economic and social changes that were occurring in the health care environment and in society as a whole. Exploding technology, cost-containment pressures, the managed care system, the health care reform, the Balanced Budget Act and economic corporate mandates amongst others, provided the impetus to look closely at the way in which patient care was being delivered and to identify alternatives to provide patients with more efficient, cost-effective services. This revolution was also part of the aftermath of the women's liberation movement, and as Lewin (1993) reveals, many nurses, armed with advanced degrees and training, were competently edging on to territories once reserved for physicians and business managers.

Today, increasingly articulate consumer groups, aided by the media, continue to raise serious questions about the quality and cost of the care they receive. As a result of the extended life expectancy and the complexity of the patient's condition, patients' demands and acuity level are rising. As the pressure to deliver more and better health care at a lower price continues to mount, extended nursing practice will become more valuable to the health care industry. Those driving forces are not about to disappear and will continue to lead nursing toward extended roles and collaborative practice.

Extended Nursing Practice: Definition, Qualifications and Role

An extended or advanced practice nurse is a registered nurse who, through study and supervised practice, has become an expert in a defined area of knowledge and practises in a selected clinical area of nursing. Whilst the health care industry embraces the concept of extended nursing practice as an attempt to respond to the multiple changes affecting health care, full consensus on the definition, qualifications and standards for the role has yet to be achieved uniformly throughout the United States.

Currently, extended nursing status may be achieved in many different ways. As Rothrock (1993) explained, qualifications may be attained through educational programmes, state or national certification programmes, specialty organizations and councils such as those of the American Nurses Association (ANA). Although most extended practice nurses are prepared at the master's degree level, there is poor understanding of the differences between the expert by experience and the advanced practitioner credentialled by formal education. Many boards, in their attempt to protect public health, welfare and safety, recognize some level of advanced nursing practice through statutes and administrative rules. However, states practice acts granting legal authority to advanced practice nurses, although similar in outline, vary widely in detail, content and specificity (Wood et al., 1996).

In an attempt to standardize the requirements for extended nurse practice, the National Council of State Boards of Nursing (NCSBN) issued a draft document in 1992 that recommended licensure of advanced practice nurses in the categories of nurse anaesthetist, nurse midwife, nurse practitioner and clinical nurse specialist. According to the NCSBN (1992), advanced nursing practice is to be 'based on knowledge and skills acquired in basic nursing education; licensure as a registered nurse; graduate degree and experience in the designated area of practice, which includes advanced nursing theory, substantial knowledge of physical and psychosocial assessment, appropriate interventions, and management of health care status' (Rothrock, 1993). The essential skills and abilities recommended by the NCSBN for advanced nursing within the designated area of practice include:

- assessing clients, synthesizing and analysing data, and understanding and applying nursing principles at an advanced level;
- providing expert guidance and teaching;
- working effectively with clients, families, and other members of the health care team;

- managing clients' physical and psychosocial health–illness status;
- utilizing research skills;
- analysing multiple sources of data, identifying alternative possibilities as to the nature of a health care problem and selecting appropriate treatment;
- making independent decisions in solving complex client care problems;
- performing acts of diagnosis and prescribing therapeutic measures consistent with the area of practice;
- recognizing the limits of knowledge and experience, planning for situations beyond expertise, and consulting with or referring clients to other health care providers as appropriate.

Another emerging category of advanced practice nurses is the Certified Registered Nurse First Assistant (CRNFA). Although the role definition for this group was not included in the 1992 NCSBN document, the Association of Operating Room Nurses (AORN, 1984) confirmed in a 1984 statement that, in the absence of a qualified physician, registered nurses with appropriate knowledge and skills are the best-qualified non-physician to act as first assistant. The definition, scope of practice, qualifications, preparation and establishment of practice privileges for the CRNFA were also outlined (AORN, 1993). Many state boards of nursing have adopted the AORN position as part of the scope of practice for CRNFAs.

Today, more than 160 000 advanced or extended practice nurses are helping to fill a growing need for medical care in the United States (Cromley, 1997). Those nurses typically work in collaboration with a physician or group of physicians. Doctors who once resisted having 'non-doctors' dispense medical care are now realizing that working with advanced practice nurses in a collaborative setting enables both sets of professionals to make better use of their time, whilst patients get the best of both (Marshall, 1994).

The treatment plan of colorectal patients, being a typically very involved process owing to the complexity of the patient's condition both physically and psychologically, benefits from the expertise of an advanced practice nurse. The advanced practice nurse or nurse clinician oversees and coordinates the patient's care from the initial visit in the physician's office through the full perioperative path. In addition to direct interaction with the patients and family acting as a coach, an advocate, an educator, a research liaison and a clinical expert, the nurse also functions as a first or second assistant in the operating room in the capacity of a CRNFA. This provides the opportunity for the advanced practice nurse to be actively involved in every aspect of the care plan and enhances communication with the patients. The nurse clinician, working in collaboration with the colorectal surgeon, has proven to be invaluable to patients, family members, consultants and the organization. The collaborative practice minimizes fragmentation and duplication of services, increases patient satisfaction and improves patient outcome.

Some feel that the nurses' move toward extended practice may create competition with physicians, especially if they were to be reimbursed for their services; however, most extended practice nurses express no desire to compete with physicians, yet identify the need for such nurses to contribute to improve patient outcome.

Extended practice nurses may carry the title of Clinical Nurse Specialist (CNS), Advanced Registered Nurse Practitioner (ARNP), Nurse Clinician (NC), Certified Registered Nurse First Assistant (CRNFA), Certified Nurse Midwife (CNM), and Certified Registered Nurse Anesthetist (CRNA), amongst others. Their role, as described in the literature, varies widely. Some extended nurses function as 'physician extenders' whereby they assume responsibilities for providing patients with expert clinical care, formerly part of medical management, in collaboration with a physician or group of physicians; hence the term collaborative practice. A more autonomous role may be assumed by others where the nurse provides 'a continuum of patient care services not only in rural and under-served areas, but also in urban communities in independent practice, practice with physicians, and, in increasing number, in nurse-run and nurse-owned clinics' (O'Malley, 1996).

One common characteristic that emerges from the states' Nurse Practice Acts is the issue of overlapping areas of practice and relationships between physicians and nurses. Nursing and medical practices are interrelated, complementary to each other, and not interchangeable either in responsibility or accountability. The physician is unanimously recognized as the expert in the medical aspects of health care, while the nurse remains the expert in nursing aspects. Therefore, a collaborative relationship between the two disciplines is advocated in order to achieve optimal patient outcome. The collaborative practice does not always imply direct physician supervision and is at times described by nursing boards as the physician being readily available for consultation when necessary.

Extended Nursing Practice: Challenges

The mere fact that extended nursing practice is identified and recognized by many as an important component of the health care delivery system does not necessarily ensure a smooth transition into that level of practice. Many issues, some originating from outside forces and others from within the nursing profession itself, continue to plague the development of extended nursing practice in the United States.

First, role ambiguity and lack of clarification on the educational requirements and the scope of practice for advanced practice nurses have created public confusion. The standards for extended practice must be articulated and implemented uniformly by the state boards of nursing across the United States. The public, government agencies, health insurance carriers, administrators, nursing educators, physicians and fellow nurses will then be educated on the role advanced practitioners play in different practice settings.

Second, traditional territorial rights as pointed out by Garcia et al. (1993) are not usually relinquished readily. In order to achieve a shared vision of extended nursing practice, it is imperative that advanced practice nurses, physicians, nursing educators and health care executives who can facilitate this process recognize that education, empowerment, self-confidence, persistence, patience and assertiveness are essential to generate mutual trust, respect, and open and honest communication which are the foundation of collaborative practice between the medical profession and nursing.

Last but not least, the issue of reimbursement for advanced nursing practice services is yet to be resolved. As cost-containment and managed care continue to impact on the financial aspect of the health care institutions, the ability to generate revenue or to implement cost-saving strategies significantly augments the value and recognition of any health care provider. Today, the extended practice nurses' contribution to the bottom line of their organization is not commonly measured and acknowledged by health care administrators. Extended practice nurses must identify ways to track and measure that financial impact. Certification in the specific area of advanced practice is a prerequisite to reimbursement; active involvement at the legislative level will also facilitate the enactment of laws to require reimbursement from the insurance carriers for services provided by extended practice nurses.

Extended Practice Nursing: Opportunities

Despite the challenges that are facing the extended nursing practice, there has never been a time as now with so much potential for the nursing profession. Throughout this tumultuous period of rapid changes, avenues and opportunities for new extended nursing roles are also emerging. According to O'Malley (1996), the benchmarks of successful health care organizations will focus on easy access, user friendliness, high quality, and low cost. Nurses in extended roles can help the health care industry achieve those objectives. The dynamics of the health care system require an interdisciplinary approach to the delivery of patient care and it is widely recognized that no one discipline can do it alone. With the increase in patient load and the proliferation of capitation plans, the contribution of extended practice nurses becomes a welcome respite for physicians. Through collaborative practice, advanced practice nurses can continue to function safely and competently in extended roles in the following areas:

- family practice;
- primary care/gatekeeper;
- preventative medicine;
- triage clinic;
- obstetrics/gynaecology;
- paediatrics;
- gerontology;
- psychiatry;
- outpatient care;
- operating room;
- specialty care;
- hospital;
- case management;
- home care;
- research;
- education;
- administration.

There is increasing evidence that successful delivery of patient care cannot be achieved through a unilateral determination of function by either nursing or medicine (Garcia et al., 1993). Extended practice nurses are providing safe, quality, cost efficient patient care and, at the same time, freeing physicians to attend to the more complicated patients. Both physicians and nurses can benefit from this relationship if it is implemented in a supportive atmosphere and a collegial way. The potential for improved morale and job satisfaction is tremendous in both groups.

Strategies for the Future

Hope for the future of health care lies in our ability to deliver coordinated, quality, cost-effective care in a collaborative setting (Miccolo and Spanier, 1993). A shift from the traditional fee-for-service, physician-dominated relationship to a more balanced multidisciplinary collaboration has occurred in the American health care industry. This new collaboration provides for improved communication, more efficient, coordinated and comprehensive care, greater patient satisfaction, improved morale and productivity amongst health care providers, and decreased cost. It is imperative that nursing comes to a consensus on the standard and qualifications of extended practice nurses in order to educate the public about their role and to position themselves to bridge the gap between quality and cost of patient care delivery.

Currently there is little argument about the contribution that the extended practice nurses can make to the health care industry and very few physicians are absolutely against the extended role. A 1986 report by the Federal Office of Technology Assessment estimated that 60–80% of the basic health care performed by doctors could be done by nurses with the same results at a lower cost (Lewin, 1993; Marshall, 1994).

Malloch (1996) reports that, generally, respect from physicians is currently high; most of them now actively seek out the advanced practice nurse to discuss the plan of care and appropriateness of resource line. But nursing must be alerted to the fact that the evolution of advanced nursing practice is similar to a race without a finish line. It will continue to evolve and be challenged as the needs of the patients, the health care industry and society as a whole continue to change.

We must continuously strive toward identifying diverse ways to affirm the importance of our role and to impact positively and efficiently on patient care. More research to analyse and document the effectiveness of extended nursing practice on patient outcome must be undertaken. As we continue to recognize, monitor and address the issues imposed on us by external and internal forces, the future will provide us with the opportunity to prove once again, as we have successfully done in the past, that nursing as a profession is an important and valuable component of the health care system.

The future is very promising; let us, as a profession, position ourselves to successfully meet its challenges!

References

Ashwell P, Saxton J (1992) On competence. Journal of Further and Higher Education 14(2): 3–25.
Association of Operating Room Nurses (1984) Official Statement on RN First

Assistants. Denver: AORN.

Association of Operation Room Nurses (1993) Official Statement on RN First Assistants. Denver: AORN.

Bowles N, Cassidy A (1997) Developing practitioners. Nursing Management 4(3): 8–9.

Castledine, G (1995) Defining specialist nursing British Journal of Nursing 4(5) 264–5.

Cromley J (1997) When your doctor is a nurse. Good Housekeeping 225(2): August 145–6.

Department of Health (1989) Working for Patients. London: DoH.

Department of Health and Social Security (1977) The Extended Role of the Clinical Nurse, DHSS HC (77) 22. London: DHSS .

Department of Health and Social Security (1989) The Extending Role of the Nurse, DHSS Circular no PL/CNO/89/10. London: DHSS.

Dimond B (1994) Legal aspects of role expansion. In Hunt G, Wainwright P (Eds) Expanding the Role of the Nurse. Oxford: Blackwell Science, pp 54–73.

Garcia M et al. (1993) Collaborative practice: a shared success. Nursing Management 24(5): May 72–8.

Humphris D (1994) The basis of nurse specialism in nursing. In Humphris D (Ed.) The Clinical Nurse Specialist: Issues in Practice. London: Macmillan.

Hunt G, Wainwright, P (1994) Introduction. In Hunt G, Wainwright, P (Eds) Expanding the Role of the Nurse. Oxford: Blackwell Science, pp x–xvi.

Koefman K (1995) Developing a new deal for nurses. Nursing Standard 9(44): 26 July 33–5.

Lewin T (1993) Nursing invades turf once ruled by doctors. New York Times 43(49,523): A1, A12.

McAlister L (1995) Why do nurses agree to take on doctors' roles? British Journal of Nursing 4(16): 948–53.

Malloch K (1996) Managed care and changing nurse practice. Aspen's Advisor for Nurse Executives 11(9): 5–6.

Marshall C (1994) Health care's 'middle managers'. Stanford Medicine 12(1): 24–8.

Miccolo M, Spanier A (1993) Critical care management in the 1990s. Critical Care Clinics 9(3): July 443–52.

Mitchinson S (1996) Are nurses independent and autonomous practitioners? Nursing Standard 10(34): 15 May 34–8.

National Council of State Boards of Nursing (1992) Position Paper on the Licensure of Advanced Nursing Practice 13 August.

NHS Management Executive (1990) Junior Doctors: the New Deal. London: NHS Management Executive.

O'Malley J (1996) Evolving roles for advanced practice nurses. Aspen's Advisor for Nurse Executives 11(9): June 7–8.

Porrett T (1996) Extending the role of the stoma care nurse. Nursing Standard 10(27): 27 March 33–5.

Rothrock J (1993) The nurse practice act and expanded roles. In Rothrock J (Ed.) The RN First Assistant. Philadelphia: Lippincott, pp 17–32.

Seifert P (1993) The RN First Assistant and collaborative practice. In Rothrock J (Ed.) The RN First Assistant. Philadelphia: Lippincott, pp 288–302.

Shaw M (1993) The discipline of nursing historical roots: current perspectives, future directions. Journal of Advanced Nursing 18: 1651–6.

Sparacino P, Cooper,D (1990) The role components. In Sparacino P, Cooper D, Minarik P (Eds) The Clinical Nurse Specialist: Implementation and Impact. Norwalk: Appleton & Lange, pp 11–40.

Tolley K (1995) Extending nurses' professional roles. Nursing Standard 9(18): 30–4.

UKCC (1992) The Scope of Professional Practice. London: UKCC.

UKCC (1994) Standards for Post Registration Education and Practice. London: UKCC.

UKCC (1997) Scope in Practice. London: UKCC.

Wainwright P (1994) Professionalism and the concept of role and extension. In Hunt G, Wainwright P (Eds) Expanding the Role of the Nurse. Oxford: Blackwell Science, pp 3–21.

Wood C et al. (1996) Clinical nurse specialist in California: who claims the title? Clinical Nurse Specialist 10(6): November 283–92.

Wright S (1995) The role of the nurse: extended or expanded? Nursing Standard 9(33): 33–5.

Chapter 2
Anatomy and Physiology of the Colon, Rectum and Anus

J. MARCIO N. JORGE MD, Director, Anorectal Physiology Laboratory, Colorectal Division, University of São Paulo, São Paulo, Brazil

Colon

The large intestine is a capacious tube which extends from the end of the ileum to the anus, and includes the colon, rectum and anal canal. In its course, the colon describes roughly an arch that surrounds the loops of small intestine and is designated according to location as: caecum, ascending colon, right colic or hepatic flexure, transverse colon, left colic or splenic flexure, descending colon and sigmoid colon (Figure 2.1). The colon can also be divided into right colon, which extends from the ileo-caecal valve to the midtransverse colon and the left colon, which travels from the midtransverse colon to the rectosigmoid junction. 'Hemi-colectomy' means removal of one of these portions. Embryologically, the right colon, including the proximal two-thirds of the transverse colon, is originated from the midgut, whereas the left colon, including the distal one-third of the transverse colon, the rectum and the anal canal above the dentate line is all derived from the hindgut.

The colon is approximately 150 cm long and its diameter decreases, gradually, from 7.5 cm at the caecum to 2.5 cm at the sigmoid. Anatomically, the colon can be differentiated from the small intestine by its greater calibre, and the presence of three distinct characteristics: the taeniae coli, the haustra and the appendices epiploicae (Figure 2.2). The three taeniae coli, anterior, posteromedial and posterolateral, represent thickened bands of the outer longitudinal muscular layer that traverses the colon from the base of the appendix

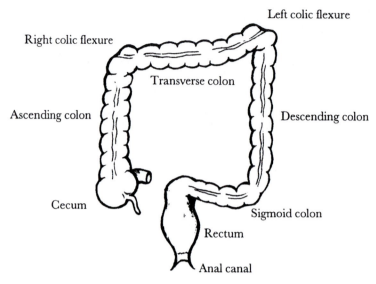

Figure 2.1: Subdivisions of the large intestine.

to the rectosigmoid junction, where they merge. The haustra or haustral sacculation are the result of outpouchings of bowel wall between the taeniae; they are attributed to the relative shortness of the taeniae compared with the length of bowel wall. The haustra are separated by crescentic folds of bowel wall, the plicae semilunares, which give the colon its characteristic X-ray appearance when filled with either air or barium. The appendices epiploicae are small appendages of fat that protrude from the serosal aspect of the colon.

Caecum

The caecum is the segment of the large bowel that projects downwards as a 'blind' pouch below the entrance of the ileum. It is a sacculated organ of 6.0–8.0 cm in both length and breadth, usually situated in the right iliac fossa. The caecum is entirely invested with peritoneum, however its mobility is usually limited by a small mesocaecum .

The ileum terminates in the posteromedial aspect of the caecum, in a narrow, transversely situated slit-like aperture, the ileocaecal valve. At either end, the two prominent semilunar lips of the valve fuse and continue as a single and narrow ridge of mucosa. The ileocaecal sphincter is a circular sphincter originated from the muscular layer of the terminal ileum. The ileocaecal valve is important in regulating the ileal emptying, as the ileocaecal sphincter seems to relax in response to the entrance of food into the stomach. Additionally, the ileocaecal

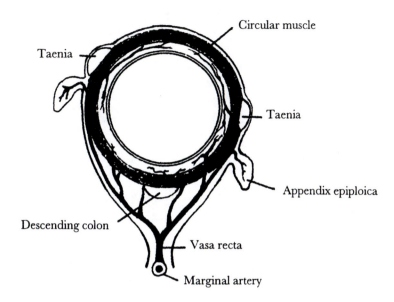

Figure 2.2: Structure of the colon.

valve is implicated in preventing reflux of colonic contents into the ileum, and a competent valve may cause, in case of colonic obstruction, a closed-loop obstruction.

The vermiform appendix is an elongated diverticulum which arises from the posteromedial aspect of the caecum about 3 cm below the ileocaecal junction. Its length varies from 2 to 20 cm and its diameter is about 5 mm. The confluence of the three taeniae can be used as a guide to locate the base of the appendix. However, due to its great mobility, the appendix may occupy a variety of positions: retrocaecal, pelvic, subcaecal, pre-ileal or post-ileal (Wakeley, 1983). The mesoappendix, a triangular fold attached to the posterior leaf of the mesentery of the terminal ileum, contains the appendicular vessels close to its free edge.

Ascending Colon

The ascending colon, extending from the level of the ileocaecal junction to the right colic or hepatic flexure, is approximately 15 cm long. It lies in the right lumbar region and ascends lateral to the psoas muscle and anteriorly to the iliacus, the quadratus lumborum and the lower pole of the right kidney. The ascending colon is covered with peritoneum anteriorly and on both sides; its posterior surface is devoid of peritoneum. At the visceral surface of the liver, the ascending colon turns sharply medially and slightly caudal and ventrally to form the right colic or hepatic flexure.

Transverse Colon

The transverse colon is approximately 45 cm long and traverses the abdomen, from the right hepatic flexure to the left colic flexure, in an inferior curve immediately caudal to the greater curvature of the stomach. The transverse colon is relatively fixed at each flexure. In between flexures it is completely invested with peritoneum and suspended by a transverse mesocolon, which provides variable mobility. The left colic flexure, or splenic flexure, is situated beneath the lower angle of the spleen and firmly attached to the diaphragm by the phrenocolic ligament.

Descending Colon

This segment of the large intestine courses inferiorly from the splenic flexure to the brim of the true pelvis, a distance usually of about 25 cm. The descending colon is narrower and more dorsally situated than the ascending colon. However, similarly to the ascending colon, it is devoid of peritoneum on its posterior aspect, and rests directly against the left kidney, and the quadratus lumborum and transversus abdominis muscles. The ureter should always be identified during resections of the right and left colon, in order to avoid injury. On either side, the ureter runs inferomedially on the psoas muscle and is crossed by the spermatic and the colic branches anteriorly, and the genitofemoral nerve posteriorly. It crosses the pelvic brim, on either side, in front of the bifurcation of the common iliac artery.

Sigmoid Colon

The sigmoid colon is approximately 38 cm long and extends from the lower end of the descending colon at the pelvic brim. It is a mobile, omega-shaped coil segment. The sigmoid colon is completely invested by peritoneum-covered mesentery, attached to the pelvic walls in an inverted V shape. The rectosigmoid junction is invariably noted during sigmoidoscopy as a narrow and sharply angulated segment. Externally, however, it is an indistinct segment comprising the last 5–8 cm of sigmoid and the uppermost 5 cm of rectum (Goligher, 1984).

Rectum

The rectum follows the sacral concavity for a distance of 12–15 cm and ends 2–3 cm anteroinferiorly to the tip of the coccyx, angulating sharply backwards and passing through the levators to become the anal canal (Figures 2.3a, 2.3b). The rectosigmoid junction is considered to be at the level of S3 by anatomists, and at the sacral promontory by surgeons. Likewise, the distal limit of the rectum is somewhat debatable, regarded as the muscular anorectal ring by surgeons and as the dentate line by anatomists.

In women, the rectum is related anteriorly to the posterior vaginal wall and in men, behind the prostate, seminal vesicles, vas deferens and urinary bladder. Posterior to the rectum lie the sacrum, coccyx,

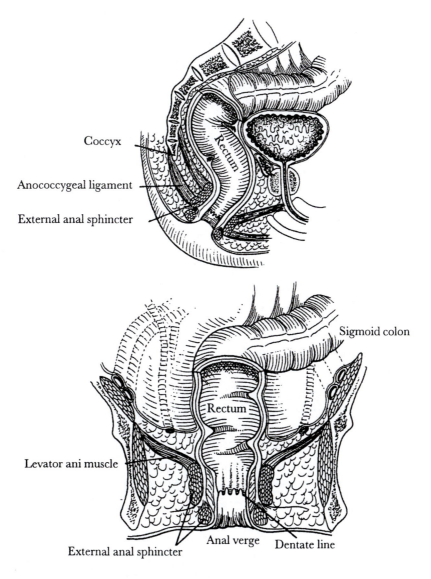

Figure 2.3: (a) Sagittal and (b) frontal diagram of the rectum and rectosigmoid junction.

levator ani muscles, the median sacral vessels, and the roots of the sacral nerve plexus. The rectum also has lateral curves, which correspond on the intraluminal aspect to the folds or valves of Houston. There are usually three folds: two on the left side (at 7–8 cm and at 12–13 cm) and one at 9–11 cm on the right side. The rectal valves represent a safe location for rectal biopsy, but they do not have any specific function.

The rectum has no taeniae, epiploic appendices, haustra or well-defined mesorectum. It is entirely extraperitoneal on its posterior aspect where an aereolar tissue containing terminal branches of the inferior mesenteric artery and enclosed by the fascia propria is referred to by surgeons as the mesorectum (Goligher, 1984; Church et al., 1987). The mesorectum may be a metastatic site from a rectal cancer and can be removed without clinical sequelae, as it contains no functionally significant nerves. The upper third of the rectum is invested anteriorly and laterally by peritoneum; more distally the peritoneum covers the rectum only on its anterior aspect. Finally, the lower third of the rectum is entirely extraperitoneal, as the peritoneum is reflected from the rectum at 9–7 cm from the anal verge. In women, the peritoneal reflection may be lower at 7.5–5.0 cm from the anal verge. The rectum has a wide, easily distensible lumen. The rectal mucosa is smooth, pink and transparent allowing visualization of the small and large submucosal vessels. This peculiar 'vascular pattern' is absent in inflammatory diseases and melanosis coli.

Fascial Relationships

The fascia propria of the rectum is continuous with the visceral pelvic fascia and invests the vessels in the posterior extraperitoneal portion of the rectum. Distal condensations of this fascia form the lateral ligaments of the rectum, which may contain accessory branches of the middle haemorrhoidal vessels. These ligaments attach the rectum to the lateral pelvic walls and therefore must be divided to promote rectal mobilization. The presacral fascia covers the sacrum, coccyx and the middle sacral artery and presacral veins. Intraoperative rupture of this fascia may cause presacral haemorrhage which, despite its venous nature, is usually severe and difficult to control (Quinyao et al., 1985). The rectosacral fascia, also known as fascia of Waldeyer, is an anteroinferior-directed thick fascial reflection from the presacral fascia at the S4 level to the fascia propria of the rectum, just above the anorectal ring. Anteriorly, the extraperitoneal rectum is separated from the prostate and seminal vesicles or vagina by a tough fascial investment, the visceral pelvic fascia or fascia of Denonvilliers. Both the rectosacral and the visceral pelvic fascia are important anatomical landmarks during rectal mobilization.

Anal Canal

In the literature, two definitions exist describing the anal canal: the 'surgical' or 'functional' anal canal extends for approximately 4 cm from the anal verge to the anorectal ring and the 'anatomical' or 'embryological' anal canal is shorter (2 cm), extending from the anal verge to the dentate line. Although representing a relatively small segment of the digestive tract, the anal canal has a peculiar anatomy and a complex physiology, which accounts for both its vital role in continence and its susceptibility to a variety of diseases.

The anus or anal orifice is an anteroposterior cutaneous slit which, at rest and with the anal canal, is kept virtually closed due to tonic circumferential contraction of the sphincters and anal cushions. The anal canal is related posteriorly to the coccyx and anteriorly to the urethra in the male, and to the perineal body and to the lowest part of the posterior vaginal wall in the female. Laterally, the ischiorectal fossa is situated on either side and contains fat and the inferior rectal vessels and nerves which cross it to enter the wall of the anal canal.

Epithelium

The lining of the anal canal consists of an upper mucosal and a lower cutaneous segment. The dentate or pectinate line represents the junction of the ectoderm and the endoderm and therefore represents an important landmark between two distinct origins of venous and lymphatic drainage, nerve supply and epithelial lining (Skandalakis et al., 1994). Above the dentate line, the intestine has sympathetic and parasympathetic innervation and the venous and lymphatic drainage and the arterial supply are to and from the hypogastric vessels. Structures distal to the dentate line have somatic nerve supply and blood supply and venous drainage derived from the inferior haemorrhoidal system. The pectinate or dentate line corresponds to a line of anal valves, which represent remnants of the proctodeal membrane (Figure 2.4). Above each valve, there is a little pocket known as an anal sinus or crypt (sinus of Morgagni). A variable number of glands, approximately 4–12, are connected to the anal crypts and traverse the submucosa to terminate in the submucosa, internal anal sphincter or the intersphincteric plane (Goligher, 1984; Pemberton, 1991). The

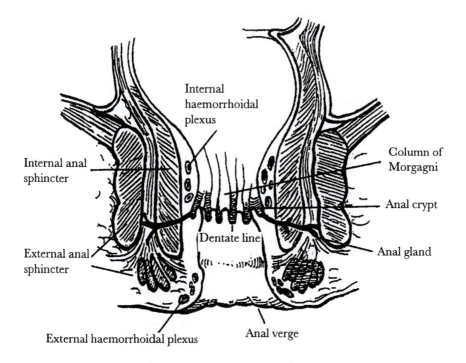

Figure 2.4: The anal canal.

anal glands are more concentrated in the posterior quadrants, and when obstructed cause perianal abscesses and fistulae.

Above the dentate line, 8 to 14 longitudinal folds known as the rectal columns (columns of Morgagni) have their bases connected in pairs to each valve at the dentate line. The mucosa in the area of the columns consists of several layers of cuboidal cells and acquires a deep purple colour. This 0.5–1.0 cm strip of mucosa above the dentate line is known as the anal transition zone. Above this area, the epithelium changes to a single layer of cuboidal columnar cells and macroscopically acquires the characteristic pink colour of the rectal mucosa. The lower cutaneous part of the anal canal consists of a modified squamous epithelium, which is thin, smooth, pale, stretched and devoid of hair and glands from the dentate line to the anal verge. The anal verge, also known as the white line of Hilton, is the lowermost edge of the anal canal, and is usually the level of reference for measurements taken during colonoscopy. Other authors prefer to evert the anus and consider the dentate line as a landmark because it is more precise (Ewing, 1954); the difference between the two is nearly 2.0 cm. Further distally, the lining becomes thicker and acquires hair follicles, glands and other histological features of normal skin.

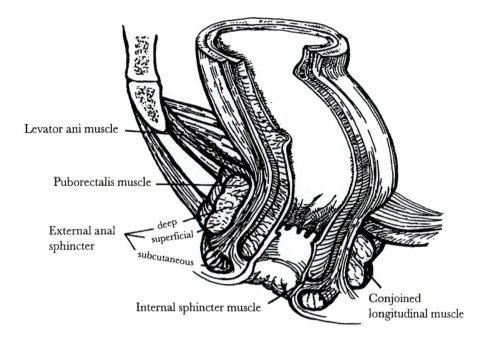

Levator ani muscle

Puborectalis muscle

External anal
sphincter
deep
superficial
subcutaneous

Internal sphincter muscle

Conjoined
longitudinal muscle

Figure 2.5: Muscles of the anal canal.

Muscles of the Anorectal Region

The muscles of the anorectal region comprise the anal canal or sphincteric group and pelvic floor or levator ani muscles (Figures 2.5 and 2.6). The anal canal group includes the internal and external anal sphincter and the conjoined longitudinal muscles.

The levator ani muscle or pelvic diaphragm comprises the major component of the pelvic floor which is 'defective' in the midline where viscera pass through it. The levator ani is a pair of broad, symmetrical sheets of striated muscle; it consists of three muscles: iliococcygeus, pubococcygeus and puborectalis (Figure 2.6). A variable fourth component, the ischiococcygeus or coccygeus, is usually rudimentary and represented by a few muscle fibres on the surface of the sacrospinous ligament (Williamson and Mortensen, 1987).

Internal Anal Sphincter

The internal anal sphincter represents a distal condensation of the inner circular muscle layer of the rectum. The lower rounded edge of the internal anal sphincter can be felt on physical examination,

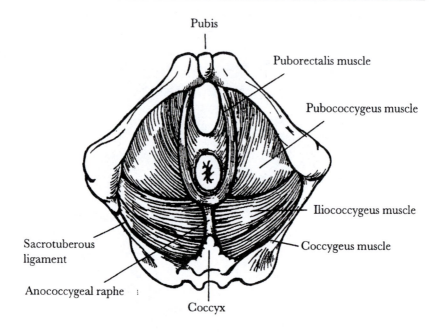

Figure 2.6: The pelvic floor muscles (perineal view).

approximately 1.2 cm distal to the dentate line; the intersphincteric sulcus, the groove between it and the external anal sphincter can be visualized or easily palpated. This sulcus is used as a reference during anorectal procedures, more specifically during sphincterotomy for anal fissure.

External Anal Sphincter

The external anal sphincter envelops the entire length of the inner tube of smooth muscle, but ends slightly more distal to the terminus of the internal anal sphincter. The external anal sphincter has been described either as a single continuous sheet or as a triple-loop system (Goligher et al., 1955; Shafik, 1975). In this three-loop system, each U-shaped loop is a separate sphincter with distinct attachments, muscle bundle directions and innervations; each loop complements the other which helps maintain continence. However, clinical experience has not supported the three-loop system theory; the external anal sphincter is more likely to be one muscle unit, not divided into layers or laminae, attached by the anococcygeal ligament posteriorly to the coccyx and anteriorly to the perineal body.

Conjoined Longitudinal Muscle

Whereas the circular layer of the rectum gives rise to the internal anal sphincter, the longitudinal layer, at the level of the anorectal ring, mixes with fibres of the levator ani muscle to form the conjoined longitudinal muscle. The conjoined longitudinal fibres descend between the internal and the external anal sphincter muscles, and ultimately some of its fibres, referred to as the corrugator cutis ani muscle, traverse the lowermost part of the external anal sphincter and merge into the perianal skin.

Levator Ani Muscles

The iliococcygeus fibres arise from the ischial spine and posterior part of the obturator fascia, and course inferiorly and medially into the lateral aspects of S3 and S4 and into the anococcygeal raphe. The pubococcygeus arises from the posterior aspect of the pubis and the anterior part of the obturator fascia. It runs dorsally alongside the anorectal junction, to fuse with fibres of the opposite side at the anococcygeal raphe; it then runs into the anterior surface of the fourth sacral and first coccygeal segments. The puborectalis muscle is a U-shaped loop of striated muscle which slings the anorectal junction to the back of the pubis. It is situated immediately cephalad to the deep component of the external sphincter; the junction between the two muscles is somewhat indistinct and consequently the puborectalis has been regarded by some authors as part of the external anal sphincter muscle and not of the levator ani complex (Russell, 1991). The puborectalis, along with the upper border of the internal anal sphincter, comprises the anorectal ring, an easily recognized boundary of the anal canal on physical examination. Despite lacking embryological significance, the anorectal ring is of clinical relevance as division of this structure during surgery for abscess and fistula will inevitably result in faecal incontinence.

Para-anal and Pararectal Spaces

The anorectal region includes several spaces of clinical significance: ischiorectal, perianal, intersphincteric, submucous, superficial postanal, deep postanal, supralevator and retrorectal spaces (Figures 2.7a, 2.7b). The ischiorectal fossa is subdivided by a thin horizontal fascia into two spaces: the perianal and ischiorectal. The ischiorectal space comprises the upper two-thirds of the ischiorectal fossa. It is a

pyramid-shaped space situated on both sides between the anal canal
and lower part of the rectum medially, and the side wall of the pelvis
laterally. The apex is at the origin of the levator ani muscles from the
obturator fascia and the base is represented by the perianal space.
Anteriorly, the fossa is bounded by the urogenital diaphragm and
transversus perinei muscles. Posterior to the ischiorectal fossa is the
sacrotuberous ligament and the inferior border of the gluteus
maximus. On the superolateral wall, the pudendal nerve and the inter-

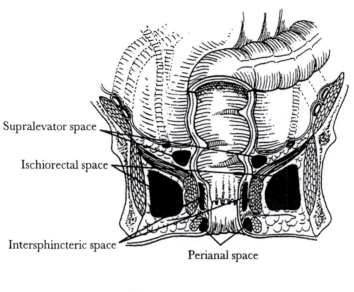

Supralevator space

Ischiorectal space

Intersphincteric space

Perianal space

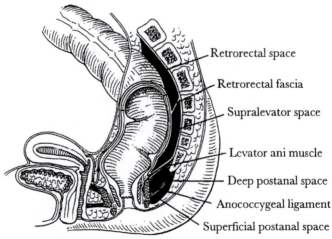

Retrorectal space

Retrorectal fascia

Supralevator space

Levator ani muscle

Deep postanal space

Anococcygeal ligament

Superficial postanal space

Figure 2.7: (a) Frontal and (b) sagittal diagram of the para-anal and pararectal
spaces.

nal pudendal vessels run into the pudendal canal or Alcock's canal. The ischiorectal fossa includes fat and the inferior haemorrhoidal vessels and nerves.

The perianal space surrounds the lower part of the anal canal. It is continuous with the subcutaneous fat of the buttocks laterally and extends into the intersphincteric space medially. The external haemorrhoidal plexus lies in the perianal space and communicates with the internal haemorrhoidal plexus at the dentate line. This space is the typical site of anal haematomas, perianal abscesses and anal fistula tracts. The perianal space also encloses the subcutaneous part of the external anal sphincter, the lowest part of the internal anal sphincter and fibres of the longitudinal muscle.

The intersphincteric space is a potential space between the internal and the external anal sphincter. Its importance lies in the genesis of perianal abscesses, as the anal glands end in this space. The submucous space is situated between the internal anal sphincter and the mucocutaneous lining of the anal canal. This space contains the internal haemorrhoidal plexus and the muscularis submucosae ani. Superiorly, it is continuous with the submucous layer of the rectum, and inferiorly, it ends at the level of the dentate line.

The superficial postanal space is interposed between the anococcygeal ligament and the adjacent skin. The deep postanal space is situated between the anococcygeal ligament and the anococcygeal raphe. Both postanal spaces communicate posteriorly with the ischiorectal fossa and are frequently sites of anorectal abscesses.

The supralevator spaces are situated between the peritoneum superiorly and the levator ani inferiorly. Medially, these bilateral spaces are related to the rectum and laterally, to the obturator fascia.

The retrorectal space is located between the fascia propria of the rectum anteriorly and the presacral fascia posteriorly. Laterally lie the lateral rectal ligaments, inferiorly is the rectosacral ligament and above, the retrorectal space is continuous with the retroperitoneum.

Blood and Nerve Supply

Blood Supply

The large intestine is entirely nourished by two of the three major gut arteries, the superior and inferior mesenteric arteries. The limit between the two territories is at the junction between the proximal two-thirds and the distal one-third of the transverse colon, which represents the embryological division between the midgut and the hindgut. Collateral circulation between these two arteries is formed by a continuous communicating arcade along the mesenteric border of the colon, the marginal artery, from which the vasa recta distribute directly to the bowel. Nevertheless, discontinuity of the marginal artery may be found, particularly at three points: the lower ascending colon, the left colic flexure and the sigmoid colon; attention to this feature is necessary during colonic resection. The anorectum is also supplied by the internal iliac artery and occasionally by the median sacral artery.

Superior Mesenteric Artery

The superior mesenteric artery originates from the aorta at the level of the superior border of the pancreas at L1 and supplies the caecum, appendix, ascending colon and most of the transverse colon (Figure 2.8). Additionally, the superior mesenteric artery supplies the entire small bowel, the pancreas and occasionally the liver.

After passing behind the neck of the pancreas, the superior mesenteric artery crosses the third part of the duodenum and continues downward and to the right along the base of the mesentery. From its

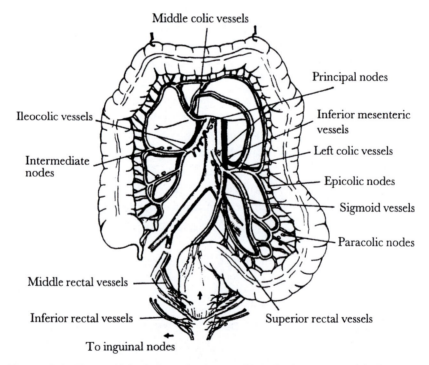

Figure 2.8: The arterial supply and venous and lymphatic drainage of the large intestine. Arrows indicate direction of lymphatic drainage.

left side a series of 12–20 jejunal and ileal branches arise. From its right side, the colic branches – middle colic, right colic and ileocolic arteries – are seen. The ileocolic is the most constant of these; it bifurcates into two branches. The ascending branch anastomoses with the descending branch of the right colic artery and the descending branch gives off the caecal and appendicular branches. Finally it continues into the small bowel mesentery as the ileal branch.

The right colic artery supplies the ascending colon and hepatic flexure through its ascending and descending branches, both of which anastomose with neighbouring vessels to contribute to the marginal artery. The middle colic artery is the highest of the three colic branches of the superior mesenteric artery, arising close to the inferior border of the pancreas. Its right branch supplies the right transverse colon and hepatic flexure, to anastomose with the ascending branch of the right colic artery. Its left branch supplies the distal half of the transverse colon. The splenic flexure comprises the watershed between midgut and hindgut supplies, the magnitude of this anastomosis (arcade of Riolan) is variable.

Inferior Mesenteric Artery

The inferior mesenteric artery arises from the aorta just above its bifurcation and runs downward and to the left, crossing the left iliac vessels, to enter the pelvis. Within the abdomen, the inferior mesenteric artery branches into the left colic artery and two to three sigmoid arteries; beyond the pelvic brim, the inferior mesenteric artery continues as the superior rectal artery (Figure 2.8). The left colic artery, the highest branch of the inferior mesenteric artery, bifurcates into an ascending branch, which runs upward to the splenic flexure to contribute to the arcade of Riolan, and a descending branch, which supplies most of the descending colon. The sigmoid arteries form arcades within the sigmoid mesocolon, in a manner that resembles the small bowel vasculature, and anastomose with branches of the left colic artery, proximally, and of the superior rectal artery, distally. The marginal artery terminates within the arcade of sigmoid arteries. The superior rectal artery or superior haemorrhoidal artery is the continuation of the inferior mesenteric artery once it crosses the left iliac vessels. The rectal superior artery descends in the sigmoid mesocolon to the level of S3, and then, on the posterior aspect of the rectum, bifurcates into right and left, and subsequently into anterior and posterior branches. These branches, once within the submucosa of the rectum, run straight downward to supply the lower rectum and the anal canal. Approximately five branches reach the level of the columns of Morgagni in capillary plexuses, mainly at the right posterior, right anterior and left lateral positions.

The superior and inferior rectal arteries represent the major blood supply to the anorectum. The contribution of the middle rectal artery varies inversely with the magnitude of the superior rectal artery. The middle rectal or middle haemorrhoidal artery, which may be absent in at least 40% of cases, originates more commonly from either the anterior division of the internal iliac or the pudendal arteries, and reaches the rectum close to the level of the pelvic floor (Ayoub, 1978). The middle haemorrhoidal artery does not traverse the lateral stalks of the rectum, but may send minor branches through those ligaments in about 25% of cases, which may account for bleeding during division of the lateral stalks (Boxall et al., 1963). The paired inferior rectal or inferior haemorrhoidal artery is a branch of the internal pudendal artery which is in turn a branch of the internal iliac artery. It arises within the pudendal canal, traverses the obturator fascia, ischiorectal fossa and the external anal sphincter to reach the submucosa of the anal canal and ultimately ascends in this plane. Although scarce in extramural anastomoses, the anorectum has a profuse intramural anastomotic network, which probably accounts for the fact that division of both the superior rectal and middle rectal arteries does not result in necrosis of the rectum (Lindstrom, 1950; Fisher and Fry, 1987). This tenet is fundamental to ileoanal reservoir surgery (Wexner et al., 1991b).

Venous Drainage

The venous drainage of the large intestine basically follows its arterial supply (Figure 2.8). Blood from the right colon, via the superior mesenteric vein, and from left colon and rectum, via the inferior mesenteric vein, reaches the intrahepatic capillary bed through the portal vein. The anorectum also drains, via middle and inferior rectal veins, to the internal iliac vein and then to the inferior vena cava.

The paired inferior and middle rectal veins and the single superior rectal vein originate from three anorectal arteriovenous plexuses. The external rectal plexus, situated subcutaneously around the anal canal below the dentate line, constitutes the external haemorrhoids when dilated. The internal rectal plexus is situated submucosally around the upper anal canal, above the dentate line. The internal haemorrhoids originate from this plexus. The perirectal or perimuscular rectal plexus drains to the middle and inferior rectal veins.

Lymphatic Drainage

The lymph drainage from any part of the colon follows its venous drainage. The submucous and subserous layers of the colon and rectum have a rich network of lymphatic plexuses, which drain into an extramural system of lymph channels and nodes. There are four groups of lymph nodes: epicolic, lying on the colon itself; paracolic, along the marginal artery; intermediate, on the main colic vessels; and principal nodes, on the superior and inferior mesenteric vessels (Figure 2.8). The lymph then drains to the cisterna chyli via a para-aortic chain of nodes. Colorectal carcinoma staging systems are based on the involvement of these various lymph node groups by the neoplasm.

Lymph from the upper two-thirds of the rectum drains exclusively upwards, via superior rectal vessels, to the inferior mesenteric nodes and then paraortic nodes. Lymphatic drainage from the lower third of the rectum follows not only the superior rectal and mesenteric nodes, but also laterally, along the middle rectal vessels to the internal iliac nodes (Figure 2.8). In the anal canal, the dentate line is the landmark for two different systems of lymphatic drainage: above, to the inferior mesenteric and internal iliac nodes; and below, to the perianal and inguinal nodes, or less frequently, along the inferior rectal artery. Lymphatic drainage of the anorectum, in the female, may also spread to the cul-de-sac, ovaries, uterus and posterior vaginal wall (Block and Enquist, 1961).

Innervation

The sympathetic and parasympathetic components of the autonomic innervation of the large intestine closely follow the blood supply (Figure 2.9).

Right Colon

The sympathetic supply originates from the lower six thoracic segments. These fibres, via thoracic splanchnic nerves, reach the coeliac, preaortic and superior mesenteric ganglia, where they synapse. The postganglionic fibres then course along the superior mesenteric artery to the small bowel and right colon. The parasympathetic supply comes from the right vagus nerve and coeliac plexus; fibres travel along the superior mesenteric artery, and finally synapse with cells in the autonomic plexuses in the bowel wall.

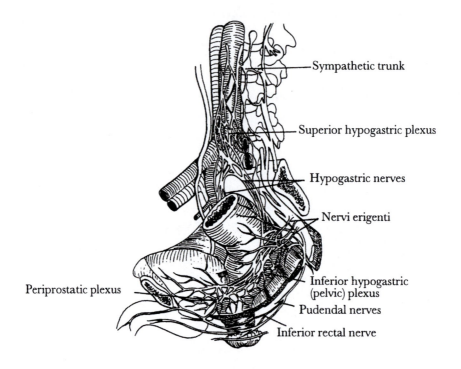

Figure 2.9: The parasympathetic and sympathetic nerve supply to the rectum.

Left Colon and Rectum

The sympathetic supply arises from L1, L2 and L3. Preganglionic fibres, via lumbar sympathetic nerves, synapse in the preaortic plexus; the postganglionic fibres follow the branches of the inferior mesenteric artery and superior rectal artery to the left colon and upper rectum. The lower rectum is innervated by the presacral nerves, which are formed by fusion of the aortic plexus and lumbar splanchnic nerves. Just below the sacral promontory, the presacral nerves form the superior hypogastric plexus. Two main hypogastric nerves, on either side of the rectum, carry sympathetic innervation from the hypogastric plexus to the pelvic plexus. The pelvic plexus lies on the lateral side of the pelvis at the level of the lower third of the rectum, adjacent to the lateral stalks.

The parasympathetic supply arises from S2, S3 and S4; these are termed nervi erigenti. They pass laterally, forward and upward to join the sympathetic hypogastric nerves in the pelvic plexus. From the pelvic plexus, postganglionic parasympathetic fibres are distributed to the left colon and upper rectum, via the inferior mesenteric plexus; to the genitals, via the periprostatic plexus; and directly to the lower rectum, upper anal canal and genitals. The pelvic autonomic plexuses lie in the plane between the peritoneum and the endopelvic fascia and are at risk during rectal surgery, especially for cancer (Church et al., 1987; Orkin, 1992).

Sexual function is regulated by cerebrospinal, sympathetic and parasympathetic components. Erection of the penis is mediated by both parasympathetic (arteriolar vasodilatation) and sympathetic (inhibition of vasoconstriction) in-flow. Sympathetic activity is responsible for emission and parasympathetic activity for ejaculation. Urinary and sexual dysfunction are commonly seen after a variety of pelvic surgical procedures, including low anterior resection, and abdominoperineal resection. Permanent bladder paresis occurs in 7–59% of patients after abdominoperineal resection of the rectum (Gerstenberg et al., 1980). The incidence of impotence is about 15% and 45% after low anterior resection and abdominoperineal resection, respectively (Orkin, 1992). The overall incidence of sexual dysfunction after proctectomy may reach up to 100% for malignant disease (Weinstein and Roberts, 1977; Balslev amd Harling, 1983); however, these rates are much lower, 0–6% (Bauer et al., 1983; Walsh and Schlegel, 1988), for benign conditions, such as inflammatory bowel disease. This occurs because dissection for benign disease is closer to the bowel wall, thus avoiding nerve injury. Sexual complications after rectal surgery are predominant in men, but are probably underdiagnosed in women. Some 30% of women have reported some discomfort and 10% report dyspareunia during intercourse after proctocolectomy and ileostomy (Metcalf et al., 1986).

Anal Canal

Motor Innervation

The internal anal sphincter is supplied by sympathetic (L5) and parasympathetic (S2, S3, S4) nerves which follow the same route as the nerves to the rectum. The levator ani is supplied by sacral roots (S2, S3 and S4) on its pelvic surface and by the perineal branch of the pudendal nerve on its inferior surface. The puborectalis receives additional innervation from the inferior rectal nerves. The external anal sphincter is innervated on each side by the inferior rectal branch (S2 and S3) of the pudendal nerve and the perineal branch of S4. Despite the fact that the puborectalis and the external anal sphincter have somewhat different innervations, these muscles seem to act as an indivisible unit.

Crossover of the fibres at the spinal cord level warrants preservation of external anal sphincter function after unilateral transection of a pudendal nerve.

Sensory Innervation

The upper anal canal contains a rich profusion of both free and organized sensory nerve-endings, especially in the vicinity of the anal valves (Duthie and Gairns, 1960). Organized nerve endings include Meissner's corpuscles (touch), Krause's bulbs (cold), Golgi-Mazzoni bodies (pressure) and genital corpuscles (friction). Anal sensation is carried in the inferior rectal branch of the pudendal nerve and is thought to play a role in anal continence.

Physiology

Anorectal physiology is complex and involves interrelation of multiple mechanisms. The high incidence of functional intestinal disorders and, more recently, the technological progress in functional testing have led to a great deal of research in this area. This research has improved our knowledge of normal and disordered physiology, and modified the therapeutic approach.

The mechanisms responsible for both faecal continence and defecation are complex and interrelated. In order to evaluate the different aspects of anorectal function, methods such as colonic transit times, anorectal manometry, defecography, electromyography and pudendal nerve latency have gained widespread popularity (Jorge and Wexner, 1993a). These methods allow better understanding of normal and disordered anorectal function. Thus, potentially disabling and highly prevalent disorders such as faecal incontinence and chronic idiopathic constipation can be stratified in several causative diagnoses with distinctive therapeutic approaches (Wexner et al., 1991a; Wexner and Jorge, 1994; Jorge and Wexner, 1993b).

Factors Maintaining Faecal Continence

Continence is maintained by the interaction of multiple mechanisms, including stool consistency and delivery of colonic contents to the rectum, rectal capacity and compliance, anorectal sensation, the function of the anal sphincter mechanism and the pelvic floor muscles and nerves.

Colon: Contractile Activity, Myoelectric Activity and Movements

Colonic motility studies are of limited use due to the relative inaccessibility of the proximal colon. Adler described three types of colonic motor patterns in humans based on colonic manometric findings (Adler et al., 1942). Type I contractions are monophasic waves of low amplitude and short duration. Type II contractions have higher amplitude and longer duration and represent about 90% of all normal manometric recording activity and correspond to combined contraction/relaxation haustral movements. Type III contractions are of low amplitude, overimpose type I or II contractions and represent a change in basal pressure. Subsequently, two other phenomena were recognized: giant motor contractions and the migrating motor complex (Kumar and Wingate, 1992). Giant motor contractions are high amplitude, rapidly propagated contraction waves, usually seen on walking and following meals, and frequently accompanied by an urge to defecate. The migrating motor complex, described only in canines, is a periodic motor activity, represented by rhythmic bursts of activity, usually with aboral migration. In humans this activity has been found only in the stomach and small bowel (Sarna et al., 1984).

Two types of activity have been detected in colonic electromyographic recordings: rhythmic slow waves and spike bursts (Pemberton, 1991). Slow waves are events of low frequency and originate in the circular muscle of the colon, representing the basal electrical activity. Spike bursts are associated with short and long-type contractions; long spike burst activity increases for two hours after each meal and is significantly reduced during sleep.

The most practical method to assess colonic transit requires ingestion of radio-opaque markers and quantification of these markers on abdominal radiographs. The mean values for normal total colonic transit time are about 32 and 41 hours for men and women, respectively. The mean segmental transit times are 12, 14 and 11 hours for right colon, left colon and rectosigmoid, respectively (Jorge and Habr-Gama, 1991).

In humans, there are three types of movements: segmentation, mass and retrograde movements (Kumar and Wingate, 1992). Segmentation, also known as haustrations or as mixing or non-propulsive movements, are large circular constrictions of 30-second duration occurring at 60-second intervals. The combined contractions of the circular layer and the taeniae coli lead to an outward bulging of the unstimulated segment of the intestine into the haustra, and the faecal bolus is 'slowly dug into and rolled over'. This movement, consisting of retrograde and anterograde movements of contents within a segment, allows gradual exposure of the faecal bolus to the surface of the large intestine, presumably to enhance colonic absorption. Mass or propulsive movements are responsible for propelling large amounts of faeces over long segments of the colon. From a constrictive ring at a distended or irritated point in the colon, a 20 cm or longer segment contracts as a unit and forces the faecal bolus distally within this segment. During a mass movement, the haustrations disappear completely. This type of movement occurs only a few times per day, and is more often seen in the transverse, descending and sigmoid colons. In fact, these segments may empty together into the rectum to elicit defecation. Finally, retrograde movements may occur, particularly in the transverse-ascending segment, and are thought to retard distal progression of the faecal bolus.

Colonic Absorption, Stool Volume and Consistency

The colon absorbs water, sodium and chloride, and secretes potassium and bicarbonate. In healthy individuals, colonic absorption of water reduces the 1000–1500 ml of fluid which enters the colon each day to about 100–150 ml (Phillips and Giller, 1973). Continence mechanisms are designed to handle the daily elimination of formed stool. Liquid stool emptied rapidly into the rectum results in great stress on the sphincters and even in normal subjects, phasic flows of liquid stool may occasionally produce urgency and incontinence.

Rectosigmoid Junction

Despite the rectum being highly capacious and compliant, during defecation a two-step pattern of emptying is usually noted; first the sigmoid empties into the rectum and subsequently the rectum evacuates. This fact has suggested an active role of the sigmoid in faecal continence, either as a reservoir or as a functional sphincter (Stoss, 1990).

Rectal Capacity and Compliance

Rectal contents must be accommodated if defecation is to be delayed. This deferral of the call to stool is possible through the mechanism of rectal compliance. The non-diseased rectum has elastic properties which allow it to maintain a low intraluminal pressure while being filled in order to preserve continence. In contrast with the high capacity and compliant characteristics of the normal rectum, significantly decreased compliance has been demonstrated in incontinent patients.

Whether poor rectal compliance is a cause or a consequence of faecal incontinence is controversial. The fact that no difference has been found in rectal compliance between patients with idiopathic and those with traumatic incontinence suggests that decreased rectal compliance is a consequence of an incompetent anal sphincter (Rasmussen et al., 1990). However, it is also plausible that if rectal compliance deteriorates, smaller volumes of faeces will result in higher intraluminal pressures causing urgency and incontinence. This mechanism was observed primarily in patients with ulcerative colitis and radiation proctitis (Denis et al., 1979; Varma et al., 1985). Sphincter-saving operations can be associated with incontinence, and loss of the rectal reservoir is thought to be the main factor; the formation of neorectal pouches, whether ileal or colonic, improves compliance (Parks and Nicholls, 1978).

Rectal Sensation

Rectal sensation involves different complex mechanisms. The rectum itself does not have receptors; proprioceptors are more probably situated in the levators, puborectalis and anal sphincters (Parks, 1975). Autonomous smooth muscle and voluntary skeletal muscles are triggered by distinct mechanisms with different thresholds. Diseases such as altered mental conditions (encephalopathy, dementia, stroke) and sensory neuropathy (diabetes) may selectively reduce conscious sensation and awareness of rectal fullness. Although these patients may not recognize or respond to threats to continence, the autonomic pathways which mediate the rectoanal inhibitory reflex may be intact. A faecal bolus in the rectum results in reflex relaxation of the internal anal sphincter. In these patients, relaxation occurs before a sensation of rectal distension, which results in both faecal impaction and overflow incontinence. High conscious rectal sensory thresholds have been observed in patients with faecal incontinence and in 28% of cases it is probably the primary cause (Buser and Miner, 1991). Although incontinence has been divided into two major groups, sphincter motor dysfunction and sensory deficiency, both disturbances probably interact.

Rectoanal Inhibitory Reflex and Anal Sensation

The rectoanal inhibitory reflex was first described by Gowers in 1877 as characterized by transient external anal sphincter contractions and pronounced internal anal sphincter reflex relaxation in response to rectal distension (Figure 2.10). This reflex enables rectal contents to

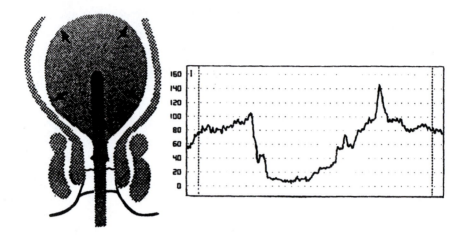

Figure 2.10: Rectoanal inhibitory reflex.

come into contact with the highly sensitive epithelial lining of the upper anal canal allowing for accurate distinction between flatus and faeces. This 'sampling' mechanism is thought to play a role in the fine adjustment of anal continence. Both reduced anal sensation and defective sampling mechanisms are probably important factors in the pathogenesis of faecal incontinence. When both are abnormal the patient may be completely unaware of impending incontinence.

Internal Anal Sphincter

The internal anal sphincter is a smooth muscle in a state of continuous maximal contraction. This tone, which provides a natural barrier to the involuntary loss of stool, is due to both intrinsic myogenic and extrinsic autonomic neurogenic properties. These properties account for 50–85% of the resting tone of the anal canal (Freckner and Euler, 1975; Lestar et al., 1989; Sun et al., 1989).

Skeletal Muscle Responses

The external anal sphincter, along with the pelvic floor muscles, maintains continuous unconscious resting electrical tone, a reflex arc at the cauda equine level. This is unlike other skeletal muscles which are usually inactive at rest. Histologic studies have shown that the external anal sphincter, puborectalis and levator ani muscles have a predominance of type I fibres, which is characteristic of skeletal muscles of tonic contractile activity (Swash, 1992). In response to conditions of threatened continence such as increased intra-abdominal pressure and rectal distension, the external anal sphincter and puborectalis muscles reflexively or voluntarily contract further in order to prevent faecal leakage. Owing to muscular fatigue, maximal voluntary contraction of the external anal sphincter can be sustained for only 40–60 seconds. The automatic continence mechanism is then formed by the resting tone, maintained by the internal anal sphincter, magnified by reflex external anal sphincter contraction. This extra pressure gradient is essential in minimizing voluntary attention to the sphincters and, consequently, optimal continence.

Puborectalis Muscle and the Anorectal Angle

The anorectal angle represents the result of the anatomic configuration of the U-shaped sling of the puborectalis muscle around the anorectal junction (Figure 2.11). Whereas the anal sphincters are responsible for closure of the anal canal to retain gas and liquid stool, the puborectalis muscle and the anorectal angle are designed to maintain gross faecal continence. Different theories have been postulated to

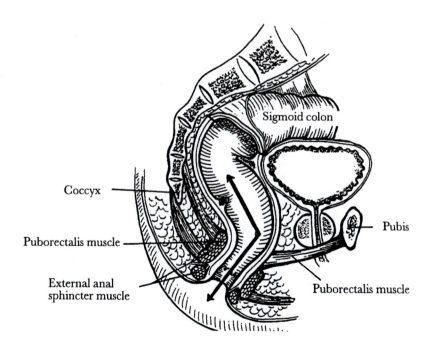

Figure 2.11: The anorectal angle.

explain the importance of the puborectalis muscle and the anorectal angle in the maintenance of faecal continence. Parks et al. (1966) considered that increasing intra-abdominal pressure forces the anterior rectal wall down into the upper anal canal occluding it by a type of flap-valve mechanism creating an effective seal. Subsequently it was demonstrated that the flap mechanism does not occur, instead a continued sphincteric occlusion-like activity attributed to the puborectalis was noted (Bartolo et al., 1986).

Sequence of Defecation

Defecation is a complex and incompletely understood phenomenon, related to several integrated mechanisms, all under the influence of the central nervous system (Figure 2.12). Defecation is triggered by filling of the rectum from the sigmoid colon. Rectal distension is interpreted, via stretch receptors located in the pelvic floor muscles, at a conscious level as a desire to defecate. Rectal distension also initiates the rectoanal inhibitory reflex. The internal anal sphincter relaxation, by opening the upper anal canal, exposes the rectal contents to the highly sensitive anal mucosa and then differentiation between flatus and stool can be made. This 'sampling' mechanism determines the urgency of defecation. Meanwhile, the simultaneous external anal sphincter reflex contraction maintains continence. If defecation is to be deferred, conscious contraction of the external anal sphincter, assisted by the mechanism of rectal compliance, yields time for recuperation of the internal anal sphincter function.

If the call to stool is answered, either the sitting or squatting position is assumed, and then the anorectal angle is 'opened'. Increase in both intrarectal and intra-abdominal pressures result in reflex relaxation in external and internal anal sphincter and puborectalis muscles; at this point, defecation may occur without straining. Nevertheless, some degree of straining is usually necessary to initiate rectal evacuation. Straining will ensure further relaxation of the anal sphincter muscles and the anorectal angle becomes even more obtuse. Consequently, pelvic floor descending and funnelling occur, and the rectal contents are expelled by direct transmission of the increased abdominal pressure through the relaxed pelvic floor.

Metabolic Function

The metabolic function of the colon is minimal compared with that of the small intestine; however, it is probably underestimated. All *in vivo*

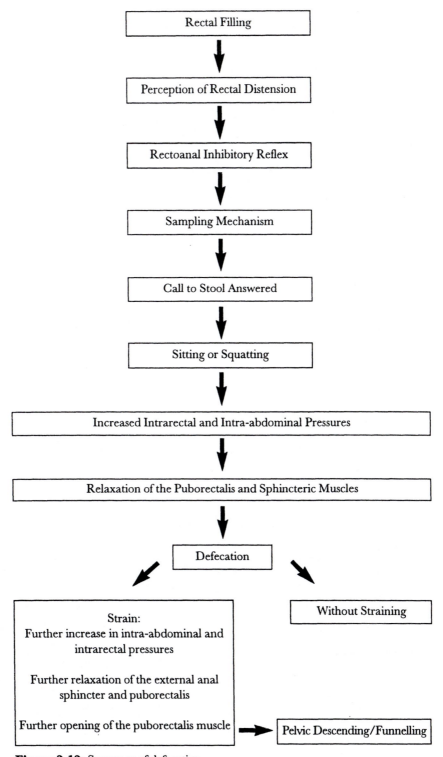

Figure 2.12: Sequence of defecation.

studies are conducted in cleansed, defunctioned colons, which have proven not to be a physiological model (Moran and Jackson, 1992).

The colon is a reservoir for bacterial metabolism and fermentation. The colonic flora, predominantly anaerobic, are estimated at over 400 different species and collectively outnumber the individual's own cells.

The colonic microflora ferment carbohydrates originated from mucus and polysaccharides which escape digestion in the small intestine. The result is the production of short-chain fatty acids (acetate, butyrate and propionate) which have been shown to stimulate growth of the colonic mucosa. Disorders of metabolism of the short-chain fatty acids have been implicated in colonic mucosal diseases, particularly in inflammatory bowel disease (Roediger, 1988). Patients with short gut but with the colon in circuit have superior nutrient absorption to those with small bowel ending in a stoma. Nightingale et al. (1991) concluded that the colon in circuit has a functional capacity in nutrient absorption similar to that of 50 cm of jejunum.

Fortunately, after total colectomy, with the bacterial colonization ileum as part of an adaptation mechanism, the remnant ileum takes over some of the metabolic functions of the colon. This, at least in part, accounts for the good functional results obtained with this operation in the vast majority of patients.

References

Adler HF, Atkinson AJ, Ivy AC (1942) Supplementary and synergistic action of stimulating drugs on motility of human colon. Surgery, Gynecology and Obstetrics 74: 809–13.

Ayoub SF (1978) Arterial supply of the human rectum. Acta Anatomica 100: 317–27.

Balslev I, Harling H (1983) Sexual dysfunction following operation for carcinoma of the rectum. Diseases of the Colon and Rectum 26: 785–8.

Bartolo DCC, Roe AM, Locke-Edmunds JC, Virjee J, Mortensen NJMcC (1986) Flap-valve theory of anorectal continence. British Journal of Surgery 73: 1012–14.

Bauer JJ, Gerlent IM, Salky B, Kreel I (1983) Sexual dysfunction following proctectomy for benign disease of the colon and rectum. Annals of Surgery 197: 363–7.

Block IR, Enquist IF (1961) Studies pertaining to local spread of carcinoma of the rectum in females. Surgery, Gynecology and Obstetrics 112: 41–6.

Boxall TA, Smart PJG, Griffiths JD (1963) The blood-supply of the distal segment of the rectum in anterior resection. British Journal of Surgery 50: 399–404.

Buser WD, Miner PB Jr (1991) Delayed rectal sensation with fecal incontinence. Diseases of the Colon and Rectum 34: 744–7.

Church JM, Raudkivi PJ, Hill GL (1987) The surgical anatomy of the rectum – a review with particular relevance to the hazards of rectal mobilisation. International Journal of Colorectal Disease 2: 158–66.

Denis Ph, Colin R, Galmiche JP, Geffroy Y, Hecketsweiler Ph, Lefrancois R,

Pasquis P (1979) Elastic properties of the rectal wall in normal adults and in patients with ulcerative colitis. Gastroenterology 77: 45-48.

Duthie HL, Gairns FW (1960) Sensory nerve endings and sensation in the anal region in man. British Journal of Surgery 47: 585–95.

Ewing MR (1954) The white line of Hilton. Proceedings of the Royal Society of Medicine 47: 525–30.

Fisher DF, Fry WI (1987) Collateral mesenteric circulation. Surgery, Gynecology and Obstetrics 164: 487–92.

Frenckner B, Euler CHRV (1975) Influence of pudendal block on the function of the anal sphincters. Gut 16: 482–9.

Gerstenberg TC, Nielsen ML, Clausen S, Blaabgerg J, Lindenberg J (1980) Bladder function after abdominoperineal resection of the rectum for anorectal cancer. American Journal of Surgery 91: 81–6.

Goligher J (1984) Surgery of the Anus, Rectum and Colon. London: Baillière Tindall, pp 1–47.

Goligher JC, Leacock AG, Brossy JJ (1955) The surgical anatomy of the anal canal. British Journal of Surgery 43: 51–61.

Gowers WR (1877) The automatic action of the sphincter ani. Proceedings of the Royal Society of London 26: 77–84.

Jorge JMN, Habr-Gama A (1991) Tempo de trânsito colônico total e segmentar: análise crítica dos métodos e estudo em indivíduos normais com marcadores radiopacos. Revista Brasiliera de Colo-Proctologia 11: 55–60.

Jorge JMN, Wexner SD (1993a) A practical guide to basic anorectal physiology. Contemporary Surgery 43: 214.

Jorge JMN, Wexner SD (1993b) Etiology and management of fecal incontinence. Diseases of the Colon and Rectum 36: 77–97.

Kumar D, Wingate DL (1992) Colorectal motility. In Henry MM, Swash M Coloproctology and the Pelvic Floor. Oxford: Butterworth-Heinemann, pp 72–85.

Lestar B, Penninckx F, Kerremans R (1989) The composition of anal basal pressure. An in vivo and in vitro study in man. International Journal of Colorectal Disease 4: 118–22.

Lindstrom BL (1950) The value of the collateral circulation from the inferior mesenteric artery in obliteration of the lower abdominal aorta. Acta Chirurgica Scandinavica 1: 677–85.

Metcalf AM, Dozois RR, Kelly KA (1986) Sexual function in women after proctocolectomy. Annals of Surgery 204: 624–7.

Moran BJ, Jackson AA (1992) Function of the human colon. British Journal of Surgery 79: 1132–7.

Nightingale JMD, Gertner DJ, Wood SR, Lennard-Jones JE (1991) Colonic preservation reduces the need for long-term intravenous nutrition, water and electrolyte therapy in the short bowel syndrome. Proceedings of the Nutrition Society 288: 678–80.

Orkin BA (1992) Rectal carcinoma: treatment. In Beck DE, Wexner SD Fundamentals of Anorectal Surgery. New York: McGraw-Hill, pp 260–369.

Parks AG (1975) Anorectal incontinence. Journal of the Royal Society of Medicine 68: 681–90.

Parks AG, Nicholls RJ (1978) Proctocolectomy without ileostomy for ulcerative colitis. British Medical Journal 2: 85–8.

Parks AG, Porter NH, Hardcastle J (1966) The syndrome of the descending perineum. Proceedings of the Royal Society of Medicine 59: 477–82.

Pemberton JH (1991) Anatomy and physiology of the anus and rectum. In Zuidema, GD Shackelford's Surgery of the Alimentary Tract. Philadelphia: WB Saunders, pp 242–73.

Phillips SF, Giller J (1973) The contribution of the colon to the electrolyte and water absorption in man. Journal of Laboratory and Clinical Medicine 81: 733–46.

Quinyao W, Weijin S, Youren Z, Wenqing Z, Zhengrui H (1985) New concepts in severe presacral hemorrhage during proctectomy. Archives of Surgery 120: 1013–20.

Rasmussen O, Christiensen B, Sorensen M, Tetzchner T, Christiansen J (1990) Rectal compliance in the assessment of patients with fecal incontinence. Diseases of the Colon and Rectum 33: 650–3.

Roediger WEW (1988) Bacterial short chain fatty acids and mucosal diseases of the colon. British Journal of Surgery 75: 346–8.

Russell KP (1991) Anatomy of the pelvic floor, rectum and anal canal. In Smith LE Practical Guide to Anorectal Testing. New York: Igaku-Shoin Medical Publications, pp 744–7.

Sarna SK, Condon R, Cowles V (1984) Colonic migrating and non-migrating motor complexes in dogs. American Journal of Physiology 246: G355–60.

Shafik A (1975) A new concept of the anatomy of the anal sphincter mechanism and the physiology of defecation, II: Anatomy of the levator ani muscle with special reference to puborectalis. Investigative Urology 13: 175–82.

Skandalakis JE, Gray SW, Ricketts R (1994) The colon and rectum. In Skandalakis JE, Gray SW (Eds) Embryology for Surgeons. The Embryological Basis for the Treatment of Congenital Anomalies. Baltimore: Williams & Wilkins: 242–81.

Stoss F (1990) Investigations of the muscular architecture of the rectosigmoid junction in humans. Diseases of the Colon and Rectum 33: 378–83.

Sun WM, Read NW, Donnelly TC (1989) Impaired internal anal sphincter in a subgroup of patients with idiopathic fecal incontinence. Gastroenterology 97: 130–5.

Swash M (1992) Histopathology of pelvic floor muscles in pelvic floor disorders. In Henry MM, Swash M (Eds) Coloproctology and the Pelvic Floor. London: Butterworth-Heinemann, pp 173–83.

Varma JS, Smith AN, Busuttil A (1985) Correlation of clinical and manometric abnormalities of rectal function following chronic radiation injury. British Journal of Surgery 72: 875–8.

Walsh PC, Schlegel PN (1988) Radical pelvic surgery with preservation of sexual function. Annals of Surgery 208: 391–400.

Weinstein M, Roberts M (1977) Sexual potency following surgery for rectal carcinoma. A follow up of 44 patients. Annals of Surgery 185: 295–300.

Wakeley CPG (1983) The position of the vermiform appendix as ascertained by an analysis of 10,000 cases. Journal of Anatomy 67: 277–83.

Wexner SD, Daniel N, Jagelman DG (1991a) Colectomy for constipation: physiologic investigation is the key to success. Diseases of the Colon and Rectum 34: 851–6.

Wexner SD, James K, Jagelman DG (1991b) The double stapled ileal reservoir and ileoanal anastomosis: a prospective review of sphincter function and clinical outcome. Diseases of the Colon and Rectum 34: 487–94.

Wexner SD, Jorge JMN (1994) Colorectal physiological tests: use or abuse of technology? European Journal of Surgery 160: 167–74.

Williamson RCN, Mortensen NJMcC (1987) Anatomy of the large intestine. In Kirsner JB, Shorter RG (Eds) Diseases of the Colon, Rectum and Anal Canal. Rochester: Williams & Wilkins, pp 1–22.

Chapter 3
Investigation and Examination of a Patient with Colorectal Problems

LAURENCE R. SANDS MD, Assistant Professor of Clinical Surgery, Division of Colon and Rectal Surgery, University of Miami School of Medicine, Florida, USA

NORMA DANIEL RN, MS, CNOR, RNFA, Surgical Nurse Clinician, Colorectal Department, Cleveland Clinic Florida, Florida, USA

Students of medicine throughout the world have traditionally been taught that a well-documented medical history obtained from the patient may provide a diagnosis as often as 90% of the time. When such a history is combined with a good physical examination, the diagnosis may well be certain. There is perhaps no greater truth to this than when one discusses the colorectal patient. Certainly, much information can be derived from a well-thought-out series of questions when obtaining the history. The physical examination, especially when combined with the modalities of office anoscopy and proctosigmoidoscopy, may well pinpoint a diagnosis with a high degree of accuracy. The goal of this chapter is to delineate the investigative techniques used to adequately evaluate the colorectal patient.

The History

The history of present illness when referring to the colorectal patient is centred around several key symptoms. These symptoms include a change in bowel habit, rectal bleeding, abdominal or anorectal pain, a history of palpable masses, and faecal incontinence.

A change in bowel habit may represent the earliest signs of colorectal malignancy. Classically, the patient will complain of a change in the calibre of the stool or will give a history of increasing bouts of constipation. These complaints should alert the clinician to pursue the additional line of questions regarding possible systemic effects of an occult malignancy; namely, weight loss, fatigue and decreased appetite. Whilst constipation itself may make one consider the possibility of a partially obstructing colonic neoplasm, one must bear in mind that this symptom in itself means relatively little. While normal bowel frequency varies greatly, most clinicians agree that the average individual has somewhere between three bowel movements per day and one bowel movement every three days. Thus, while the history of having one bowel movement every three days may be generally normal, it certainly represents a significant change for the individual who is having two to three bowel movements per day. It is this change that is important to consider.

Rectal bleeding is a relatively frequent symptom. While the patient's fear associated with rectal bleeding is most commonly that of a colorectal neoplasm, in fact, bleeding may occur for a variety of benign reasons. Anal fissures, haemorrhoids, and diverticular disease are just a few of the other causes of rectal bleeding. In obtaining the history of passing blood per rectum, it is important to characterize both the quality as well as the quantity of bleeding. For instance, there is a considerable difference between streaks of blood lining the stool, which may be indicative of haemorrhoidal bleeding or bleeding from an anal fissure, and passing large amounts of bright red blood with clots, which may be attributed to diverticular bleeding or an arteriovenous malformation of the colon. Alternatively, the stool may appear as dark black in colour, and may only test positively for blood on a haemoccult test. This may be suspicious for a right-sided colonic neoplasm or even a slowly bleeding duodenal ulcer.

Rectal bleeding may often be seen in patients with inflammatory bowel disease. This type of persistent bleeding typically accompanies frequent bouts of diarrhoea with or without crampy abdominal pain. Weight loss may be seen in conjunction with inflammatory bowel disease and, in extreme cases, the patient may even appear toxic, with episodes of severe inflammation. It is thus the responsibility of the clinician to obtain an accurate history pertaining to rectal bleeding in order to develop a plan that will lead to the appropriate tests that will result in the correct diagnosis.

Anorectal pain may be associated with a number of anorectal problems; most notably, perianal abscess, anal fissure, levator spasm or coccydynia. The type of pain as well as its duration may lead one toward the proper diagnosis. Acute anal pain associated with bright red blood coating the stool is quite characteristic of anal fissure; a tear of the perianal skin, often the result of the passage of a hard stool. A smouldering sort of discomfort that develops into intense pain with or without fevers may indicate an abscess. Pain that is exacerbated with movement may well relate to coccydynia, while a deep-seated and intermittent pain may be related to levator spasm.

Abdominal pain may be related to a variety of different conditions. A diffuse, crampy and spasmodic pain associated with bloody diarrhoea may in fact be due to Crohn's disease, mucosal ulcerative colitis, or an infectious gastroenteritis, while an intense, steady pain may be secondary to peritoneal irritation. Peritoneal irritation may be the result of any sort of inflammatory process such as acute diverticulitis, acute appendicitis, or acute cholecystitis. Understanding and eliciting the symptoms of abdominal pain will enable the clinician to conduct a physical examination to locate the site of discomfort as well as its severity and arrive at the correct diagnosis.

Patients often describe a lump or bulging of the perianal or rectal area. Often, they are referring to prolapsing haemorrhoidal disease. Alternatively, a protrusion of the rectum that either reduces spontaneously or with gentle pressure may be due to rectal prolapse. Occasionally, condyloma or skin tags may be the cause of a perianal mass. Condyloma acuminata is caused by the human papilloma virus and is often a sexually transmitted disease that is seen more commonly among the homosexual community. By asking the appropriate questions, including a detailed sexual history, the clinician may yield a great deal of information with regard to the diagnosis of perianal masses.

Faecal incontinence may be due to a variety of factors, including trauma to the perineal area, prior episiotomies with damage to the sphincter mechanism, neurologic injury, which may occur from chronic diabetes mellitus, or faecal impaction. Once again, a careful history consisting of appropriately asked questions, including other systemic diseases, may add great insight into the causes of faecal incontinence.

Physical Examination

The history, no matter how accurate, is never complete without an adequate physical examination. It has been said that 'diseases often escape the attention of the family physician simply because he fails to make an examination' (Keen, 1987). It has also been said 'the physician should never forget that his examining room constitutes a cancer detection center, the potentialities of which rest within his own hands' (Nesselrod, 1957). These quotations seem so simple in their words, yet it cannot be overstated how important a good physical examination is to the patient. All too often, patients present with advanced diseases simply because the physician failed to perform an adequate examination.

The Abdominal Examination

The colorectal patient should be examined thoroughly, as with any other patient. There is special emphasis placed on the abdominal examination especially when one elicits symptoms of abdominal pain, bloating, or change in bowel habits. This highly specialized examination includes careful inspection, palpation, percussion, and auscultation of the abdomen.

The patient is placed supine on the examining table exposing the entire abdominal and inguinal regions. First, an initial inspection may reveal scars, stomas, or obvious abdominal distension. These scars may reveal clues as to the previous types of abdominal surgery, even if the patient is unable to provide this information in the history. For example, a right upper quadrant subcostal incision may alert the examiner to a prior cholecystectomy whilst a small right lower quadrant scar may suggest a prior appendectomy. Also, a lower midline incision in a female classically suggests either a prior caesarian section or hysterectomy.

Auscultation may reveal normal, hypoactive, or high-pitched bowel sounds. High-pitched rushes may be suggestive of a partial intestinal obstruction or an intestinal stricture whilst hypoactive bowel sounds may be present in a late intestinal obstruction.

The examiner should then proceed with a careful and systematic palpation of the abdomen. This includes feeling all four quadrants of the abdomen in an attempt to elicit tenderness or detect abdominal masses. Tympany suggests air-filled loops of intestine whilst dullness may suggest signs of abdominal ascites or fluid-filled loops of bowel.

The abdominal exam is then concluded by a careful inspection of both inguinal regions searching for enlarged lymph nodes or masses. Lymphadenopathy may be present in patients with metastatic disease from anorectal cancer or a variety of inflammatory or infectious conditions.

The Anorectal Examination

The anorectal exam may well be performed in a variety of positions. Each position has relative advantages and disadvantages for the patient, as well as the physician (Figure 3.1).

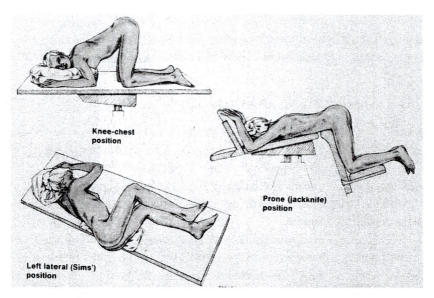

Knee-chest
position

Prone (jackknife)
position

Left lateral (Sims')
position

Figure 3.1: Positions commonly used for performing anorectal examinations.

The prone (jackknife) position may be the least comfortable position for the patient, though it affords the physician the best view of the anorectal region. It requires the use of a specialized examination table that may be expensive to buy.

The left lateral (Sims') position may be the most comfortable position for the patient. This position places the patient on his/her left side with the buttocks extending slightly over the edge of the table, while the patient's hips are flexed upwards and the knees slightly extended. This position is slightly more inconvenient for the examiner to view the anorectal region. However, sigmoidoscopic examination may be easily performed in this position.

The knee–chest position may also be used. This position may be more comfortable for the patient than the jackknife position, but it is certainly more awkward for the examiner.

The entire examination should be explained to the patient well beforehand. This will certainly ease the patient as to what is to be expected during the examination. First, the examiner will inspect the perianal area. The area should carefully be examined for lesions such as anal fissure, condyloma, skin tags, perirectal abscesses, perianal Crohn's disease, perianal rashes or dermatitis. A variety of diseases may be seen initially on inspection that may give the physician ideas for treatment. After inspection, a digital examination should be performed. This examination will assess the tone of the anal musculature. It will also examine the prostate in males and assess whether there are any distinct masses, nodularity or diffuse enlargement. It will also determine whether there are any masses or polyps in the anorectal canal. In addition, digital examination may determine whether there is any tenderness of the anorectal region that may indicate anal fissure or abscess. Also, pelvic inflammatory conditions such as pelvic inflammatory disease or appendicitis may be suspected with a careful rectal examination. If a prior coloanal or ileoanal anastomosis has been performed in the past, this area may be carefully palpated to ensure patency while examining for stricture, stenosis or recurrent tumour.

The rectal examination also tests the quality of stool present and may test for both gross or occult blood in the stool. In a recent study at the University of Minnesota determining the validity of the faecal occult blood test, it was determined that the mortality from colorectal cancer decreased by 33%, while the test itself was found to be about 90% sensitive (Church et al., 1997).

The rectal exam may also note any abnormalities along the rectal–vaginal septum in women, while a bi-manual examination and a pelvic examination may also provide additional information. While this is done, one may also note the thickness of the sphincter muscle, particularly if the patient complains of faecal incontinence. The cul-de-sac may also be palpated for any firm masses, particularly noting whether there exists a Blumer's shelf, or a hard mass along the pelvic floor that may be indicative of metastatic cancer.

Presacral masses or extrinsic lesions may also be noted on rectal examination. These rare lesions may present as a bulge in the posterior rectal wall. These lesions may represent cysts, tumours or chordomas.

Proctoscopy

After digital examination, proctoscopy is usually the first instrument examination used in assessing the colorectal patient. Proctoscopy affords the clinician the best view of the anorectal region, while one carefully inspects for fissures, fistulas, skin tags, haemorrhoids or hypertrophied papilla.

There are many proctoscopes available, some of which may be seen in Figure 3.2. Some of these instruments shown may best be used in the operating room with proper sedation rather than in the office because of their large size and the discomfort they may cause the non-sedated patient.

While performing proctoscopy, an adequate light source must be used. This light source may be either a head-lamp or a wall-mounted

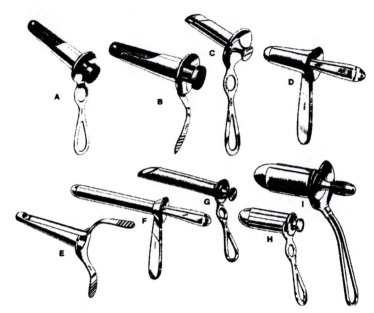

Figure 3.2: Different types of instruments used for anorectal examinations.

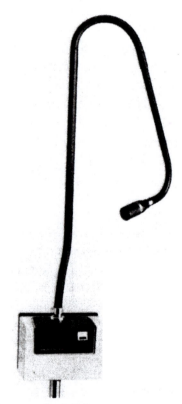

Figure 3.3: The wall-mounted unit light source.

unit (Figure 3.3). Other proctoscopes have an adaptor that may allow the attachment of the light source directly into the anoscope. The clinician should carefully document any anorectal pathology that is seen with anoscopy by stating whether the lesions are anterior, posterior, to the right or left side of the anal canal. This sort of documentation obviates the use of the o'clock positions that are commonly used, as these positions require a known patient position when examined.

Sigmoidoscopy

The examination may be performed as either a flexible or rigid sigmoidoscopy (Figures 3.4a, 3.4b). The major advantage of the flexible instrument rests in the fact that this tool may be inserted further than the rigid sigmoidoscope. This, however, should not underestimate the value of rigid sigmoidoscopy to evaluate the entire rectum as well as the distal sigmoid colon. This instrument is classically 25 cm in length and may be disposable or reusable. One of the advantages of the rigid sigmoidoscope is in its ability to accurately measure distances from the anal verge. This becomes extremely important in low-lying rectal cancers, when a restorative proctectomy is contemplated.

Both examinations have the ability to evaluate the rectal and colonic mucosa, as well as to evaluate for polypoid lesions or masses. These examinations may be performed in the left lateral or jackknife positions after an appropriate bowel preparation consisting of two Fleet's enemas. The instrument is gently inserted past the anal sphincter muscles and advanced under direct vision through the anal canal with minimal air insufflation. The instrument is advanced as far as possible or until patient discomfort prohibits further examination. A careful inspection is performed upon withdrawal of the sigmoidoscope. The instrument should be withdrawn in a circular motion, with visualization of all the walls of the bowel, as well as the three valves of Houston, which may be seen in the rectum. These valves simply represent mucosal folds that may help one identify the position within the rectum.

A variety of procedures may be performed through the sigmoidoscope, including biopsies, fulguration of rectal lesions, as well as snare excision of polyps. Biopsies are most often performed on the posterior rectal wall or on a valve of Houston to minimize the risk associated with perforation. In any event, the risk of perforation associated with sigmoidoscopy remains quite low (Gilbertson, 1974).

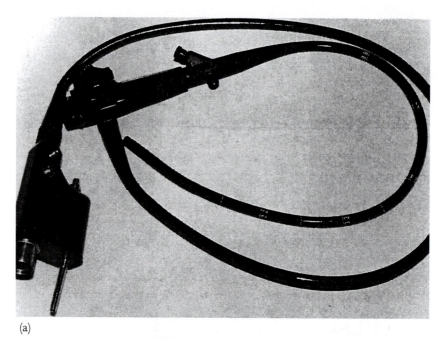

(a)

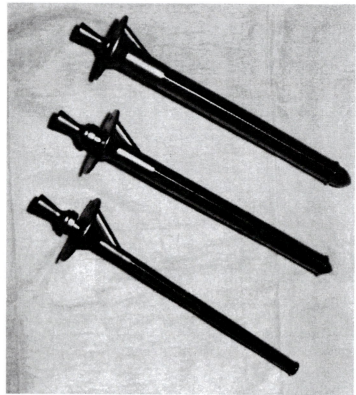

(b)

Figure 3.4: (a) The flexible fibreoptic sigmoidoscope; (b) the rigid proctoscope.

Screening sigmoidoscopies should be performed for asymptomatic individuals aged 50 and over and colonoscopy every 3 to 5 years in high-risk groups (Columbo et al., 1997). Adherence to these recommendations will surely reduce the risk of developing colorectal cancer.

Colonoscopy

A colonoscopy is indicated under a variety of circumstances. Patients at high risk for developing colorectal malignancies may benefit from a colonoscopy (Figure 3.5). Other indications may be seen in Table 3.1. Colonoscopy is classically performed in either a gastrointestinal unit or some type of monitored setting. The patient must prepare for the examination by first cleansing the bowel the day prior to the study with an electrolyte solution of sodium sulphate with the osmotic agent of polyethylene glycol. This solution consists of a 4-litre dose that is usually consumed over several hours. An alternate solution of 45 cc of Fleet's phosphosoda may be given the day prior to the exam with a repeat dose on the early morning of the exam. In addition to this the patient is to consume a clear liquid diet the day prior to the exam. This solution may be better tolerated than the large volume associated with the 4-litre solution of polyethylene glycol.

The patient is then placed on the left side with the appropriate nasal cannula oxygen and with monitors in place for observing the heart rate, blood pressure and oxygen saturation (Fleischer, 1989).

Table 3.1: Indications for colonoscopy

(1)	Confirmation or refutation of suspected or equivocal radiologic abnormality
(2)	Evaluation and follow-up of inflammatory bowel disease
(3)	Differential diagnosis of diverticular disease or malignancy
(4)	Presence of a rectal polyp or other colonic polyps
(5)	GI symptoms (bleeding, anaemia, abdominal pain)
(6)	Follow-up after colon resection surgery
(7)	Acute lower GI bleeding
(8)	Persistent diarrhoea of unexplained origin
(9)	Endoscopic polypectomy for colonic polyps
(10)	Reducing a sigmoid volvulus
(11)	Decompression of a dilated colon
(12)	Intraoperative use to locate the site of a lesion

Source: Adapted from: Corman ML (1993) Colon and Rectal Surgery. Philadelphia: JB Lippincott.

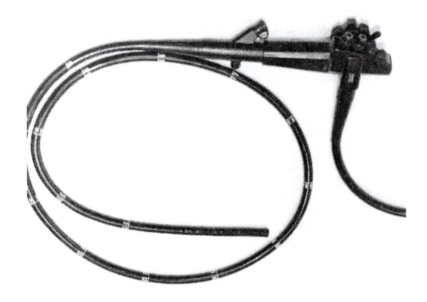

Figure 3.5: The fibreoptic colonoscope.

The patient is then given sedation with intravenous medication usually consisting of a combination of Demerol and Versed. The colonoscope is introduced into the rectum after a digital examination. It is then advanced under direct vision all the way to the caecum. A detailed examination is then performed while removing the colonoscope. Any suspicious lesions or polyps may be removed by biopsy forceps or with the use of a snare and electrocautery. A nurse must be present for this study in order to assist with the procedure as well as to monitor the patient's vital signs. In addition to this important role, the nurse may help reassure the patient during the procedure.

The greatest risks associated with colonoscopy include bleeding, perforation, and post-procedure distension. Bleeding, although rare, is the most frequent complication encountered. Perforation occurs half as often as bleeding with an incidence in one study of 0.33% (Berci et al., 1974). However, when perforation occurs, it may pose a serious and possibly life-threatening complication. Post-colonoscopic distension may be most dramatic. Fortunately, however, it is rather benign and often resolves with conservative management.

Blood-work

Routine blood-work is not often obtained in an initial visit to the colorectal surgeon. However, if a there is a history of anorectal bleeding and the patient complains of generalized fatigue, it may be prudent to check a complete blood count to assure that the patient is not anaemic. Coagulation factors may also be checked prior to performing any procedure where bleeding may be encountered in order to ensure adequate haemostasis.

For patients being followed for colorectal malignancy, one may obtain a carcinoembryonic antigen (CEA) level. CEA concentrations may reflect the extent of tumour spread and recurrence (Lewis, 1984). A rising CEA level may well be indicative of tumour recurrence and may precipitate a search for such recurrence.

Radiologic Studies

Plain X-rays of the abdomen may be somewhat helpful in determining whether a normal bowel gas pattern exists. These films often add little to the routine evaluation of the colorectal patient. However, such X-rays may, in fact, suggest various abnormalities including colonic or small bowel distension, bowel perforation, or even colonic volvulus.

Barium enema remains an excellent study in determining colonic pathology. This examination may be done as either a single or double air contrast study. The double contrast study offers the advantage of finer detailing of the colonic mucosa with perhaps more accuracy in diagnosing inflammatory bowel disease as well as smaller polyps. Most radiologists would agree that the double air contrast study is superior to the single contrast study (DeRoos et al., 1985). Multiple angles are observed and X-ray pictures taken during the study in order to best visualize all the twists and turns of the colon.

A barium enema is contraindicated if a patient has recently undergone a polypectomy for fear of perforation and possibly causing barium peritonitis. This study should also not be performed in the face of acute conditions such as acute fulminant colitis, active diverticulitis or colonic obstruction. Acute or sub-acute situations such as these may best be studied with a water-soluble contrast medium such as hypaque or gastrograffin. These solutions must still be used with caution but will not precipitate as violent a peritoneal response as barium in the event of perforation.

Both examinations are performed by placing a balloon catheter into the rectum and instilling barium. Because the balloon will occupy the majority of the rectum, the lower portion of the gastrointestinal tract must be studied by some form of endoscopy in order not to miss a low-lying rectal lesion. The patient is rolled back and forth on the table while the radiologist uses fluoroscopy to obtain X-ray pictures of the colon. The major disadvantage of the barium enema is that once a polypoid lesion is found in the colon, the patient must then be subjected to a colonoscopy in order to retrieve the polyp or biopsy the lesion, thereby subjecting the patient to two examinations. However, the barium enema remains a highly accurate test in detecting colonic polyps and should be considered in evaluating the colon (Warden et al., 1988). The test becomes extremely valuable when used for considering surgery in the patient with refractory chronic diverticular disease. The muscular hypertrophy may be seen clearly in many cases studied with barium enema. The test may also be useful in evaluating the patient with rectal prolapse in order to see the amount of redundancy in the sigmoid colon.

Computed Tomography (CT Scan)

CT scan of the abdomen may be helpful in a variety of situations. This test may be performed routinely in some centres for all colorectal malignancies in an attempt to define metastatic disease and preoperatively stage the cancer patient. The CT scan will provide a detailed image of the liver as well as the urinary system. This may be particularly helpful in the patient with a rectosigmoid carcinoma that can cause obstructive uropathy. A CT scan may also aid in the diagnosis of inflammatory conditions such as Crohn's disease or complicated diverticulitis. Abscesses may also be drained with CT-guided placement of a percutaneous catheter, thereby obviating the need for emergent operative intervention which otherwise might require a temporary colostomy. Percutaneous drainage of an abdominal abscess can be followed by elective colon resection with primary anastomosis in the setting of properly prepared bowel.

Pelvic magnetic resonance imaging (MRI) with an endorectal coil is now utilized in some centres for patients with rectal cancer. This study may provide detailed imaging of a tumour with information about the depth of invasion which might assist in preoperative planning.

Anorectal Physiology

The pelvic floor can be studied with the use of anal manometry and electromyography. These tests are useful in evaluation of the patient with faecal incontinence, defecatory disorders, rectal prolapse and anal stenosis. They may also help in the decision of performing either an ileoanal or coloanal anastomosis.

Anal manometry is performed by placing a water-perfused catheter within the anal canal. This catheter is then connected to a computer

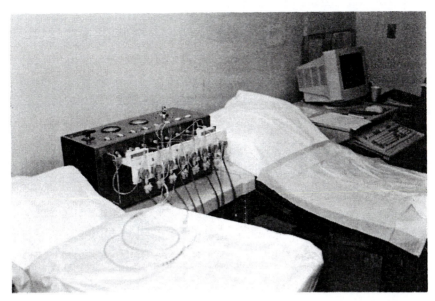

Figure 3.6: Anal manometry unit (Arndorfer Medical Specialties Inc, Greendale, WI).

recording device (Figure 3.6). The patient is asked to relax and squeeze the anal sphincter while the catheter is withdrawn from the anal canal. The resting pressures recorded are a measure of the internal anal sphincter, while the squeeze pressures reflect the activity of the external anal sphincter. As one might expect, the pressures generated will be considerably lower than normal in an individual who is suffering from faecal incontinence secondary to a sphincter disruption (Jorge and Wexner, 1993).

Manometry is a relatively easy and painless test to perform. It simply requires having the necessary equipment available. The perfusion machine along with the software and computer is quite expensive. However, combining the use of this machine with the gastroenterologist who may also use it for upper gastrointestinal (GI) manometric studies will make this cost more justifiable.

Electromyography (EMG) may prove helpful in determining the innervation of the pelvic floor. Both concentric needle and single-fibre EMG studies show external anal sphincter defects and may complement ultrasound findings. Electrical stimulation of the pudendal nerves may also be performed to help in deciding if the sphincter complex is properly innervated. This may determine a possible neurogenic cause of faecal incontinence such as might be seen in the patient with diabetes mellitus with a peripheral neuropathy.

Colonic transit studies may be performed in the evaluation of patients with colonic inertia and severe constipation. The patient is instructed to avoid use of all laxatives for one week prior to the study. After the ingestion of a capsule containing radio-opaque markers, abdominal X-rays are obtained on days 3 and 5. A normal study shows that 80% of the markers have been passed in 5 days. If more than 20% of the markers are distributed evenly through out the colon, there is strong evidence for colonic inertia.

Cinedefecography is performed to evaluate the pelvic floor musculature and to evaluate the relaxation of the pelvic floor during defecation. This test is performed by placing a contrast medium in the rectal vault while the patient is placed on a special commode. As the contrast is expelled from the rectum, radiographs are taken under fluoroscopy. It may also aid in the diagnosis of internal prolapse or intussusception, the precursor to rectal prolapse as well as obstructive defecatory disorders. This test is usually performed at specialty centres that have the proper equipment.

These tests provide an objective measurement of the pelvic floor musculature and its innervation. They may add some insight into the evaluation of the colorectal patient who presents with specific disorders.

Anorectal Ultrasound

Anal ultrasound may provide a detailed picture of the internal and external sphincter muscles. This test may clearly show a sphincter laceration resulting from perineal trauma, previous anorectal surgery, or an obstetric injury. The test is performed using an ultrasound scanner, with an endoscopic ultrasound probe which is placed in the anal canal in order to obtain the visual images (Figures 3.7a, 3.7b). It is usually performed with the patient in the left lateral position on the examination table. The examination is relatively painless yet mildly uncomfortable.

Rectal ultrasound is slightly more uncomfortable than anal ultrasound. This test also requires a good understanding of the rectal anatomy. It is particularly useful in evaluating low-lying rectal tumours as the ultrasound may accurately stage the tumour in order to determine whether the lesion may be excised trans-anally or transabdominally. The ultrasound probe is placed proximal to the lesion through a rigid sigmoidoscope while the patient is in the left lateral position. A balloon is then inflated around the probe and the instrument is manipulated to visualize the tumour. The depth of tumour invasion into the bowel wall as well as the presence or absence of mesorectal lymph nodes may be seen. This may stage rectal tumours with a great deal of accuracy.

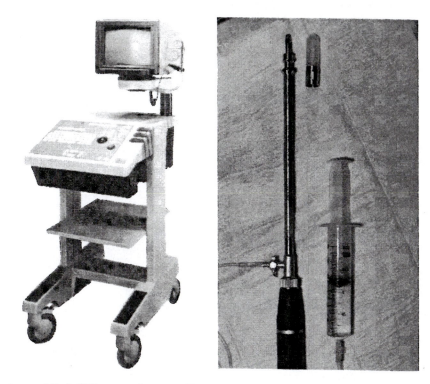

Figure 3.7: (left)Ultrasound scanner Type 2001 (B & K Medical Systems, Massachusetts USA); (right) the endoscopic ultrasound probe and transducer for transrectral scanning.

Nursing Considerations

The examination and investigation of the patient with colorectal problems remains a threatening event, regardless of the confidence the patient may have in the physician and health care professionals managing his or her care. Fear of the outcome of radiological or invasive procedures can evoke extreme anxiety. This emotional response can result in inappropriate behaviours, which may form barriers to obtaining accurate assessment and valuable information in arriving at a diagnosis. Bearing in mind that patients vary in their ability to cope with stressful situations, overt reaction during examination and investigation is not usually consistent with their internal feeling.

Because illness disrupts normal equilibrium and activities of daily living, a patient's ability to think critically and make decisions may be decreased. As a result, there is an exaggerated response of normal coping ability (Atkinson, 1992). Nurses should not only focus on the physical health of the patient, but the emotional well-being should be of equal concern. An understanding of basic human needs should equip nurses to provide educational and emotional support to patients undergoing investigative anorectal procedures. Preparatory information has been found to have a positive effect on anxiety (Fullhart, 1992). How an individual responds to his or her health influences preoperative response, and that response can contribute significantly to postoperative recovery.

The Initial Encounter

A nurse–patient relationship begins with the initial encounter. While collecting specific data, the patient should be thoroughly assessed. This is an opportune time for the nurse to establish rapport with the patient in order to become acquainted and to have knowledge of the associated colorectal problems. Initially the patient's reaction to the illness may be irrational, but the nurse should demonstrate patience and understanding to allay any fears and anxieties.

Some individuals find it difficult to talk about colorectal-related problems and are sometimes so embarrassed that they refrain from volunteering pertinent information which may be vital to their plan of care. In taking the history, the nurse should be tactful, taking into consideration culture, religion and socioeconomic factors, which can have an impact on the patient's interpretation of his or her illness.

Patients presenting with functional disorders, such a rectal prolapse, prolapsing haemorrhoids and faecal incontinence, may have suffered silently for years before seeking medical attention. Coming out of social isolation, and exposing 'private' parts of their bodies to a total stranger could be extremely distressing and embarrassing. The thought of undergoing invasive anorectal examinations can also reactivate fears of childhood abuse. The jackknife position most commonly used for anorectal examination has been considered by many patients to be very undignified and embarrassing, at the same time generating great anxiety.

The care of the patient should be individualized, with the nurse exhibiting a confident professional attitude and a humanistic approach to his or her responsibilities as a patient advocate. Because the patient is seeking help to cope with a disease or disability, the nurse should give the assurance that he or she is the focus of attention at all times.

Pre-investigative Preparation

Before the patient actually undergoes the proposed examination or investigation, a brief review should be given, explaining in clear simple language the nature, purpose and extent of the procedure. The position to be used for the examination should also be explained, as this helps the patient to be better prepared and more compliant. It may be wise to keep all instruments covered to avoid undue anxiety. Reassurance should be given that the examination is not expected to hurt, but would involve the use of instruments, which may cause some individuals to experience temporary minor discomfort.

When undergoing a rigid proctoscopy or flexible sigmoidoscopy, the enemas for cleaning the lower rectum can be done 1 hour prior to the examination. This can be done at home, at the clinic or at the doctor's office if the facilities are appropriate. Administering the enemas more than 1 hour before the examination can result in the movement of stool from the proximal colon into the distal colon and rectum, making the examination inadequate (Beck, 1997). Because of the possibility of taking biopsies, the nurse should ascertain that the patient does not have a history of a bleeding disorder, or has not taken any aspirin, aspirin-containing products or anticoagulants within the last 10 days.

Safety Precautions During Examination

During the abdominal examination, the patient is positioned supine, and dignity is maintained by draping the patient's body with a sheet, exposing only the abdomen and inguinal areas. Assistance should be given to older patients who require removal of stoma appliances during the examination.

As seen in Figure 3.1, the prone jackknife position is usually used for anorectal examination, using the movable table. These office examinations could be a simple digital, anoscopy, rigid proctoscopy or fibreoptic flexible sigmoidoscopy. The nurse assisting the physician must have an understanding of the function and trouble shooting of the equipment. The parts should be properly assembled to provide clear vision, and the instrument must be in excellent working condition. Instead of the conventional sigmoidoscope, some facilities use the channel-free sigmoidoscope and disposable EndoSheath (Vision Sciences Inc, Natick, MA) (Figure 3.8). This unit has been found to be safe, cost effective and requiring less reprocessing time, thus reducing the possibility of endoscopic contamination (Sardinha et al., 1996). The nurse should have available specimen containers and biopsy forceps.

For the prone jackknife position, the patient kneels on the platform to avoid slacks or trousers falling to the floor, then leans forward with the abdomen resting on a soft pillow and chest on the table, arms

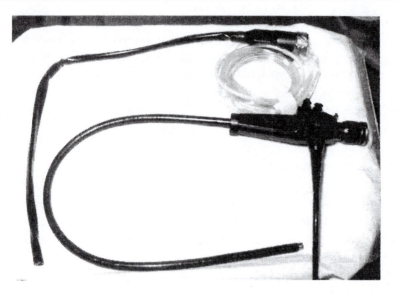

Figure 3.8: The S-F 100 Sigmoidoscope and disposable Endosheath System (Vision Sciences Inc, Natick, MA).

stretched forward with hands in front or holding on to the table's edge. To provide for patient modesty, a sheet is draped around the patient's back and legs. When the patient is positioned the table is raised and tilted forward, the sheet is then discreetly lowered and the buttocks exposed to facilitate the examination. At that time, the patient is given constant reassurance and a step-by-step explanation of the procedure. Changing positions of the examination table should be done only after the patient is warned. Patients who are pregnant or have a history of hip replacement, arthritis or cardiovascular disease may not tolerate the prone jackknife position. Therefore alternative positions such as Sims' or modified left lateral decubitus positions should be used (Perry, 1997).

The nurse closely monitors the patient during the procedure, as he or she may become faint, diaphoretic or experience a vasovagal attack that could have serious complications. If this occurs, the nurse should immediately notify the physician, then the table should be tilted to the horizontal position. The patient who becomes unresponsive should be placed in the supine position and oxygen administered (Beck,1997). A crash cart should be in close proximity, in case there is a need for resuscitation

The nurse should also be aware of any pre-existing medical conditions, which could have a negative effect on positioning. As the examination progresses, the patient should be instructed to take slow deep breaths to prevent hyperventilation (Beck, 1997), and told that the sensation of fullness, cramping or the desire to evacuate is normal. Sitting on the toilet after the procedure has been found helpful to eliminate gas and relieve discomfort. After the procedure, the patient should be informed of the possibility of abdominal pain, bloating and gas. Should abdominal pain persist, intensify or the patient complain of fever or rectal bleeding of more than a teaspoon, the physician should be notified immediately. If biopsies were taken some physicians advise patients to avoid all aspirin, aspirin-containing medications and all non-steroidal anti-inflammatory drugs (NSAIDs) for 7 days. If the patient's medical condition warrants blood thinners, the prescribing physician should be notified regarding restarting the medication.

When preparing for a colonoscopy, the patient should be told that this investigation is more extensive, that it usually involves the administration of intravenous sedation, and someone should be available for transportation home. The nurse must ascertain that the patient followed the pre-procedure instructions similar to those of sigmoidoscopy regarding aspirin and blood thinners. Other instructions include bowel cleansing preparation and following usual medication regimen for cardiopulmonary disease, diabetes or seizures.

The endoscopy nurse is responsible for assembling and trouble shooting the colonoscope so that it is in excellent working condition before its use. Biopsy forceps, snares and containers, cautery machine and pad should be assembled for biopsy or the removal of polyps.

During the procedure, the nurse must vigilantly monitor the patient, constantly checking the heart rate, blood pressure and oxygen saturation. Resuscitative equipment must be in close proximity, in the event of an emergency. The intravenous sedation is given slowly in small increments to keep the patient conscious but comfortably relaxed during the procedure. In the event of an adverse effect of the intravenous sedation, the following drugs should be available: naloxone (Narcan) for reversal of meperidine and flumazenil (Romazicon) for reversal of Versed.

Post-procedure instructions for colonoscopy are the same as those given to patients who have had sigmoidoscopy. In addition, patients should be instructed to refrain from driving, operating dangerous machinery for the remainder of the day, and should abstain from alcohol for the next 24 hours. The patient can resume regular diet and normal activities.

Before the patient undergoes any radiological or anorectal physiologic studies, the procedure and what it hopes to achieve should be explained. An enema to clean the lower rectum should be

performed, if the tests include cinedefecography and anorectal ultrasound.

Preoperative Preparation

When the patient and surgeon make a decision about the surgical
procedure, the nurse must assist the patient in preparing for the surgical experience. Thoughts of the proposed surgery and its implications
can generate tremendous stress, and it is to the nurse that the patient
looks for support and reassurance. The nurse needs to know that the
patient understands the surgeon's explanation of the surgical procedure, the risks, benefits, possible complications and alternatives.
Despite the fact that modern technology is providing better ways to
enhance patient care, one factor remains constant – the patient
(Gillette, 1996). Therefore preoperative counselling provides a perfect
opportunity for the nurse to use excellent communication skills to
establish and promote a therapeutic relationship with the patient and
family. This will encourage more effective communication as the
patient prepares for the surgical event. This relationship sometimes
may be the most memorable part of the patient's perioperative experience (Dunn, 1997) so it is imperative that the patient be prepared
physically and emotionally. All the preoperative routines should be
explained, as preoperative preparation can dispel fears and doubts
derived from lack of knowledge of the proposed procedure. Studies
have shown that a well-informed patient is less anxious, more confident, is a more active participant and experiences a more positive
surgical outcome (Brumfeld et al., 1996). Team approach to patient
care is invaluable as it fosters collaborative care. Family involvement at
this time helps the patient tremendously, as the patient is concerned
not only with the hospitalization and surgical procedure, but the
potential complications that can result. As a result the support of loved
ones during a vulnerable time of a patient's life is very important.
During the preoperative preparation, the nursing process is utilized to
collect data, make a nursing diagnosis and prepare nursing care plans
to meet the specific needs of the patient. Patient assessment involves
the collection of subjective information from the patient, and objective
evaluation by the nurse in order to ascertain needs and establish goals.
Patients preparing for colon and rectal surgery entertain many fears.
Body image disturbance is a major factor especially to patients whose
surgery requires a stoma. It is then that the enterostomal therapist is
consulted to give the appropriate information and support necessary
to ensure a satisfactory quality of life. It is the stoma nurse's responsi-

bility to educate the patient by adhering to the guidelines as approved by the National Digestive Diseases Board for Enterostomal Patient Education. The patient should understand the structure, function and care of the stoma; the physiological changes related to the stoma; the potential impact of body image and self-esteem; and sexual and social adjustment. The appropriate site for stoma marking, the reason for the site selection and the patient's expectation of self-care is explained. It is at this time that the patient is shown an array of appliances and choices are made. It is during this time as well that doubts and fears are dispelled, as the length of hospital stay and stoma-related complications are directly related to quality of the patient preparation (Wicks, 1996).

Numerous professional and voluntary organizations are available to assist patients with ostomies. Manufacturers and ostomy equipment suppliers are willing to provide educational materials. Hospital support groups and independent community groups from local chapters can provide counselling, and are excellent resources for the ostomy patient. In the United States, a variety of organizations are available for information, these include:

- American Cancer Society, Ostomy Rehabilitation Program
- American Society of Colon and Rectal Surgeons
- Crohn's and Colitis Foundation of America Inc
- American Urological Association Allied Inc
- United Ostomy Association
- International Association for Enterostomal Therapy
- Wound Ostomy and Continence Nurses Society
- American Dietetic Association
- Association of Rehabilitation Nurses
- National Digestive Diseases Information Clearing House.

After the surgeon has initiated a candid discussion of sexual dysfunction following procedures that involve deep pelvic dissection, sexually active males may become concerned about impotence or retrograde ejaculation. It is then that the nurse offers information regarding sperm banking and sexual prosthetic devices.

Summary

Although the investigation and evaluation of the patient with colorectal disorders may lead to a variety of tests and procedures, one must remember the importance of starting with a detailed history and physical examination. This stands as the cornerstone in determining the proper series of tests to perform. If the clinician simply listens to the patient, then determining the correct diagnosis becomes a relatively easy task. However, amidst all the battery of tests and procedures the care of the patient must not be lost. Patients need physical and emotional preparation as they undergo such investigations, and should surgical intervention be planned, a positive surgical outcome depends greatly on the preoperative preparation given.

References

Atkinson LJ (1992) Perioperative nursing. Berry and Kohn's Operating Room Technique 7th edn. St Louis: Mosby's Year Book.

Beck DE (1997) Endoscopy. In Beck DE (Ed.) Handbook of Colorectal Surgery. St Louis, MO: Quality Medical Publishing.

Berci G, Panish JF, Schapiro M, Corlin R (1974) Complications of colonoscopy and polypectomy. Gastroenterology 67: 584.

Brumfeld VC, Kee CE, Johnson JY (1996) Perioperative patient teaching in ambulatory surgery settings. AORN Journal 64 (6) 941–52.

Church TR, Ederer F, Mandel JS (1997) Fecal occult blood screening in the Minnesota Study: sensitivity of the screening test. Journal of the National Cancer Institute 89 (19): 1440–8.

Columbo L, Corti G, Magri F et al. (1997) Results of pilot study of endoscopic screening of first degree relatives of colorectal cancer patients in Italy. Journal of Epidemiology and Community Health 51(4): 453–8.

DeRoos AD, Hermans J, Shaw PC, Kroun H (1985) Prospective comparison of the single and double contrast examination in the same patients. Radiology 154: 1–13.

Dunn D (1997) Responsibilities of the Preoperative Holding Area Nurse. AORN Journal 66 (5): 820–37.

Fleischer D (1989) Monitoring the patient receiving conscious sedation for gastrointestinal endoscopy: issues and guidelines. Gastrointestinal Endoscopy 35: 262.

Fullhart JW (1992) Preparatory information and anxiety before sigmoidoscopy: a comparative study. Society of Gastroenterology Nurses and Associates 14(6): 286–90.

Gilbertson VA (1974) Proctosigmoidoscopy and polypectomy in reducing the incidence of rectal cancer. Cancer 34: 936.

Gillette UA (1996) Applying nursing theory to perioperative nursing practice. AORN Journal 64 (2): 261–8.

Jorge JMN, Wexner SD (1993) A practice guide to anorectal physiology. Contemporary Surgery 43: 214–24.

Keen WW (1987) Treatment of Cancer of the Rectum with a Report of Twenty-five Cases. Detroit: George S Davis.

Lewis H, Blumgart LH, Carter DC et al. (1984) Preoperative carcinoembryonic antigens and survivals in patients with colorectal cancer. British Journal of Surgery 71: 206–8.

Nesselrod JP (1957) Clinical Proctology. Philadelphia: WB Saunders.

Perry BW (1997) History and physical examination. In Beck DE (Ed.) Handbook of Colorectal Surgery. St Louis, MO: Quality Medical Publishing.

Sardinha TC, Wexner SD, Gilliland J, Daniel N, Kroll M, Lee E, Wexler J, Hudzinski D, Glass D (1996) Efficiency and productivity of a sheathed fiberoptic sigmoidoscope compared with a conventional sigmoidoscope. Diseases of the Colon and Rectum 40 (10): 1248–53.

Warden MJ, Petrelli N, Herrera L, Mittleman A (1988) Endoscopy versus double contrast enema in the evaluation of patients with symptoms of colorectal cancer. Americal Journal of Surgery 155: 224–6.

Wicks LJ (1996) Treatment modalities for colorectal cancer. Seminars in Oncology Nursing (4): 242–8.

Chapter 4
Common Anal Conditions

PETER J. LUNNISS BSc, MS, FRCS, Senior Lecturer & Honorary Consultant, Queen Mary and Westfield College, The Royal London Hospital and Homerton Hospital, London, UK

THERESA PORRETT RGN, Nurse Practitioner in Coloproctology, Homerton Hospital, London, UK

Anal conditions constitute a considerable proportion of the complaints of patients presenting to general surgical clinics as well as colorectal clinics and therefore will commonly be seen by nurses for advice, dressings, support and follow-up. The majority of such patients fall into two categories; those with a history of the passage of blood per rectum, in whom exclusion of the diagnosis of colorectal cancer is often foremost in the patient's mind, and those with a local anal condition which is often referred to by both patient and referring primary care physician as 'piles' (pertaining to prolapse) or haemorrhoids (pertaining to bleeding). In addition to bleeding or the presence of a lump, patients may also present with pain, discharge and soiling, and it is essential to elicit a thorough history of the complaint such that the clinician is sure he/she understands the nature of the complaint before proceeding with clinical examination, investigations, etc. Examination in the clinic must be both general and local, the latter involving correct positioning of the patient in the left lateral position (Figure 4.1) (in the USA the knee–elbow position is often used), and then careful inspection of the perineum (state of the skin, presence of soiling, position of the perineum in relation to the ischial tuberosities, presence of lumps, external openings, etc.) at rest and on straining. Soiling may result from incontinence or poor local hygiene. Anal seepage secondary to haemorrhoids, fistula, proctitis, rectal polyp, prolapse or malignancy, as a result of previous surgery, and liquid stool from whatever cause can lead to itching and excoriation. Excoriation can also result from primary skin disorders affecting the perineum, fungal, viral and parasitic infections as well as from hypersensitivity to a wide variety of agents including soaps, washing powders and topical agents applied to try to alleviate the itching. A story suggestive of prolapse may require asking the patient to bear down whilst seated on a lavatory for the prolapse to become evident, the patient crouched forward so the examiner can lean over to look from behind.

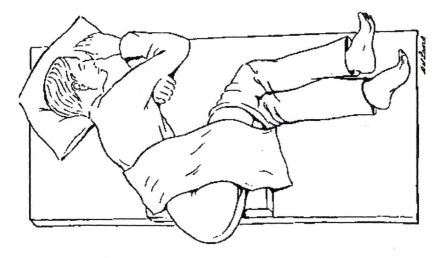

Figure 4.1: The left lateral position.

Inspection is followed by palpation with an adequately lubricated digit (the lubricant preferably containing a local anaesthetic), starting perianally and then within the anorectum. The index finger is introduced from the posterior aspect, the pulp of the finger facing anteriorly. Pain sufficient to prevent full examination means that arrangements should be made for the patient to undergo an examination under anaesthetic (EUA) as a matter of urgency. Palpation must be methodical and include an assessment of the resting tone and squeeze attainable; integrity of the sphincters; the length of the anal canal; and the presence of any palpable abnormality within the anal canal and then the lower rectum. The levator sling should be assessed on each side and the presence of induration sought. Anteriorly in the male the prostate gland should be assessed; in the female the cervix uteri can be felt. Above the prostate or cervix uteri the rectovesical pouch or pouch of Douglas should be assessed digitally. The presence, volume and consistency of the stool in the rectum should be recorded, and on withdrawal of the examining finger, colour of the stool on the glove noted.

The rectum should then be assessed using the rigid sigmoidoscope. Failure to get good views circumferentially to the limit of comfort with the scope means that the patient should have an enema inserted and the examination repeated with the rectum empty. The sigmoidoscope is used to visualize the rectal mucosa and to assess the rectum beyond the limit of the examining finger. Examination is completed after careful inspection of the anorectal lumen with a proctoscope.

Haemorrhoidal Disease

Haemorrhoids may be regarded as pathological anal cushions. Anal cushions, which can be seen well in sections from foetal anal canals (Figure 4.2) are important structures whose distensibility affords a complete seal to the anal canal at rest; the distensibility being brought about by the presence of vascular plexuses contained within them. The positions of the cushions are maintained by subepithelial smooth muscle and connective tissue, these in turn connected to the ramifying supporting tissues which cross the internal and external anal sphincters. An attractive hypothesis is that with ageing, and in an accelerated manner in people with symptomatic haemorrhoids, shearing and other forces act to disrupt the supporting mechanisms and allow caudal displacement of the cushions. Although constipation is often associated with haemorrhoidal symptoms, there are few prospective studies to support this. Certainly, however, prolonged straining at stool, or even prolonged sitting on the lavatory with a relaxed perineum would favour anal cushion displacement. Thus what may be considered as simple re-education of bowel habit becomes an important nursing intervention in the symptomatic long-term control of these patients.

The proctoscopic diagnosis of haemorrhoids far exceeds the prevalence of symptoms. This is important, because, as with most benign problems, treatment should be directed at symptoms, as all interventional treatments carry some degree of risk. Patients may complain of a variety of symptoms. Bleeding is usually characteristic, bright red in colour, separate from the motion, and seen on the paper on wiping after defaecation or as a fresh splash or drip into the pan. Bleeding from haemorrhoids may coexist with a more proximal malignancy, and the threshold for further investigation should be low. Pain is not usual, and suggests the possibility of another diagnosis, unless caused by congestion by a hypertonic sphincter. Perianal itching and soreness

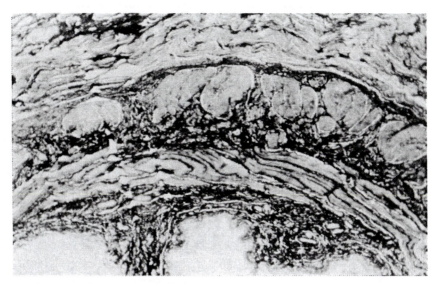

Figure 4.2: Transverse section of part of the wall of a foetal anal canal. The anal cushions are well developed. Deep to the submucosa lie the internal sphincter, the longitudinal muscle of the anal canal (more prominent in the foetus than adult) and the external anal sphincter. See colour section.

may arise either from mucous discharge from displaced rectal mucosa, or from the leakage of flecks of stool and liquid along the gutters between the prolapsing masses which have lost their action of effecting a watertight seal to the anal canal.

Difficulty in cleaning after defaecation is often associated with the aftermath of haemorrhoidal disease, in which the internal components have abated leaving enlarged external skin components (tags), presumably the result of repeated congestion and oedema.

Haemorrhoids are classified as first degree (those which bleed); second degree (bleeding associated with lumps which appear at the anal margin during defaecation but which reduce spontaneously); third degree, which have to be manually replaced, and fourth degree, which lie permanently outside the anus (although often it is the external cutaneous component which the patient erroneously tries to insert into the anal canal). They may be also classified anatomically, into primary haemorrhoids, corresponding to the positions of the anal cushions, and secondary haemorrhoids, those being haemorrhoidal tissue lying between the cushions and which may cause problems if dealt with surgically by the inexperienced. Strangulated piles usually present via the emergency department with severe unremitting pain associated with large pile masses protruding from the anal orifice with oedema and later ulceration.

Management of Haemorrhoids

Exclusion of other causes of rectal bleeding must be foremost in the mind of the clinician. Any concern that the bleeding is not truly anal means that investigation of the proximal colon, preferably by colonoscopy, should be instituted. It must be remembered that colonoscopy may miss lesions picked up by sigmoidoscopy, just as sigmoidoscopy may miss lesions seen at proctoscopy.

The spectrum of treatments available for symptomatic haemorrhoids is ample evidence that none carries any particular advantage. Careful assessment of defecatory habits and education of the patient into passing soft, bulky stool with minimum effort often yields more relief in the long term than interventional treatments. Many people find adjustment of diet too much of a change in lifestyle, and the addition of supplementary dietary fibre and ensuring an adequate fluid intake are more acceptable. It is in this non-invasive management support that nurses can have a large part to play (Table 4.1). Initially patients require reassurance regarding their diagnosis as many are alarmed when they pass blood, fearing cancer. Sensitive history taking needs to focus on bowel function. The frequency and ease of defecation along with the calibre of stools passed need to be ascertained. It is also important to elicit straining and sitting on the toilet for long periods of time. Education is paramount, because if patients fully understand the causal factors associated with their problem, they feel empowered to manage their bowel habit thus minimizing further episodes of straining and constipation. It is essential that written information is given to reinforce information delivered verbally (Figure 4.3). If patients are to be compliant in taking medication they need to be aware of how the medication works, for example bulking agents are commonly used to increase the calibre of the stool but are only truly effective if fluid intake is increased to around 2 litres per day. Patients with a history of straining need advice and support. For many there is a belief that if they do not have their bowels open daily they are constipated. Re-education is required, as straining daily to pass stool will further exacerbate their problems. Patients should aim to have their bowels open with ease. A good guide is if in the time it takes them to micturate they cannot have their bowels open they should not strain but leave the toilet and retry later when the urge to open their bowels returns.

First and second degree piles may be treated by injection sclerotherapy, rubber banding, cryotherapy or infrared coagulation. Whichever method is adopted, it is essential that the patient understands the risks involved and what they might expect to feel, both immediately after and over the ensuing days.

Table 4.1: Nursing management of haemorrhoids

History	Sensitive history taking , focus on bowel function
Education	Written information should be given to reinforce advice
Advice	Diet, fibre, fluid intake. Bowel habit, especially straining should be covered
Support	Encouragement in lifestyle alterations

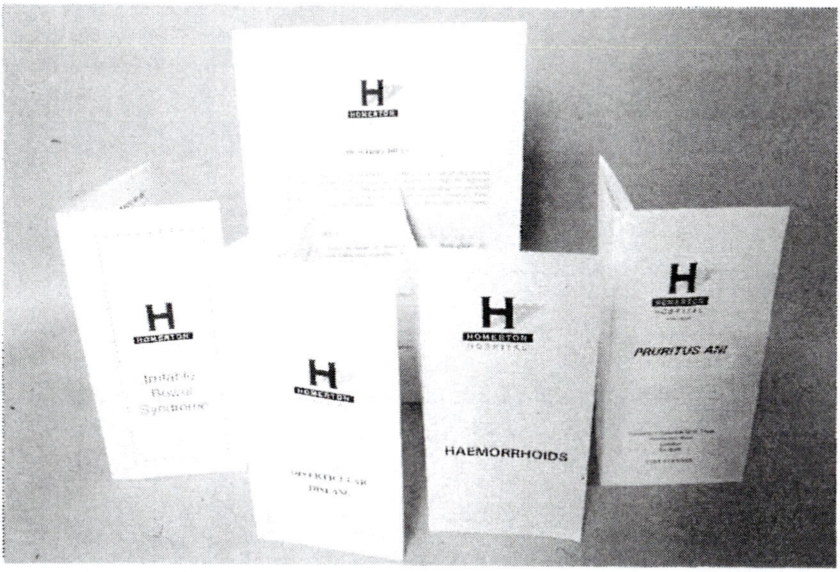

Figure 4.3: Patient information leaflets.

Any doubt about the diagnosis of haemorrhoids when the patient is seen in the clinic means that arrangements should be made for urgent admission, EUA and biopsy. The other strong indication for surgery is bleeding sufficient to cause anaemia (other causes having been excluded). Beyond these, indications for surgery are relative. Failure of clinic treatments and symptomatic third degree piles are best managed by surgery. The benefits of surgery must be weighed against the risks, which must be fully explained, including disturbance to continence, stenosis and recurrence. Surgery should be avoided in those with a patulous anus perhaps associated with pudendal neuropathy, in whom removal of haemorrhoidal tissue may result in frank incontinence. If there is doubt about sphincter strength, anorectal physiological assessment should be performed. The operation of manual dilatation of the anus, with the aim of reducing sphincter spasm, should be condemned as it may be associated with widespread sphincter muscle disruption, with incontinence resulting. The other procedure which aims to lower distal anal canal resting pressure, lateral internal anal sphincterotomy, is advised only when a fissure coexists with haemorrhoids. In the UK, open haemorrhoidectomy, based on that described by Milligan et al. (1937), under general anaesthesia in the lithotomy position is the commonest procedure. In the USA, closed haemorrhoidectomy in the prone jackknife position under regional anaesthesia is more commonly used. Haemorrhoidectomy carries a bad reputation for postoperative pain among the public, the two components of the pain being the background wound pain and that associated with defaecation (Table 4.2). Preoperative counselling and honest advice about expectations can do much do reduce anxiety; preoperative use of laxatives, continued postoperatively, eases defecatory discomfort; and wound pain can be significantly reduced with appropriate analgesia and the avoidance of an intra-anal dressing.

Anal Fissure

An anal fissure is a tear in the ectodermal segment of the anal canal, usually in the posterior or anterior midline, presumably because the epithelium at these sites is more firmly tethered to the subepithelial tissues and is thus less elastic and more susceptible to shearing forces. It commonly occurs after a bout of constipation; the anticipation of defecatory and post-defecatory pain inhibits normal bowel habit and a vicious circle develops. Bleeding is usually not marked, and is noticed as fresh blood on the paper, the patient often noticing a particularly tender area. Most acute fissures resolve spontaneously; some become chronic when they may be associated with an external skin tag

Table 4.2: Nursing implications following haemorrhoidectomy

Education	Patients must be aware of: post-operative complications, need for high fibre, analgesia
Hygiene	Twice daily baths. Thorough cleaning of area following bowel action. Ensure perianal region is thoroughly dried
Diet/fluids	High fibre. Increase fluid intake to 2 litres daily to facilitate action of stool bulking agents
Compliance with medication	Patients need to understand the function and importance of medication, especially bulking agents. Will require clear instructions for mixing and taking bulking agents
Management	Patients usually need to remain in hospital until after their first bowel action

('sentinel pile') distally and a fibroepithelial anal polyp proximally. The history is usually characteristic. Full examination in the clinic may be impossible because of pain, but the diagnosis can often be made on gentle parting of the buttocks. Fissures as part of perianal Crohn's disease are often very florid, and may be painless.

Acute fissures are managed conservatively with stool softeners and advice about constipation and topical anaesthetic agents (Hancock, 1993). Twice-daily dilatation of the anal canal using an appropriately sized anal dilator is used with success in some patients, but not tolerated by all. Recently, excellent healing rates have been achieved using topical glycerine trinitrate ointment, 0.2%, applied thrice daily. This has a local effect on the internal sphincter to reduce spasm and resting tone, and thus allow the fissure to heal. There is the potential side-effect of severe headaches but the occurrence of these can be reduced if patients are advised to use the ointment around the anus only and to wash their hands immediately they have applied the ointment. Any headache that the patient may experience with initial use normally wears off if treatment is continued.

Patients with persistent symptoms despite conservative approaches and those with chronic fissures benefit from surgery, the aim being to reduce distal anal canal tone. Manual dilatation has already been discussed and should not be performed. Lateral anal sphincterotomy, with division of the internal sphincter to the level of the upper limit of the fissure, usually the dentate line, combined with excision of the tag and polyp, is extremely effective. Division of the internal sphincter is of course not without risk. In patients with normal-length anal canals, and increased tone, the risks of disturbance to continence (flatus incontinence, soiling) are remote. Some patients develop fissures (presumably from a different aetiology) in canals where spasm and high pressures are not a feature, however, and any interference with the sphincters may have significant effects on function. In such patients, excision of the fissure with a sliding advancement flap of perianal skin into the wound is a sensible option.

Pilonidal Disease

A pilonidal sinus is a chronic inflammatory tissue-lined track extending from a midline epithelialized pit in the natal cleft, usually cephalad, to end either blindly or at another orifice. The aetiology is unproven, and may be congenital or acquired through local trauma, but the sinus almost invariably contains a nest of hairs. It is rarely seen before puberty and beyond the fifth decade of life. Secondary infection causes abscesses which cannot drain through the skin directly overlying because of the presence of fibrous septa, and the pus tracks laterally. Caudal spread towards the anus may make the clinical findings similar to hidradenitis suppurativa or anal fistula (both of which may coexist with pilonidal disease).

Treatment depends upon symptoms. Acute pilonidal abscesses are incised and drained; multiple operations have been described for eradication of the chronic condition, ranging from simple lay open and curettage, to excision with healing by secondary intention, by primary closure, or by rotation flap closure. Selection for more radical approaches should be careful, as classically such patients are not always the most compliant. Crucial to success in management is avoidance of hair regrowth into the wound, and regular attendance (weekly) to the clinic postoperatively for shaving is often mandatory (Stephens and Stephens, 1995).

As outlined, the surgical treatment options are many (Khaira and Brown, 1995), but whatever the treatment pathway chosen the nursing implications remain the same: how to support a young patient through treatment, minimizing disruption to work and social activities whilst promoting wound healing. People are often too embarrassed to consult their doctor and many present only after acute infection has resulted in abscess formation (Gould, 1997). Therefore a number of patients will require wide local excision, with its resulting wound which will heal slowly by secondary intention. (Table 4.3). These deep cavity wounds require a dressing for a number of reasons:

1. Comfort. A wound dressing keeps the wound edges apart and prevents friction damage when mobilizing.
2. To aid healing. Keeping the wound edges apart ensures that superficial skin bridges do not form.
3. Hygiene. Dressings will absorb exudate and aid drainage.

The more comfortable and easy the dressing is, the better it is for the patient, who is able to mobilize in comfort and manage the wound dressing independently. Depending on the size of the cavity, the wound may take months to heal and therefore the restriction on work and social activities can be considerable if these factors are not taken into account (Bale and Jones, 1997). For the first 2–3 days following wide excision the wound is dressed with an alginate dressing. This dressing is then soaked with saline and removed. A foam elastomer dressing is then made to fill the cavity (Berry et al., 1996). The patient lies flat in the prone position. Two nurses will be required, one to ensure the cavity is clearly exposed, the other to insert the foam solution. The foam mould is then held in place with tape. The patient is advised to bathe twice daily, remove the foam, rinse under the tap and reposition. Patients will require weekly outpatient appointments to shave the area and renew the foam dressing. Research (Wood and Hughes, 1975) has shown that although there was no difference in wound healing, patients with a foam dressing were in less pain and distress.

Table 4.3: Principles of wound management

Hygiene	twice daily baths
Comfort	the dressing should prevent the two skin edges from touching. Firm packing will cause discomfort
Dressing	wound not to be tightly packed as this prevents drainage
Prevention of premature bridging and skin pockets	digitation of wound, use of foam cavity dressing
Ensure hair does not become enmeshed in wound	weekly shaving of perineal/natal cleft area
Wound observation (Foster and Moore, 1994)	Exudate – amount Wound – granulating, epithelializing, sloughy, necrotic, inflamed, infected Surrounding skin – healthy, dry, macerated

Pruritus Ani

Pruritus ani or anal itching is a common condition which is most noticeable at night and results in an irresistible urge to scratch the skin around the back passage. Often the underlying cause cannot be identified but in many cases it may be related to haemorrhoids, fissures, diabetes, infection or skin disease.

Nurses are often the first people that patients confide in about this socially embarrassing problem. Although investigation of the cause is required there are a number of nursing interventions/advice which can be offered to lessen the problem.

The most important thing is patient reassurance. Usually patients fear that the condition is caused by a lack of cleanliness and hygiene but this is rarely the case. More often once the condition has occurred patients clean the anal area excessively, vigorously and often using soap. This can result in an exacerbation of the problem as the skin is damaged and natural protective oils are washed away (Jones, 1993).

Excessive moisture around the anus is another exacerbating factor, therefore patients should be advised to keep the area dry; talcum powder can be applied to the skin around the back passage but it must be unfragranced. Cotton underwear rather than man-made fibres is preferable. Soap should not be used and, when washing, the area should not be rubbed but patted dry. The perianal area should be cleaned after each bowel action. Certain drinks and foods have been noted to aggravate the problem. These include beer, milk, drinks with caffeine, chocolate, tomatoes and nuts. If patients comply with these simple lifestyle changes they will often experience marked improvement in their symptoms over a number of weeks.

Hidradenitis Suppurativa

Hidradenitis is a chronic suppurative condition that may affect the apocrine glands of the axillae, groin and perineum. Although the condition overall is more common in women, perianal hidradenitis involving the circumanal glands of Gay is seen more often in men. The aetiology is unclear, but obesity, excessive sweating, poor hygiene and endocrine disturbances (relative androgen excess or increased androgen target organ sensitivity) have been implicated. The condition is not seen before puberty, and rarely after the fourth decade of life. Apocrine gland occlusion leads to bacterial proliferation, gland rupture and spread to adjacent glands; secondary infection causes further extension, scarring and fibrosis. The initial appearances are multiple tender raised red lesions, but in the chronic state multiple communicating sinuses are evident, with variable scarring and deformity. Extension into the anal canal has been observed, but never above the dentate line.

Treatment of the mildest early forms is with antibiotics, which should be prescribed until all inflammation has fully settled. Acute abscesses need to be drained. Formal surgery is necessary for the chronic burrowing disease, the surgical alternatives dependent upon the magnitude of the problem. Wide lay open of all tracks with healing by secondary intention, excision, excision and marsupialization, excision and primary closure, and excision with skin graft closure have all been used. The type of wound dressing used will depend on the size of the wound and position of the wound. The mainstays of nursing intervention continue to be patient education, scrupulous wound hygiene and wound dressing. All disease must be dealt with if recurrence is to be avoided. The presence of multiple lesions close to the anus may necessitate raising a temporary stoma to allow adequate local surgery.

Anal Fistula

In Western Europe the incidence of idiopathic anal fistula is approximately 10:100 000, and is seen in men much more than women. The majority are thought to arise through intersphincteric anal gland (cryptoglandular) infection, which presents acutely as a perianal or ischiorectal abscess, or chronically as persistent discharge through an external opening somewhere on the perineum, the track usually communicating at some point with the anal canal lumen. Anal fistulae may also be seen in association with specific conditions, the most common of which are Crohn's disease, trauma and tuberculosis, as well as in relation to fissures and previous anal surgery.

Patients with anal fistulae usually complain of intermittent perianal pain and discharge from the external opening, the severity of the two symptoms often inversely related, pain building up as tissue tension increases until relief is brought about by discharge of pus. Patients with large internal openings and those where the communication with the bowel is above the anal sphincters (e.g. an extrasphincteric fistula) may pass flatus and stool through the external opening. If the external opening is in the vagina (i.e. an anorecto-vaginal fistula) the patient will have vaginal symptoms. The majority of fistulae are simple, and can be cured surgically with little morbidity. A minority of patients, however, have many years of symptoms, multiple failed operations, increasing incontinence, and may be totally incapacitated by the condition. It was for this reason, amongst others, that St Mark's Hospital was founded, so that experience and expertise in dealing with such cases could be gained.

Treatment of cryptoglandular anal fistula is nearly always surgical, and is a balance between eradication of pathology and preservation of continence. This in turn depends upon the level and course of the fistula (and any secondary extensions) through the sphincter muscle complex, and thus depends upon accurate assessment. Previous surgery, the complexity of some fistulae and personal experience are factors which can make assessment difficult or inaccurate; inaccuracy can have disastrous consequences. Although clinical examination remains the mainstay of assessment, several imaging modalities have been used to delineate fistulae: fistulography is of limited value but is useful in detecting and imaging extrasphincteric fistulae; ultrasound is fairly accurate in looking at pathology within the sphincter complex, but does not demonstrate well tracks lateral to or above the sphincters (the latter of great surgical importance); and CT has many drawbacks. MRI, however, has been shown to be extremely accurate and demonstrates tracks which may be missed at surgery and which are the cause of persistent chronic sepsis, and is the investigation of choice in difficult fistulae.

Clinical examination involves five essential points, recognized at the turn of the century by Goodsall and Miles: the location of the internal and external openings, the course of the primary track and any secondary tracks, and the presence of other diseases complicating the fistula. Examination must be systematic, careful and thorough, and may be complemented by examination under anaesthesia. Anorectal physiological assessment is usually reserved for those in whom the sphincters are thought to be compromised before surgery, in those who have had previous failed surgery, and for research purposes.

Anal fistulae are usually ranked according to the classification devised by Sir Alan Parks. The importance of classification and accurate documentation of operative findings (best drawn on a St Mark's Hospital fistula operation sheet: Figure 4.4) cannot be overemphasized. Parks subdivided fistulae according to the relation of the primary track to the external sphincter, the source of the fistula, the intersphincteric anal gland, lying medial to the voluntary muscle. Thus, there are four main fistula types: intersphincteric (confined to planes medial to the external sphincter), trans-sphincteric (in which the track crosses the external sphincter at a variable level), suprasphincteric (in which the track passes cephalad in the intersphincteric space to a level above the sphincters, and then curls downwards through the levators and ischiorectal space to reach the perineal skin), and extrasphincteric (which runs without relation to the sphincters and may be caused by pelvic disease or iatrogenically through overzealous probing. Each of these primary tracks may be further subdivided according to the presence and course of any secondary extensions and abscesses, which may run in a vertical, horizontal or circumferential plane (Figure 4.5).

Surgical Management of Anal Fistula

Up to 90% of anal fistulae are relatively easy to treat, being either intersphincteric or low trans-sphincteric, which can be most effectively dealt with safely by lay open, cutting down on to the track to convert the fistula 'tunnel' into an open wound which is allowed to heal by

ST. MARK'S HOSPITAL
FISTULA OPERATION NOTES

Name   Hospital Number   Date

DESCRIPTION

PRIMARY TRACK
superfical
intersphincteric
trans-sphincteric
suprasphincteric
extrasphincteric

INTERNAL OPENING
Site   O'clock
Level –   below
            at   dentate line
            above
            rectum

EXTERNAL OPENING (S)

Number

Sites   O'clock

HORSE-SHOEING
intersphincteric
infralevator (in ischiorectal fossa)
supralevator

ABSCESS
superficial
intersphincteric
infralevator (in ischiorectal fossa)
supralevator

OTHER ANAL CONDITIONS
Fissure
Haemorrhoids

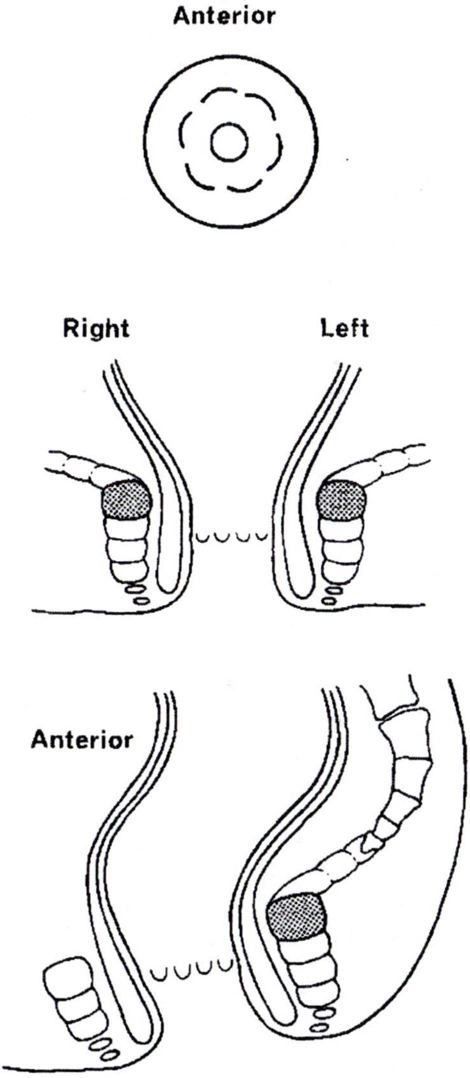

Anterior

Right   Left

Anterior

Figure 4.4: The St Marks Hospital Fistula Operation Sheet.

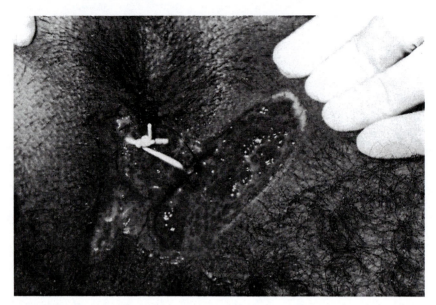

Figure 4.5: Trans-sphincteric fistulae with intersphincteric horeshoe and high
ischiorectal extension. See colour section.

secondary intention. The track is curetted and granulation tissue sent
for histological appraisal (to look for evidence of Crohn's disease,
tuberculosis, etc.). A careful search is made for any secondary extensions, usually marked at the site where granulation tissue cannot be
curetted away completely; these tracks must be followed to their limits,
and either laid open or curetted fully. In order to allow optimal healing, extensions in the ischiorectal fossa must be laid open widely, sometimes with the formation of wounds of alarming size; careful wound
design and expert postoperative care, however, allow remarkable rates
of healing and minimal residual deformity. In the USA, the placement
of catheter drains through incisions and counter incisions is sometimes
preferred – this certainly reduces wound size, but eradication of sepsis
may not be so successful. When laying open intersphincteric fistulae,
the back-cut technique of Salmon is a useful way of ensuring a flat
shallow wound that can be easily digitated and dressed, thereby avoiding the problem of bridging. Wound size after lay open can be reduced
by marsupialization, the suturing of the laid open track to the wound
edges.

The wound should be dressed using an alginate dressing laid into
the apices of the wound. Postoperatively, the patient should be asked to
bathe daily and after each bowel action, and the wounds then digitated
and irrigated with saline to ensure healing from the base and prevention of deep collections. The necessity for these regular dressings can

cause many problems for patients wishing to return to work and social activity, therefore if at all possible the patient, spouse, partner or friend should be taught to perform the dressing. Dressings need to be practical, easy to use and comfortable (see Table 4.4). The wound will require weekly review and any seton sutures mobilized to ensure they do not become embedded in the wound. Digitation is the mainstay of fistula wound management. It involves the insertion of a gloved and lubricated index finger into the wound. The purpose is to break down any bridging tissue preventing pockets from forming in the cavity/track. Therefore it is essential that gentle pressure is exerted on all the walls of the cavity. It makes it much easier to assess wound healing if there is continuity in the nurses undertaking the wound dressing. Any wound that does not show signs of good healing should be re-examined under anaesthesia to make sure no secondary tracks have been missed.

Table 4.4: Perineal cavity wounds: dressing choice

Dressing	Wound
Alginates (Thomas, 1992)	Large cavities Moderate to heavy exudating wounds Some desloughing properties Loosely placed in cavity
Hydrogels	Shallow cavities Light exudate Some debridement properties
Foams (Macfie and McMahon, 1980)	Deep cavities Will not absorb large amounts of exudate
Hydrogels	Shallow cavities Light to moderate exudate
Hydrocolloid paste	Shallow cavities Can be used in infected wounds

For those fistulae in which the primary track crosses the sphincters at a level where fistulotomy carries the risk of functional morbidity, other strategies need to be employed. These of course are not as successful as lay open at getting rid of the fistula. Such strategies include the use of setons (loose, tight or cutting, or chemical), core-out fistulectomy, advancement flaps, intersphincteric approaches, etc., each of which may have advantages in different circumstances, and which therefore should be in the armamentarium of the surgeon. In general, acute sepsis must have been fully eradicated (often by partial lay open and loose seton insertion) before these more complex procedures can be contemplated. Bowel preparation and antibiotic prophylaxis are also indicated. Secondary extensions should be treated as in simple fistulae. Wounds outside the sphincters may be closed primarily or left open, and postoperative toilet depends on which has been employed.

Whatever strategy is employed, it is imperative that the patient understands the potential risks of faecal incontinence. Patients react differently and one patient's minor staining of the underwear is devastating incontinence to another, therefore it is essential that this is discussed preoperatively. Most patients, however, are happy to put up with minor disturbances of continence if they are rid of the disabling symptoms that fistulae may give.

Anal Conditions Presenting as Emergencies

Acute Anorectal Sepsis

Acute anorectal sepsis is common, and constitutes a considerable proportion of patients attending the emergency department. Most cases arise spontaneously in otherwise fit individuals; occasionally they may be seen as part of an established underlying disorder, either gut pathology such as inflammatory bowel disease, or non-specific depression of immunity, as in diabetes, HIV infection, etc. An understanding of the anatomy and aetiologies is paramount for correct management, and it is unfortunate that a condition which may result in considerable morbidity is often relegated to the most junior surgical trainee to deal with in the middle of the night after all other emergencies have been dealt with. Basically, acute anal sepsis can be divided into that which has nothing to do with the anus, the sepsis arising there by chance, and that which is intimately related to the presence of the anorectum. Hidradenitis and pilonidal disease presenting as abscesses are usually easily recognizable. Sepsis presenting near the anus may arise through (presumably) simple folliculitis or may arise as a result of spread of infection from an acute abscess originating in an anal gland in the intersphincteric space of the anal canal. Both may present as perianal (within the confines of the terminal inferior ramifications of the conjoined longitudinal muscle layer of the anal canal) or ischiorectal abscesses. Folliculitis tends to be confined to the superficial ischiorectal space (i.e. cutaneous) whereas cryptoglandular sepsis passes through the deep ischiorectal space. The incidence of simple follicular infection is equal among men and women. Cryptoglandular sepsis is, however, much more common in men, for reasons which remain unclear. Of great significance to management is microbiology. The majority of simple abscesses yield skin organisms on culture of the pus drained at surgery, although a minority will yield gut organisms (30–40%); cryptoglandular sepsis is always associated with gut organisms and never with skin organisms. Microbiology is therefore highly sensitive but not particularly specific for underlying fistula. A history of previous sepsis at the same site is also indicative, but not diagnostic, of a communication with the anal canal.

Patients with acute anorectal sepsis usually present with a history of pain and a lump. If the abscess is perianal, the history is relatively short and there is little constitutional upset. Patients with ischiorectal sepsis present later, as pus may accumulate in much greater quantities in the relatively avascular, areolar-filled ischiorectal space, the history of a lump is less constant, and there is often associated fever. Patients with sepsis high up in the anorectum may not notice a lump, but have vague deep pelvic discomfort, and possibly urinary symptoms or dyspareunia. Spontaneous rupture of the abscess into the gut lumen brings immediate relief of symptoms, and the patient notices pus per rectum.

Examination of the patient with acute anal sepsis is usually limited to inspection because of the pain, and arrangements must be made for immediate examination under anaesthesia in the lithotomy position. After skin preparation (with a clear solution which does not stain the skin) the perineum is shaved. Inspection will show whether the abscess is perianal or ischiorectal. Careful palpation with a lubricated digit, initially externally and then internally, should allow the relation of the abscess to the anal sphincters and the presence of supralevator sepsis (either intermuscular or pararectal) to be ascertained. After sigmoidoscopy and conventional proctoscopy, a search for an internal opening (if not already felt on palpation or seen at the site of efflux of pus) can often be more adequately performed with an Eisenhammer proctoscope. Gentle external pressure over the abscess may lead to pus appearing at the internal opening.

The safest surgical management is simply to incise and drain the abscess, leaving the resulting wound shaped to allow optimal healing. Pus should be sent for culture, and biopsies of the abscess wall sent for histological appraisal. Loculi should be broken down digitally, and instrumentation avoided as it carries the risk of creating false tracks and even iatrogenic openings into the rectum. Any form of manipulation should be accompanied by the opposite index finger placed in the anorectal lumen so that the anatomy can be felt. Further management depends on the results of culture and clinical course. If skin organisms are cultured the patient can be reassured that there is no fistula. If gut organisms are cultured, there will be a possibility of failure of healing, recurrence, and chronic fistula formation. Some advocate a further EUA in patients in whom a fistula is suspected once the acute inflammatory changes have settled; others simply wait and see.

An anatomical approach, in determining whether sepsis is present in the intersphincteric space, is more specific than the results of microbiological culture in prediction of fistula, and of course can be performed at initial EUA (Lunniss and Philips, 1994). In the USA, more surgeons are keen on primary fistulotomy, and there is certainly a lower recurrence risk if this policy is pursued. However, it certainly leads to sphincter division in a proportion of patients in whom simple drainage would be curative, and in the hands of anyone without much experience in this speciality carries significant risk. If a more aggressive approach is entertained, the patient must be fully counselled beforehand.

Strangulated Haemorrhoids

Prolapsed strangulated haemorrhoids usually present as an emergency after a period of straining at stool. The internal haemorrhoidal tissue prolapses through the sphincter ring, and then swells as a result of vascular congestion, and sphincter spasm. The external cutaneous component becomes oedematous, and on examination this part of the pile mass may obscure the underlying, often necrotic prolapsed haemorrhoid. The swelling, pain and sphincter spasm prevent spontaneous and often manual reduction. Most cases can be managed conservatively, with bed rest, analgesics, laxatives, and the application of cold (crushed ice in a rubber glove or a bag of frozen peas). The patient must be advised that it will take several days for symptoms to subside. Some patients will continue to have symptoms from their piles and will ultimately undergo haemorrhoidectomy. Others, however, have no symptoms subsequently. There is evidence that emergency haemorrhoidectomy is a safe procedure in experienced hands, but as in acute anal sepsis, it seems logical to postpone surgery until the acute inflammatory changes have resolved.

Thrombosed External Haemorrhoid

This is a spontaneous thrombosis in one of the vessels of the external or superficial haemorrhoidal plexus which form a circumferential ring around the anal margin (and is therefore unrelated to internal haemorrhoids arising from the superior or internal haemorrhoidal plexus). It presents as a painful, blue, olive-shaped swelling at the anal margin. If the patient presents within 24 hours of the onset of symptoms, simple incision and evacuation under local anaesthesia gives immediate relief. Once the thrombus begins to organize, evacuation becomes more difficult and conservative management is pursued, the possible sequel being a residual skin tag which can be removed if troublesome.

Anal warts, perianal Crohn's disease, sexually transmitted diseases of the anus and rectum, and perianal disease in the HIV positive patient are all covered in Chapter 14 .

Anal conditions are common and although in many cases are minor in severity they can cause patients a disproportionate amount of pain, embarrassment and interruption to work and social activity. It is through the sensitive and knowledgeable intervention of the nurse that the management of these conditions can minimize inconvenience, pain and recurrence.

References

Bale SJ, Jones V (1997) Wound Care Nursing: A Patient Centred Approach. London: Bailliere Tindall.

Berry D, Bale S, Harding K (1996) Dressings for treating cavity wounds. Journal of Wound Care 5 (1):10–13.

Foster L, Moore P (1994) The management of recurrent pilonidal sinus. Nursing Times 93 (32): 63–5.

Gould D (1997) Pilonidal sinus. Nursing Times 93 (32): 59–62.

Hancock BD (1993) ABC of Colorectal Diseases. London: BMJ Publishing Group.

Jones DJ (1993) ABC of Colorectal Diseases. London: BMJ Publishing Group.

Khaira HS, Brown JH (1995) Excision and primary suture of pilondial sinus. Annals of the Royal College of Surgery 77 (4): 242–4.

Lunniss PJ, Philips RKS (1994) Surgical assessment of acute anorectal sepsis is a better predictor of fistula than microbiological analysis. British Journal of Surgery 81: 368–9.

Macfie J, McMahon J (1980) The management of the open perineal wound using a foam elastomer dressing: a prospective clinical trial. British Journal of Surgery 67: 74–8.

Milligan ETC, Morgan C, Naughton Jones LF, Officer R (1937) Surgical anatomy of the anal canal and the operative treatment of haemorrhoids. Lancet ii: 1119–24.

Stephens FD, Stephens RB (1995) Pilonidal sinus; management objectives. Australian and New Zealand Journal of Surgery 65 (8): 558–60.

Thomas S (1992) Alginates. Journal of Wound Care 1(1): 29–32.

Wood RAB, Hughes LF (1975) Silicone foam sponge for pilonidal sinus: a new technique for dressing granulating wounds. British Medical Journal 4 (5989): 131–3.

Chapter 5
Colorectal Cancer

ERIC G. WEISS, MD FACS, FASCRS, Staff Physician, Colorectal Surgery, Cleveland Clinic Florida, Florida, USA

THELMA E. JOHNSON RN, CNOR, RNFA, Surgical Nurse Clinician, Colorectal Surgery, Cleveland Clinic Florida, Florida, USA

Introduction

Colorectal cancer is one of the most common tumours occurring in humans, ranking third worldwide. Of 6.35 million invasive neoplasms occurring annually (American Cancer Society, 1984), 570 000 are in the colon or rectum. It is the second most common malignant tumour in females and the third most common tumour in males. Despite increased awareness, improved surgery and screening techniques, it remains the second leading cause of cancer deaths overall, following lung cancer.

The aetiology of colon and rectal cancer is multifactorial, with links to the environment, genetics and other exposures. The vast majority of cancers seem to arise from a benign, although neoplastic, precursor lesion. These precursor lesions are adenomatous polyps and the underlying theory is coined the 'adenoma to carcinoma sequence'. Almost all patients with colon or rectal cancer will have synchronous polyps found elsewhere within the colon. In addition, patients who have had adenomatous polyps removed in the past have a lower risk of developing colon cancer (Winawer et al., 1987).

More recently, specific genetic abnormalities have been found that are strongly linked to the development of colorectal cancer. These include APC gene, K-ras, and others. These specific genetic disorders are associated with very high risks of developing colorectal cancer.

Despite the above-mentioned increased understanding of the causes of colorectal cancer, the overall death rate and incidence has not decreased. Increased and earlier screening and improved surgical techniques have improved surgical morbidity and mortality, but long-term outcome is relatively unchanged.

Incidence and Prevalence

Colorectal cancer accounts for 9% of the 6.35 million invasive cancers occurring throughout the world annually. The ratio of colon to rectal cancer is approximately 10:1. Whether this is secondary to more tissue being at risk in the colon as compared with the rectum, or whether they are two separate disease entities, is unknown. There is a slight female predominance of colon and rectal cancers, and the prognosis in females is slightly better. There has been a proximal shift in colon cancer development with an increasing proportion of right-sided cancers and a decrease in rectal cancers. This is thought to be due to improved screening methods.

The incidence of colorectal cancers varies depending on the population base with western countries in general having a higher incidence than less developed countries. The highest incidences are reported in North America, Australia and New Zealand. The lowest rates occurred in El Salvador, Poland and Mexico. Western European countries hold an intermediate position.

In the United States there are 165 000 new cases of colorectal cancer annually, amongst which 150 000 are located within the colon and 15 000 within the rectum. These account for 60 000 deaths annually in the United States alone. Similar percentages occur in Canada with an annual cancer prevalence of 15 000 cases annually regularly distributed in a 10:1 colon to rectal location. Other factors, such as race, religion and occupation, do play a minor role in the development of colon and rectal cancer.

Signs and Symptoms

Presenting signs and symptoms of colorectal cancer vary widely in relationship to site and extent of disease. Generally, signs and symptoms may be of an acute or chronic nature, related either to local or systemic manifestations.

The most common symptom of colon and rectal cancer is rectal bleeding. Visible bleeding occurs more commonly with left-sided colonic or rectal lesions, as opposed to the right-sided or more proximal lesions, which may bleed occultly but less often visibly. Although most patients with rectal bleeding do not have colon or rectal cancer, many with these cancers will have symptoms of rectal bleeding.

Change in bowel habit is probably the second most common presenting symptom of colon and rectal cancer. Constipation, change of stool calibre or consistency, or diarrhoea are all common when one has colorectal carcinoma. These symptoms occur earlier when the lesions are left sided, whereas they are more insidious and occur later in those patients with right-sided lesions.

Abdominal pain, although rather non-specific, is exceedingly common in patients with colorectal carcinoma. It is doubtful that it is always associated with the tumour and may be of other, long-standing GI pathology such as irritable bowel syndrome. Classic pain attributable to GI neoplasms occurs secondary to partial obstruction resulting in colicky, crampy, rhythmic pain. Isolated pain in the rectum in association with rectal cancer is usually representative of sacral nerve root involvement, as is back pain with colon cancer. Other local symptoms include tenesmus, urgency and mucus discharge.

Generalized symptoms may also occur and are usually manifestations of advanced disease with either liver metastases, carcinomatosis or obstruction. Anorexia, weight loss, nausea and vomiting may occur from any of the above-mentioned conditions. Fever may also be present due to local perforation, tumour bulk and/or involvement of adjacent organs such as the bladder.

Laboratory evaluation is relatively non-specific but iron deficiency anaemia with characteristic microcytic indices may often be seen. In addition, abnormal liver function studies, hypoalbuminaemia and elevated sedimentation rates can be seen with advanced disease.

Physical Examination and Diagnostic Studies

A detailed history is imperative when questioning a patient with regard to diagnosing colon and rectal cancer. Questions pertaining to the classic symptoms of colon and rectal cancer need to be asked. These include the presence or absence of rectal bleeding and, if present, its nature. Whether the bleeding is bright red, melanotic or haematochezic is important as it may imply the location of the tumour. Associated changes in bowel habit, abdominal pain and its nature should also be searched for. Generalized questions regarding the pertinent review of systems, including the absence or presence of nausea, vomiting, anorexia, weight loss, lethargy, shortness of breath and chest pain, may indicate advanced disease, anaemia or malnutrition. Family history, especially first-degree relatives, is extremely important. Trying to create a family tree of all persons with cancers in a given family may allow the proper diagnosis of a family cancer syndrome patient, which has various treatment implications.

Physical examination should focus on associated findings that may occur with colon and rectal cancer. Scleral icterus may be seen with jaundice secondary to metastatic disease, pale conjuctiva, or other mucous membranes may be seen with anaemia. Enlarged supraclavic-ular or inguinal lymph nodes may be seen with colon or rectal cancer. Tachycardia and functional heart murmurs can be detected in patients with significant anaemias. Abdominal examination should focus on any abdominal masses, the presence or absence of ascites, whether the liver is palpable, and the nature of the liver itself. Identification of previous incisions to help plan future surgery, and possibly to place stomas, is important.

Lastly, digital examination of the rectum should be performed in all patients. This should include examination of the stool for occult blood. In addition, females should undergo pelvic examination and mammography to rule out either continuous involvement or concomi-tant pathologies in those regions. Men should also have prostate exams and PSA levels sent to rule out concurrent prostate cancer.

Further diagnostic studies are usually required to diagnose colon and rectal cancer with the exception being low rectal cancers that are palpable on digital examination. These would include all lower-third rectal cancers and some middle-third rectal cancers which make up less than 10% of all colon and rectal malignancies.

Imaging studies would indicate proctoscopy, sigmoidoscopy, barium enema and/or colonoscopy. In symptomatic patients, sigmoi-doscopy or proctoscopy alone are not sufficient to rule out colon cancer completely. However, one-third of all colon and rectal malig-nancies are diagnosable using flexible sigmoidoscopy (Hertz et al., 1960).

Typically, when one is concerned about colorectal cancer in a differential diagnosis, a test that will allow complete examination of the colon is favoured. Colonoscopy, or the combination of flexible sigmoidoscopy and barium enema, will both provide complete exami-nation of the colon. Colonoscopy has several advantages over sigmoi-doscopy and barium enema. Colonoscopy allows for visualization and removal of synchronous polyps if a polyp or tumour is identified and occurs in approximately 40% of patients (Eddy, 1990). Colonoscopy allows for biopsy of a suspicious lesion as well as the opportunity to remove the index lesion, if possible. Colonoscopy, however, is more expensive and more risky in that there is a low, albeit present, risk of perforation in less than 1% of patients (Smith and Nivatvongs, 1975; Smith, 1976).

Staging

Staging, or the determination of the extent of disease, is an important component in the management of patients with cancer. Staging may have relevance to the type of initial treatment offered as well as the use of subsequent adjuvant therapy. However, the most important role of staging lies in its prognostic abilities, allowing for the prediction of long- and short-term outcomes in patients with cancer. There are many models of staging, including pathological, radiologic and clinical. Typically, pathological staging is the most reliable; however, it is only available after complete examination of a specimen occurs following surgical removal.

Staging for colon and rectal cancer has traditionally been approached by a pathological staging system. The most well-known and widely used system is Dukes' staging system, reported by Cuthbert Dukes in 1932. This staging system, applicable to both colon and rectal malignancies, is based on two prime considerations: depth of tumour invasion, and extent of lymph node metastases, if any. Originally, there were three Dukes' stages described: Dukes' A – where the tumour was confined to the bowel wall; Dukes' B – where the tumour had invaded full thickness into the bowel wall after spread into the serosa or fat; and Dukes' C – where lymph node metastasis was present. Many modifications of Dukes' system have occurred since its inception.

One of the more common modifications is that by Astler and Coller (1954). The modified A patient has a tumour that is confined to the mucosa. The B category has been divided into B1 where the tumour invades the muscularis propria and B2 where the tumour invades through the entire bowel wall. Similarly, the C category was subdivided so that the B1 or B2 with positive lymph node metastasis was defined as a C1 or C2, respectively. The aim of such a modification was to allow better prognostication.

Lastly, the use of the TNM system has been attempted to standardize reporting, but continues to fall prey to the above-mentioned systems (Hermanek and Sabin, 1995). Although the above staging systems require pathological evaluation, preoperative staging with radiological assessment can be utilized. The determination of metastatic disease, typically to the liver, can be made with either ultrasound or CT scan. CT scan is more sensitive and can image liver lesions at a resolution of about 1 cm whereas ultrasound limits are slightly larger, in the order of 2 cm. It has been estimated that CT will show some liver abnormality in approximately 35% of patients, consistent with the number of patients with metastatic disease as shown in other studies.

For rectal cancer, the use of endoanal ultrasound can also offer preoperative staging with good sensitivity. Although a technically demanding and highly skilled procedure, endoanal ultrasound is 90–95% sensitive for determining the depth of tumour invasion and 80–85% in determining positive lymph node metastasis. This has particular relevance in offering patients transanal approaches or preoperative adjuvant therapy (Sentovich et al., 1993).

Genetics and High-risk Patients

The genetic abnormalities associated with the development of colorectal carcinoma continue to be elucidated by basic science researchers and clinicians. It was felt that 85% of colorectal cancers occur secondary to somatic mutations, whereas 15% occur secondary to germline mutations and are inherited, being passed down from generation to generation. As most carcinomas are sporadic, and not inherited, mechanisms occur that protect one's vulnerability to developing cancer. Mutations occur on a daily basis but the body has corrective mechanisms to override these mechanisms; typically, more than one mutation is required for cancer to develop. This mechanism is known as Knudsen's two-hit hypothesis (Knudsen, 1971).

The highest risk individuals are those with either familial adenomatous polyposis (FAP) or hereditary nonpolyposis colorectal cancer syndromes (HNPCC). HNPCC, which accounts for 5% of all colorectal cancers, has a germline mutation occurring in one of two genes coding for genes which repair mutations. These genes are hMSH2, hMLH1, and hPMS1 (Fishel et al.,1993). A second defect, which is acquired, occurs, allowing for progression to cancer in those patients.

FAP is caused by a germline mutation of the APC gene. Although 20% of cases can occur sporadically, 80% are hereditary. Other genes such as Kras, P53, DCC and MCC, as well as the previously described APC, and mismatch repair genes (hMLH2, hMLH1) all play roles, becoming more evident with further research in the formation of colon cancer.

Treatment

The treatment of colon and rectal cancers must be considered separately from each other. There are relatively standard procedures for the treatment of colon cancer and few surgical options, whereas the treatment of rectal cancer is more difficult and requires multiple considerations.

Colon cancer treatment typically requires segmental resection of the colon. As in all cancer operations, adequate margins, with the removal of all gross disease, as well as adequate lymph node basin removal, is primary in the treatment of colon cancer. Segmental colectomy, typically in the form of right hemicolectomy, left hemicolectomy or sigmoid resection, is the primary procedure performed for the vast majority of colon cancers. These distinctions are based on where the tumour resides in the colon and on the location of the vascular supply, and lymphatic drainage.

For tumours involving the caecum, ascending colon and/or hepatic flexure a right hemicolectomy is performed (Figure 5.1). This resection entails removal of 5–10 cm of terminal ileum, the caecum, ascending colon and hepatic flexure. The blood supply to this segment includes the ileocolic artery, right colic artery and the right branch of the middle colic artery. These arteries, with their concomitant lymph nodes and lymphatics, are removed with the colon. Anastomosis occurs between the ileum and transverse colon. Tumours involving the descending colon, splenic flexure or sigmoid colon are usually managed by left hemicolectomy (Figure 5.2). Left hemicolectomy entails removing the colon from the middle transverse colon to below the sigmoid colon. Again the blood supply includes the left branch of the middle colic artery, the left colic artery, the sigmoid vessels, and the superior haemorrhoidal artery. Anastomosis entails attaching the transverse colon to the upper rectum.

Occasionally for sigmoid tumours, only a resection of the sigmoid colon may be performed (Figure 5.3). Some discrepancies for transverse colon tumours and splenic flexure cancers exist. Some advocate total abdominal colectomy with ileoproctostomy for transverse colon lesions as multiple blood supplies and lymphatics may be involved.

Rectal cancer is much more complex. Traditionally, rectal cancer was treated by the Miles procedure described by Miles in 1908. This procedure entailed the removal of the pelvic rectum from both an abdominal and perineal approach, resulting in removal of the sphincter complex and the formation of a permanent colostomy. All treatments of rectal carcinoma are judged against this 'Gold Standard'.

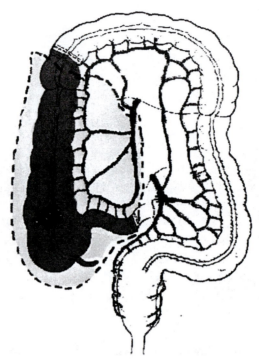

Figure 5.1: Right hemicolectomy depicted by shaded area.

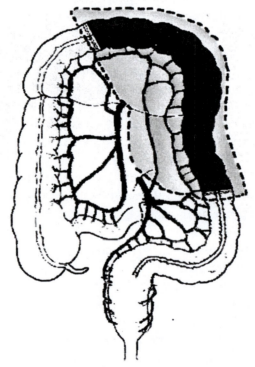

Figure 5.2: Left hemicolectomy depicted by shaded area.

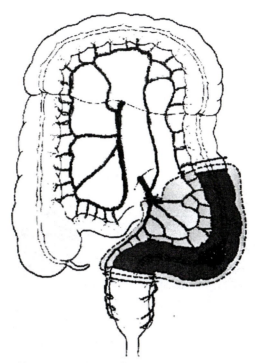

Figure 5.3: Sigmoid colectomy depicted by shaded area.

Current views of rectal cancer have changed significantly in the past one to two decades. The extent of resection, ability to perform an anastomosis and save the sphincters, and the use of transanal approaches have become much more common recently. Primarily, from an oncologic standpoint, there have been several changes in the understanding of rectal cancer. It was initially thought that rectal cancer would spread through lymphatics involving the sphincter muscle. This fact, and the technical inability to perform a safe low anastomosis resulted in the use of Miles's abdominoperineal resection (APR) for the treatment of rectal cancer. The need to sacrifice the sphincter for the above reasons is now refuted. Anterior resection, first advocated by Dixon in 1948 and Wangersteen in 1945, showed that a 5 cm distal margin, if achievable, would not require removing the sphincters and would provide adequate oncologic results in combination with preservation of function. Further studies by Williams and Quirke challenged the 5 cm rule and lowered that to 2 cm or less (Williams et al., 1983; Quirke et al., 1986).

Currently tumours of the rectum at least 2 cm from the dentate line can be managed by sphincter-sparing techniques with adequate oncologic results compatible with those achieved with APR. Relative contraindications do exist and not all patients are candidates for sphincter-sparing surgery. These contraindications include poor sphincter function, patient preference, co-morbidity and technical ability.

Further refinements of surgical technique as described by Heald (Heald et al., 1982) have even further broadened sphincter-saving surgery and improved oncologic results. Total mesorectal excision (TME) is now favoured by many as the method of treating middle-third, or lower, rectal cancers.

Local therapy for rectal cancer also has a role. Tumours that are exophytic, well to moderately well differentiated, posteriorly based, mobile, and less than or equal to 3 cm in size may be managed by local techniques. Local techniques include fulguration, radiotherapy, cryoablation and transanal excision. Transanal excision is the most commonly used procedure and can be performed on lesions to about 8 cm from the dentate line. Lesions above this level, with the above criteria, may be approached using the technique described by Buess called transanal endoscopic microsurgery (Buess et al., 1989). Endoanal ultrasound aids in selecting patients for this technique, by identifying patients with tumours confined to the mucosa or submucosa.

Reconstruction following rectal cancer surgery has progressed from the straight anastomosis to the use of a colonic reservoir, as first described by Parc (see Parc et al., 1986). Currently, many favour the use of a colonic J-pouch for the treatment of restorative surgery in rectal cancer. Improved function is the primary benefit of this technique.

Prognosis and Outcome

As mentioned earlier, overall outcome in colon and rectal cancer is based on stage. Numerous studies exist and overall Dukes' staging continues to be the best prognosticator of outcome. Patients with Dukes' A have a 95% chance of 5-year survival without cancer, whereas Dukes' B patients 5-year survival rate is in the order of 75%, and for those patients with Dukes' C disease it is in the order of 50%. Overall, one-third of patients with colorectal cancer will succumb to the disease. Patients with metastatic disease to the liver typically die within 2 years of diagnosis.

Adjuvant Therapy

Adjuvant therapy for colorectal cancer involves the addition of chemotherapy and/or radiation therapy. Again, as in the surgical treatment, colon cancer and rectal cancer need to be considered separately. For colon cancer, radiotherapy is rarely indicated. Only in cases where advanced loco-regional disease exists may there be a role for radiation therapy. However, the addition of chemotherapy is routinely used in patients with lymph node metastases. The North Central Cancer Treatment Group (NCCTG) combined 5-flourouracil (5-FU) with levamisole for Dukes' B and Dukes' C patients (Laurie et al., 1989). In that trial, significant benefit was shown for Dukes' C patients. Subsequently, the Intergroup study confirmed these findings and currently, in Dukes' C patients, this combination is the standard of care. A reduction by 39% in recurrence rate as well as a reduction in cancer-related death rates by 32% was shown. This combination requires weekly chemotherapy for 12 months.

Comparison with combination therapy with 5-FU and folinic acid showed similar results and both regimens are commonly used (O'Connel et al., 1993).

For rectal cancer, combination chemotherapy and radiotherapy is advocated for patients with full-thickness tumours and those involving lymph nodes. The landmark paper by Krook et al. in 1991, which represented the NCCTG trial, showed a significant reduction in local recurrence to about 14% using chemo- and radiation therapy with a 5-year survival rate of 58%. Currently, the NIH and NCI consensus recommends that all patients with Dukes' B or C rectal cancer should receive 4500–5000 Rads over 4 to 6 weeks, with concomitant 5-FU and methyl CCNU. Subsequently, methyl CCNU has been dropped and continuous infusion 5-FU advocated.

The use of adjuvant radiotherapy for the reduction of local recurrences must be balanced against surgical treatment alone. Given results such as those published by Heald and others, where local recurrences alone are 5–7%, the addition of chemo-/radiation therapy must be used in highly selected patients rather than 'blanketed' by stage alone.

Surveillance and Follow-up

No single strategy for surveillance or follow-up has been agreed upon. Although most surgeons will follow patients with some combination of physical examination, endoscopy, tumour markers, and radiographic exams, no single routine is followed.

At our institution, clinical examination, along with CEA determination, is performed every 3 months following surgery for the 1 year. At 1 year following surgery, colonoscopy is performed to rule out synchronous or metachronous tumours or polyps.

In patients who did not have complete colonoscopy preoperatively, it is performed 6 months following surgery rather than at 1 year. At

1 year, additional studies of liver function and chest X-rays are obtained. Routine follow-up is then spread out to 6 months, and then finally, annually. Follow-up endoscopy is typically done on an every-3-year basis. Routine radiologic follow-up with liver CT or liver ultrasound is not used and any that is ordered is based on symptoms or other abnormalities.

With the incidence of colorectal cancer (CRC) deaths increasing at such an alarming rate, nurses have been responsive to the need for public education. Nurses are challenged to collaborate with physicians and other members of the medical team to promote and employ methods of prevention and early detection, which are the keys to curing CRC.

Successful management of CRC requires skilled nursing care. Nurses should prepare themselves by gaining knowledge of the disease process and advances in treatment options. A strong foundation for high-level patient education and nursing intervention can be achieved through attendance at lectures and seminars, as well as by acquiring reading material on the subject.

The importance of nursing in all aspects of care and treatment of patients diagnosed with CRC cannot be understated. In many medical facilities, a nurse is the first member of the medical team that the patient encounters. If this experience is positive, the patient who is concerned about symptoms or potential procedures may find the initial visit with the physician a less stressful event. Nurses should be cognizant of the fact that, to many patients, cancer is a word that is surrounded with many myths and misconceptions. Therefore, the need for effective communication skills is very important in patient understanding and education.

A nursing staff that is caring and supportive can provide significant assistance to a patient trying to cope with a diagnosis, or possible diagnosis, of CRC.

Health Education

Health education, as it relates to colorectal cancer, is an important nursing responsibility.

Knowledge of health habits that promote or prevent CRC can help millions of individuals protect themselves against cancer-causing agents, thus lowering incidence rates.

Dietary Considerations

Diet has long been recognized as playing an important role in colorectal carcinogenesis. Consumption of excess fat, cholesterol, large amounts of alcohol (especially beer), as well as inadequate intake of fruit, vegetables and cereals figure prominently in this process. Dietary habits differ greatly between countries and change with people's migration to other countries (Amarnath and Wexner, 1996).

Intake of a diet high in animal fat is associated with a high incidence of left colon cancer and is also associated with increased bile acids. These acids cause bacteria in the colon to increase secondary bile acid production. In turn, these secondary bile acids cause increased intestinal cell turnover, thus promoting tumour formation.

Studies have shown a relationship between serum cholesterol levels and the rate of colorectal adenomas in both male and female patients. Recently, the association has been made between women whose diet consisted of increased saturated fat and decreased fibre with a high incidence and recurrence of CRC (Amarnath and Wexner, 1996).

Nurses can encourage inclusion of oleic (olive oil) and omega-3 (fish oil) fatty acids in the diet, as these are associated with low risk of cancer.

It is believed that high intake of dietary fibre is the primary factor responsible for the low incidence of CRC in African natives (Corman, 1993). Dietary fibre, especially wheat bran, protects against CRC by increasing intestinal transit time. This increase causes a more rapid excretion of carcinogens. It also dilutes bile acid concentration and faecal mass, as well as any carcinogens, partly by the alteration of colonic flora and faecal pH (Amarnath and Wexner, 1996).

Fibre is that part of a plant food that is not digestible; otherwise known as roughage. It contains very few calories and adds bulk to the diet by absorption of water. Some fibres are soluble and others are insoluble. Examples of foods high in soluble fibre are oats, barley, peas, beans and citrus fruits. High insoluble fibre sources include wheat, bran and some vegetables. Daily fibre intake can be supplemented by various fibre products. Konsyl, Metamucil and Citrucel are some of the fibre products often recommended for daily use (Figure 5.4).

Dietary fluids should be increased to 8–10 cups daily with increased fibre intake; alcohol and caffeinated drinks are not included. Usually, several decades have elapsed between response to a carcinogen and a diagnosis of cancer, giving rise to the speculation that a diet consumed in childhood and middle age may be responsible for cancer in later years (Amarnath and Wexner, 1996). It follows, therefore, that healthy dietary habits are as important for a child as they are for an adult. Public education on dietary fibre issues should include the entire family, especially where there is a history of CRC.

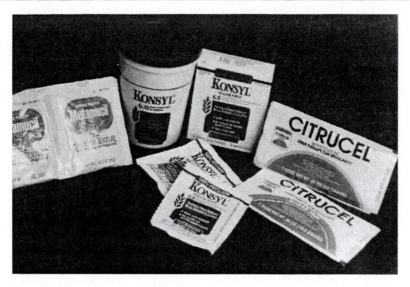

Figure 5.4: Some types of fibre products.

Much study has been directed towards the antioxidant factors of micronutrients. Vitamins A, C, D, calcium and selenium are shown to provide some benefit in the prevention of CRC.

In a study of female registered nurses, it was found that with regular aspirin use for 10 years or more, at doses similar to those used for cardiovascular disease prevention, the risk of CRC was substantially reduced. Other studies indicate a similar benefit for men (Giovanucci et al., 1995).

During patient education, consideration should be given to botanical medicines and herbs used for cancer prevention. Often patients will approach the physician or nurse with questions or articles they have read on the subject. Some epidemiological studies have shown that the risk of stomach and colon cancer is reduced in people who consume garlic (Allium stratum). Onion (Allium cepa) has also been credited with reduced risk of gastrointestinal cancer, although it is not clear by what level of intake cancer is reduced in a significant way.

Green tea, used in Japan, China and other parts of Asia, is shown in studies to reduce risk of many types of cancer, including colon cancer. The fact that some anti-cancer drugs (Vincristin and Taxol) are derived from plants gives some credibility to the cancer-prevention properties of some foods. Nurses should review information on these medicinal herbs and, with reasonable scepticism, help patients make safe decisions about maintaining good health (Yarnell, 1997).

Patients should be made aware of inherited conditions that predispose to CRC. Information should be available on familial adenomatous polyposis – characterized by multiple adenomatous polyps of the colon, and hereditary nonpolyposis colorectal cancer (HNPCC) – a syndrome which is manifested by family history of colon cancer at an early age (Wexner and Nogueras, 1995).

Other patients at higher risk for CRC are those with inflammatory bowel disease (IBD). The cancer risk of patients with mucosal ulcerative colitis (MUC), and Crohn's disease increases with time and severity (Amarnath and Wexner, 1996).

The following recommendations have been made by the American Cancer Society (Winawer et al., 1995):

- Reduce fat intake to less than 30% of daily calories.
- Increase fibre intake to 30 g daily, with an upper limit of 35 g.
- Include a variety of vegetables and fruits in your daily diet.
- Avoid obesity.
- Consume alcoholic beverages in moderation, if at all.
- Minimize consumption of salt-cured, salt-pickled and smoked foods.
- If possible, reduction of fat intake to 20–25% of daily calories would be beneficial.

Nurses should utilize teaching materials – pamphlets, charts and posters – for patient education. They should be prominently displayed and accessible to patients. This information and product samples should be given to them whenever possible.

Early Detection and Screening

Although there is no curative treatment available, early detection of CRC offers the best possibility of reduced mortality. Treatment of this disease is most effective when diagnosed at an early stage. The 5-year survival rate for localized lesions is 80–90%. This rate drops to 35–65% once the disease has spread to adjacent structures and lymph nodes. Five-year survival for patients with distant metastases is rare (Wexner and Nogueras, 1995).

The importance of public education regarding early symptoms of CRC and the need for routine screening of asymptomatic individuals is emphasized by these statistics.

Nurses should be aware that the rationale for screenings in a population that has no symptoms of CRC is to detect the lesion at a stage where it will be most responsive to treatment. An effective screening programme should be highly sensitive and specific with positive predictive value. The tests employed should have a low rate of false positive and false negative results.

Documentation from CRC screening trials indicates 70% higher diagnostic yield in the screened group than in the controlled group. It is important to note that 60% of the cancers found in the screened group had no positive lymph nodes. However, only 45% of the controlled group were node negative. Additionally, more pre-cancerous adenomas were found in the screened group.

Currently, the American Cancer Society recommends, for asymptomatic individuals, an annual digital rectal examination beginning at age 40 years, a sigmoidoscopic examination every 3 to 5 years and a faecal occult blood test annually after age 50 years. In addition, colonoscopy every 5 years, starting at age 35–40, is recommended for patients whose first-degree relative has been diagnosed with CRC at an age younger than 55 years (Wexner & Nogueras, 1995). The increasing number of right-sided colon cancers, which can be detected only by colonoscopy or barium enema, may warrant screening change from sigmoidoscopy to colonoscopy every 3 to 5 years after age 50 (Witt, 1993).

Some screening procedures are simple and require very little patient preparation, such as rectal examination and faecal occult blood. However, others like sigmoidoscopy and colonoscopy require enemas or laxatives which some patients find difficult to tolerate. The most commonly used occult blood test is the Hemoccult test which consists of a filter-paper slide impregnated with guaiac. When hydrogen peroxide is added to stool placed on this slide, a colour change occurs. Blue indicates a positive test for blood in the stool. The sensitivity of the test is reduced by ingestion of fresh fruits, such as bananas, and vegetables, such as broccoli and radishes. Agents such as ascorbic acid can produce a false negative effect even when haemoglobin is present. These problems are reduced by testing and retesting patients after imposition of dietary restrictions (Williams, 1996).

Nurses are relied upon to prepare the patient psychologically as well as physically for these procedures. Very often patients are prepared upon arrival in the physician's office, with enemas. These are administered by nurses or by patients with nursing assistance.

It is usual for patients to require reassurance to allay fears and anxiety, as well as an explanation of what the procedure entails. A patient who has an understanding of the procedure is more likely to cooperate, which then promotes relaxation and facilitates comfort during the procedure.

A nurse should be in attendance while the procedure is in progress, providing assistance to the physician, assessing patient tolerance and comfort, and ensuring patient privacy.

At the completion of the procedure, when the physician relays the findings to the patient, the nurse should be present to provide support, and to give patients post-procedural instructions.

Presentation of CRC

Usually patients with symptomatic CRC tumours have advanced disease. More frequently, patients complain of changes in bowel habits. This change may be insignificant, therefore very little emphasis is placed on this observation until the change is more profound.

A left-sided lesion creates more obvious symptoms than a right-sided lesion. This occurs because the stool in the narrower left colon is more formed and therefore passes through with more difficulty than the relatively liquid stool in the wider lumen of the right colon. Other symptoms of left-sided lesions are bleeding, pain and discharge.

CRC often presents as rectal bleeding which can be either overt or occult, bright red, purple, mahogany, black, or not apparent. The blood will often appear redder or less altered in a more distally located lesion. Many people assume that all rectal bleeding is caused by haemorrhoids and so do not seek medical attention, but this can be very dangerous (Corman, 1993).

Other signs and symptoms of CRC are anaemia and weakness due to blood loss and weight loss. In 5–15% of individuals the presenting symptom is abdominal pain which suggests an obstructing or partially obstructing lesion. Any of these signs and symptoms should prompt a complete work-up (Corman, 1993).

Support and Follow-up for Patients Diagnosed with Colorectal Cancer, and their Families

By the time a patient receives a diagnosis of colon or rectal cancer, a nurse/patient relationship has usually been formed. The patient has, after all, allowed various probing questions and accepted assistance with many private bodily functions and examinations. Patient and nurse have probably shared the occasional unpleasant or anxious moments and most likely some embarrassing ones as well, during which some amount of trust and belief in the nurse's professional ability has developed. Thus the nurse, in the majority of situations, would be the person most acceptable to the patient and, therefore, most effective in providing psychological support and other assistance.

Psychological Support

To facilitate the grieving process, the nurse should provide the patient and family members with time to discuss feelings and concerns. This is the first level of supportive counselling and encourages ventilation of feelings. Patients may feel like crying, yelling, lapsing into deep thought, or have continuous talking spells. Reassurance that these behaviours are acceptable and that expressing confusing, conflicting or negative emotions is normal, helps in dealing with grief.

The patient may request information or clarification about the disease or treatment plan. This gives the nurse the opportunity to help the patient confront the diagnosis and have understanding of the issues by providing accurate information and classification about CRC and treatment. The physician's explanation about the diagnosis and treatment options should be reinforced at this time.

Treatment options may include surgery, pre- or postoperative radiation, chemotherapy, or a combination of these. Curative surgery may not be an option for some patients. If symptom control is the only option, the nurse should explain the rationale and specific treatment procedures or guidelines and their effectiveness (Doughty and Broadwell, 1993).

Sexual concerns are common in patients undergoing colorectal surgery. Changes in body image and sexual performance are important considerations. Nurses are encouraged to discuss with the surgeon how surgery may affect the individual's sexual performance. With adequate information the nurse can provide the support and counselling the patient and their significant other may need.

Family members must adapt to changes in the patient's health status, income reduction, or potential fatal outcome, and may require some assistance. Nurses can assist in promotion of open communication between patient and family members. This will reduce misunderstandings and improve coping skills. Family counselling and referral to appropriate organizations may be suggested when indicated.

An important area of concern is the possibility of wearing a 'bag' as is necessary with abdominal perineal resections performed for rectal tumours less than 8 cm from the anal verge. Some patients become extremely distressed by the thought of disfigurement and lifestyle changes. Nurses should provide explanations to patients and family members regarding the purpose of a colostomy or ileostomy and discuss basic management and refer the patient to an Enterostomal Therapist (ET) Nurse for in-depth management. Family members should be encouraged to participate in these patient care activities and treatment.

Community Support

Recognizing that patients may experience a sense of isolation, nurses should refer patients with CRC to organizations for counselling and assistance as needed. Cancer societies provide resources and rehabilitation programmes including support groups, equipment loans, transportation, education materials, and free supplies. Ostomy associations offer help on a one-to-one basis with home visits and supplies. Support and information is also available from individual patients who have had a similar surgical procedure.

While many patients are surrounded by loving family, friends and organizations to assist with physical care and provide emotional support, some patients ultimately must come to terms with their disease alone. Many tools are available to aid in this coping process which are beneficial to even those patients with family support. These basic tools are books and audiotapes, and they are available in many varieties. Some help patients relax by use of a technique called 'guided imagery'. Others strengthen or enhance spirituality, while many others help the patient focus on the positive and assist in the acceptance of the hand they have been dealt (McGannon, 1995).

Guided imagery is also known as visualization and is a method of deliberately creating images of sights, sounds, smell, taste and feelings in the mind via audiotapes. It is a method of promoting communication with the mind and body for restoration of balance, relaxation and fighting disease. Patients can use visualization to control anxiety, decrease stress and possibly strengthen the immune system (Tusek, 1995). Some institutions presently enrol patients in self-help classes preoperatively. Various audiotapes are provided for preoperative and intra-operative listening – which has been shown to provide a better postoperative outcome.

Colorectal Nurse Specialists

In some situations in the USA colorectal surgery patients receive support and total patient care from specialist nurses known as Surgical Nurse Clinicians. These nurses are involved in all aspects (pre-, intra- and postoperative) patient care. Responsibilities include preoperative history and physical, step-by-step explanation of the surgical procedure, and bowel preparation instructions. They discuss the hospitalization process including treatment plan, discharge from hospital and rehabilitation. Surgical Nurse Clinicians are experienced surgical assistants who are involved in postoperative rounds, coordination of home care with a home health nurse and follow-up with the patient and family at home via phone calls. Postoperative care includes office visits with the patient for staple removal, and assisting JB physician with follow-up visits.

Conclusion

The diagnosis of colon or rectal cancer is devastating news to most patients, especially those patients with very little information about the disease. The shock of this discovery sometimes results in confusion and despair, not only for the patient but also for family members. Patients in such a mental state have a reduced capacity to accept and process information. Most patients, after consultation with the physician, will refer to the nurse for support, reassurance and additional information. The nurse who is knowledgeable and caring can be of considerable help in reducing the patient's anxiety level and increasing coping skills.

Summary

Although colorectal cancer is a frequent malady affecting a significant portion of the population on an annual basis, improved understanding of aetiology and pathogenesis, together with improved surgical and adjuvant therapy, will hopefully allow for better outcomes in these patients.

References

Amarnath B, Wexner SD (1996) Etiologic and clinical implications of colorectal cancer. In Contemporary Surgery. California: Bobit Publishing.

American Cancer Society (1984) Nutrition, Common Sense and Cancer. Booklet 84.25mm-Rev/93 – No. 2096-LE.

Astler VB, Coller FA (1954) The prognostic significance of direct extension of carcinoma of the colon and rectum. Annals of Surgery 139: 846–51.

Buess G, Theiss R, Gunther M (1985) Endoscopic surgery in the rectum. Endoscopy 17(1): 31–5.

Corman M (1993) Colon and Rectal Surgery. 3rd edn. Philadelphia: JB Lippincott.

Dixon CF (1948) Anterior resection for malignant lesions of the upper part of the rectum and lower part of the sigmoid. Annals of Surgery 128: 425.

Doughty D, Broadwell D (1993) Gastrointestinal Disorders. Mosby's Clinical Nursing Series. Missouri: Mosby-Year Book.

Dukes CE (1932) The classification of cancer of the rectum. Journal of Pathology and Bacteriology 35: 323–32.

Eddy DM (1990) Screening for colorectal cancer. Annals of Internal Medicine 113(5): 373–84.

Fishel R, Lescoe MK, Rao MR et al. (1993) The human mutator gene, homolog MSH2, and its association with hereditary nonpolyposis colon cancer. Cell.

Giovanucci U, Egan KM, Hunter DJ, Stampfer MJ, Coldiz GA, Willett WC, Speizer FE (1995) Aspirin and the risk of colorectal cancer in women. New England Journal of Medicine 333(10): 609–14.

Heald RJ, Husband EM, Ryal RD (1982) The meso rectum in rectal cancer surgery: the clue to pelvic recurrence. British Journal of Surgery 69(10): 613–16.

Hermanek P, Sabin LH (1995) Colorectal carcinoma. In Prognostic Factors in Cancer. Berlin: Springer-Verlag, pp. 64–79.

Hertz RE, Deddish MR, Day E (1960) Value of periodic examination in detecting cancer of the rectum and colon. Postgraduate Medicine 27: 290.

Knudsen AGJ (1971) Mutation and cancer: statistical study of retinoblastoma. Proceedings of the National Academy of Science, USA.

Krook JE, Moertal CG, Gunderson LL et al. (1991) Effective adjuvant therapy for high risk rectal carcinoma. New England Journal of Medicine 324(11): 764–7.

Laurie JA, Moertel CG, Fleming TR et al. for the National Center Cancer Treatment Group and the Mayo Clinic (1989) Surgical adjuvant therapy of large bowel carcinoma: an evaluation of levamisole and the combination of levamisole and fluorouracil. Journal of Clinical Oncology 7(10): 1447–56.

McGannon E (1995) Family Matters: Information for People with Colorectal Cancer in their Family. Vol. 1. Cleveland: Cleveland Clinic Foundation.

Miles WE (1908) A method of performing abdomino-perineal excision for carcinoma of the rectum and of the terminal portion of the pelvic colon. Lancet.

O'Connell M, Malliard J, Macdonald J et al. (1993) An intergroup trial of intensive course 5-fu and levamisole as surgical adjuvant for high risk colon cancer. Abstracted. Proceedings of the American Society of Clinical Oncology.

Parc R, Tiret E, Frileux P et al. (1986) Resection and coloanal anastomosis with colonic reservoir for rectal carcinoma. British Journal of Surgery 73(2): 139–41.

Quirke P, Durdey P, Dixon MF, Williams NS (1986) Local recurrence of rectal adenocarcinoma due to inadequate surgical resection. Histopathological study of lateral tumor spread and surgical excision. Lancet 2(8514): 996–9.

Sentovich SM, Blatchford GJ, Falk PM et al. (1993) Transrectal ultrasound of rectal tumors. American Journal of Surgery 166(6): 638–41.

Smith LE (1976) Fiberoptic colonoscopy: complications of colonoscopy and polypectomy. Diseases of the Colon and Rectum 19(5): 407–12.

Smith LE, Nivatvongs S (1975) Complications in colonoscopy. Diseases of the Colon and Rectum 18(3): 214–20.

Tusek D (1995) Family Matters: Information for People with Colorectal Cancer in their Family. Vol. 1. Cleveland: Cleveland Clinic Foundation.

Wangersteen OH (1945) Primary resection (closed anastomosis) of rectal ampulla for malignancy with preservation of sphincteric function together with further account on primary resection of colon and rectosigmoid and note on hepatic metastases. Surgery for Gynecology and Obstetrics 81: 1.

Wexner SD, Nogueras JJ (1995) Malignant diseases of the colon and rectum. In Rakel R (Ed.) Conn's Current Therapy. Philadelphia: WB Saunders.

Williams NS (Ed.) (1996) Colorectal Cancer. New York: Churchill Livingstone.

Williams NS, Dixon MF, Johnson D (1983) Re-appraisal of the 5 cm rule of distal excision for carcinoma of the rectum: a study of distal intramural spread and of patients' survival. British Journal of Surgery 70(3): 150–4.

Winawer SJ, O'Brian MJ, Waye JD et al. (1990) Risk and surveillance of individuals
    with colorectal polyps. WHO Collaborating Centre for the Prevention of
    Colorectal Cancer. Bulletin of World Health Organization 68(6): 789–95.
Winawer SJ, Zauber AG, Diaz B (1987) The National Polyp Study: temporal
    sequence of evolving colorectal cancer from normal colon. Gastrointestinal
    Endoscopy.
Witt ME (1993) Current management of adults with colorectal cancer. Medical
    Surgical Nursing 2(2).
Yarnell E (1997) Prevention of cancer with botanical medicines. Alternative and
    Complementary Therapies 3(6): 427–32.

Chapter 6
Inflammatory Bowel Disease: The Nursing Implications

JACQUELINE JOELS RGN, Colorectal Nurse Specialist, Southend
  Hospital, Essex, UK

Introduction

Ulcerative colitis and Crohn's disease are chronic, incurable inflammatory bowel diseases (IBDs) whose specific causes remain unknown.
The unpredictable and complex nature of IBD, together with the
personal and distressing symptoms the illness can produce, poses a
great challenge for nurses involved in the care of this client group.

This chapter will present an understanding of IBD, and the affects it can
have on all aspects of the individual's life physically, psychologically and
socially. It will include quotes from patients who were interviewed for a
research study and explore ways in which the health care team may
provide the support, understanding and practical advice to help them cope.

Aetiology

The unknown aetiology of IBD is distressing for its victims; patients
want to know 'Why has it happened to me?' and often experience feelings of guilt, blame or frustration when searching for a cause.

Extensive research is under way, but to date only a few theories of
possible contributing factors exist. For example, smoking has long
been known to protect people from ulcerative colitis but conversely
increases the risk of developing Crohn's (Pullan, 1996). There have
also been connections between the measles virus (Thompson, 1995)
and pasteurised milk predisposing to Crohn's but these as yet are
unconfirmed. It is, however, thought that individuals may have a

genetic predisposition to developing IBD, and in particular Crohn's disease (Kamm, 1996).

Incidence and Disease Pattern

IBD most commonly occurs during early adulthood with both diseases mentioned above being slightly more prevalent in women than men. In the western world the number of people affected by ulcerative colitis is 1 in 1000 and by Crohn's disease 1 in 1500, with the incidence, particularly of Crohn's, having risen during the last 40 years (Kamm, 1996.)

Ulcerative colitis and Crohn's have a disease pattern of exacerbation followed by a period of remission during which time the patient often feels quite well. The symptoms each produce during an acute phase are similar, namely profuse diarrhoea often accompanied by passage of mucus and blood, weight loss, abdominal pain, lethargy and anaemia. In addition to affecting the gut each can exhibit extra-intestinal manifestations. There are, however, specific differences between the two and it is important for a definitive diagnosis to be made as treatment, in particular surgical intervention, will vary accordingly.

Ulcerative Colitis

Ulcerative colitis occurs only within the colon and rectum. Their function is to store and absorb water from its content so that at the end of transit the waste matter is formed into normal faecal consistency. Ulcerative colitis affects the mucosa, which is the inner lining of the bowel. This becomes swollen, inflamed and may lead to ulceration – hence the presenting symptoms of diarrhoea, mucus and bleeding (Figure 6.4).

The disease originates within the rectum and in 50% of patients it will remain at this stage (Brian and Ferguson, 1993a). However, for others it can extend to the left side of the colon, involving the sigmoid and descending colon, or affect the large bowel completely, which is described as total colitis.

Some 20% of patients will experience only one episode of colitis but 25% will suffer chronic active disease. A feature of concern to many who have had active extensive colitis for 8–10 years is the marked risk of their developing malignant changes within the colon. It is important that these individuals are made aware of this and hence understand the recommendation of many physicians for such patients to undergo an annual colonoscopy to detect any dysplasia and facilitate early treatment.

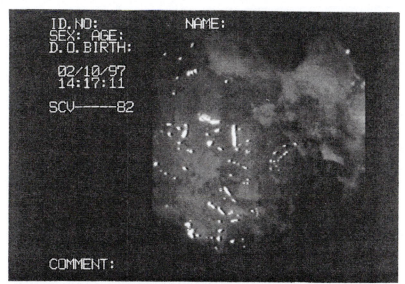

Figure 6.1: Ulcerative colitis. See colour section.

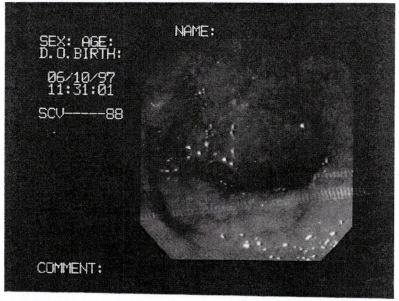

Figure 6.2: View of normal bowel mucosa. See colour section.

Crohn's Disease

Of the two inflammatory bowel diseases Crohn's can prove the more cruel. Although it most commonly presents in the ileocaecal area, Crohn's disease can affect any part of the gastrointestinal tract from the mouth

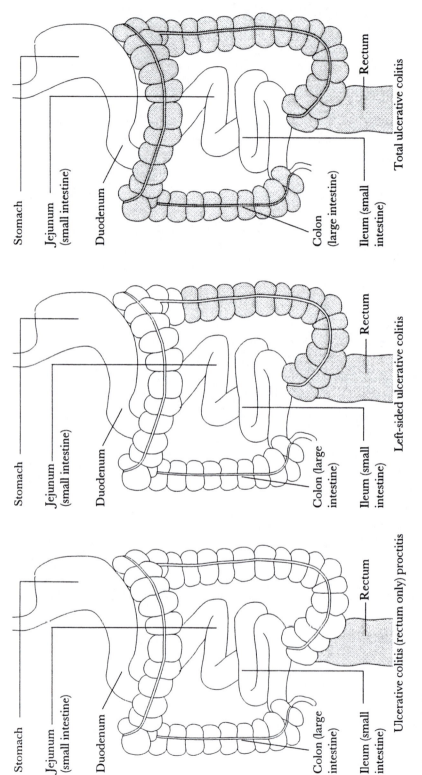

Figure 6.3: Diagrammatic representation of varying degrees of ulcerative colitis within the colon.

Commonly experienced symptoms of ulcerative colitis	Extra-intestinal manifestations associated with ulcerative colitis
Diarrhoea	Arthritis
Abdominal pain/cramping	Iritis/conjuctivitis
Urgency	Ankylosing spondylitis
Passage of mucus and blood	Erythema nodosum (present as painful swellings mainly on the shins)
Long-term effects	Pyoderma gangrenosum (affects lower legs or parastomal) treated with steroids or colectomy
50% may have minor liver abnormalities	
Increased risk of sclerosing cholangitis	
Increased risk of colonic cancer after 8–10 years	

Figure 6.4: Symptoms and associated manifestations of ulcerative colitis.

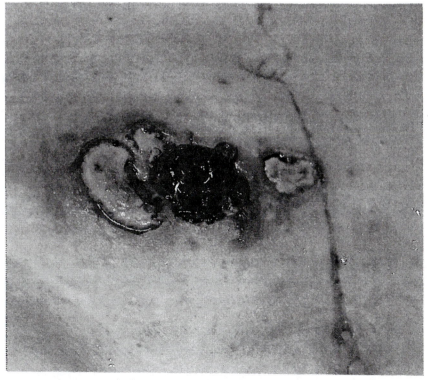

Figure 6.5: Parastomal pyoderma gangrenosum. See colour section.

Commonly experienced symptoms of Crohn's	Manifestations associated with Crohn's
Diarrhoea (particularly	Fistulae
Bleeding if colonic disease)	Abscesses
Pain – more common if small	Anal tags
bowel affected	Fissures
Anorexia	Granulomas – may affect skin,
Weight loss	epiglottis, vocal chords or lips
Fever	Growth retardation in children/
	adolescents

Figure 6.6: Symptoms and associated manifestations of Crohn's disease.

to the anus, and patients can therefore never be offered a surgical cure.

Unlike colitis, Crohn's inflammation penetrates the full thickness of the intestinal wall (transmural) which becomes inflamed and thickened with intraluminal narrowing, sometimes affecting passage of food through the tract. In addition its transmural nature can predispose to other distressing presentations.

The progression of Crohn's is not continuous but has classical skip lesions, that is areas of diseased bowel with healthy sections in between. Around 20–40% of patients will also have perianal disease and within 10 years of diagnosis approximately half will have had a bowel resection, especially if the small bowel is affected.

Symptoms of Crohn's disease are often quite non-specific and may differ according to the part of the bowel affected. For example, pain is symbolic of small bowel disease, with passage of blood and diarrhoea being associated with colonic inflammation.

Diagnosis

On referral to the gastroenterologist investigations will be performed in order to obtain a diagnosis and to initiate appropriate treatment. Clinical assessment and history will establish symptom pattern, severity and the general health of the individual. Stool analysis will exclude bowel infection such as *Clostridium difficile* or *Helicobacter* which can imitate symptoms of IBD in causing bloody diarrhoea (Pullen, 1997).

Endoscopic Investigations

The rigid or flexible proctosigmoidoscope is used to view the rectum and sigmoid colon. Colonoscopy involves passage of a fibreoptic scope

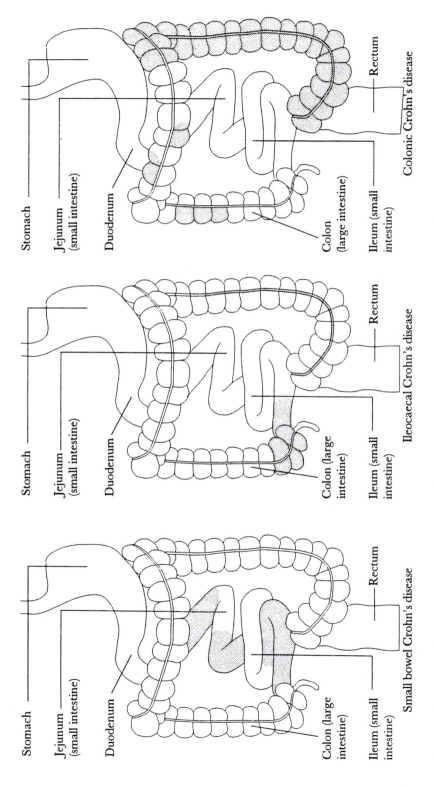

Figure 6.7: Diagrammatic representation of how Crohn's disease may present through the gastrointestinal tract, with classical skip lesions.

to permit observation of the whole colon and terminal ileum from which biopsies can be obtained for histology to confirm a suspected diagnosis.

Radiology

Contrast X-rays necessitate radio-opaque liquid barium being taken orally in order to view the upper gastrointestinal tract, or this may be administered as an enema to determine the extent of bowel affected.

Haematology

Blood chemistry and haematology tests may include:

- haemoglobin level: iron deficiency anaemia can result from large or chronic blood loss;
- erythroycte sedimentation rate (ESR) may be raised if there is active inflammation;
- albumin concentration: hypoalbuminaemia often indicates severe disease (Jewell et al., 1992);

Information on Diagnosis

Diagnosis of inflammatory bowel disease may generate a multitude of feelings, fears and questions within the individual and is a time during which a sensitive, empathetic approach is required. Considering the chronic nature of IBD and the need for treatment compliance, the lack of information about the disease sometimes provided to patients at diagnosis is a cause for concern:

> Then they told me I had Crohn's disease, but I didn't really know what it was … I mean I still don't know fully … They sort of said 'It's like inflammation of the bowel' they didn't explain what to expect or what was normal.

In recognizing the pressures upon medical time Probert (1991) suggests that there is potential for nurses to provide this crucial education and counselling. In his autobiographical account of having ulcerative colitis, Kelly (1986) stated that more opportunity should be given for patients to express their anxieties, fears and doubts about what is happening to them. Patients also relate having wanted practical advice and information to equip them in coping with the disease.

Few people have much knowledge or understanding of the 'normal' functioning of their 'insides' and showing a basic diagram of the gastrointestinal tract, indicating the process of digestion, pointing out which part of the bowel is affected by the disease and why they are experiencing such symptoms, will help to put it all into perspective. Knowing what may happen, such as rectal bleeding, will also help prevent panic situations and fear of the unknown.

Sometimes diagnosis can actually prove to be a relief for the patient after months of feeling unwell and not having known what was wrong. A variety of well-written and comprehensible booklets about living with IBD as well as a video series are available from voluntary organizations and pharmaceutical companies in the UK. These are ideal for patients to take home so that they may absorb the information in their own time and share this with other members of the family, who may themselves be feeling worried and helpless.

Psychological Effects of IBD on the Individual

> It is mental as well ... there have been times when I've felt such hatred for other people because they're leading a normal life.

Emotions that the individual may experience are many and diverse but the most commonly expressed are those of embarrassment, nervousness, fear and depression (Joachim and Milne, 1985).

As a culture we tend not to discuss our bowels, maintaining them as fulfilling a discreet function conducted in the privacy of one's own bathroom. But for patients with IBD this for them suddenly becomes public, not only in respect of having to endure unpleasant and undignified investigations but in daily life having to use lavatories when in public or at work, often with explosive and noisy diarrhoea and then having to face people afterwards. It is little wonder therefore that patients often have low self-esteem.

> How do I feel about myself? ... I don't really know, I probably try not to think about it too much.

IBD remains a little known disease which is rarely publicized during medical television programmes or in media sources, thus making it less easy for victims to discuss or for the general public to understand its distressing symptoms. Nurses can help redress this by demonstrating acceptance and helping the patient understand that it is by no means an uncommon condition.

Patients may develop a feeling of isolation following diagnosis. Meeting a fellow sufferer can be both helpful and encouraging: to know that he/she is not 'the only one' and to be able to speak to another person who has experienced the same emotions and difficulties can provide tremendous support and help the individual to cope.

It can be beneficial within a gastrointestinal unit to recruit a network of 'voluntary visitors' who have a positive attitude to living with IBD, trying to match people closely if possible in gender, age and lifestyle. Also, patients need to be aware of the National Association for Crohn's and Colitis (NACC), which is a support group in the UK producing factsheets and newsletters. It also organizes local meetings and runs a telephone helpline service. Although not every individual will want to discuss their illness with others, to have the information and contact number if they should need it is empowering.

It is important to be sensitive to patients' needs when they visit hospital by ensuring that they are aware of the location of the nearest toilets, or for an inpatient, providing a bed positioned close to a bathroom.

Body Image

The feature of IBD as most commonly affecting people in their early adult life can itself generate many difficulties, being a stage when the individual will be experiencing major life events such as starting at college or embarking on a career, and developing sexual relationships, and it is a time when one is particularly concerned with how one looks and appears to others. Self-esteem and body image are inextricably linked. We are living in a visual age when how we look matters; feeling attractive fills us with confidence and facilitates a positive approach to others, which is thus reciprocated.

IBD is not always invisible and can negatively affect the individual's body image. The dramatic weight loss that often accompanies active disease is distressing. Patients may say that they cannot bring themselves to look at their body in a mirror, and I also recently had experience of nursing a woman in her thirties who had lost most of her hair because she had become so malnourished.

It is not only the illness itself which causes changes to the individual's appearance: for example, the side-effects of steroids can produce acne and weight gain, and in particular a 'moon-shaped face'. A teenage girl who had undergone ileostomy formation reported that the stoma had affected her body image less than the striae covering her thighs and abdomen that were the result of steroids.

Children and Adolescents

Children and adolescents are in danger of the illness causing growth retardation, particularly if it is undiagnosed for some time and puberty is delayed. In years past adults who had developed IBD in childhood sometimes never developed fully.

This aspect can generate enormous distress, especially in boys. Children need to fit in and be accepted by their peers, and if they appear years younger than their age it is traumatic. Nowadays treatment ideas have altered. Patients may have overnight nasogastric feeding and early surgical intervention is commonplace to avoid stunted growth.

It may help if the nurse is able to prepare the family for the possible psychological effects on their child and make them aware of the emotions that he/she may demonstrate such as being angry, awkward or withdrawn. The child may also find increased tiredness difficult to cope with, especially combined with pressures of school and joining in an active social life.

A child can also feel very embarrassed at school if it is necessary to leave the classroom, and if he/she is conscious of odour. Liaison with the school nurse and teacher helps provide understanding and support.

Whilst trying to maintain as normal a life as possible it is important for affected children to be encouraged to eat a healthy, well-balanced diet, to take their medication regularly and to ensure they have adequate rest during an exacerbation.

Relationships and Sexual Issues

Each person affected by IBD will react to having the disease in an individual way and this will determine whether he/she tells others about it, and if so whom. Some adopt a cavalier approach in that others must accept them as they are, or not at all, but conversely others report actively avoiding people and in particular abstaining from developing relationships with members of the opposite sex.

Ignorance on the part of the public concerning IBD can increase awkwardness when discussing the disease. There does, however, appear to be a gender division with females generally feeling quite comfortable in talking about it with their girlfriends whereas men tend to have less of an intimate closeness with their peers. For example, one young man's reaction was:

> It's not like a rash on the arm or something; it's perhaps a subject people, or young men, don't like talking about.

It should be recognized that a chronic illness such as this affects far more lives than that of the individual sufferer:

> He was just so worried about me, he said he felt so helpless that there was nothing he could do for me, he got so frustrated ... he found it hard to come to terms with, I think, more than I did.

At the point of diagnosis, or at subsequent hospital appointments, the partner should be encouraged to attend so they can be given support and advice to understand the pattern of the disease, what to expect and how he/she can help. Research studies indicate that patients who are already involved with someone when they develop IBD do not feel their relationship is adversely affected because of it, although when symptoms are severe with accompanying tiredness and the patient feels unwell, feelings can become strained.

In adopting a holistic approach to nursing assessment, the individual's sexual health is integral but unfortunately often is omitted, perhaps due to hesitancy on the professional's part in not wanting to cause embarrassment or to embarrass him/herself.

Sex life was found to be one of the most important areas about which patients want to ask questions (Scholmerich et al., 1987) and to address this would be a relief to many, giving them 'permission' to talk and express their concerns. Although having IBD is no contraindication to an active and fulfilling sex life, both physical and psychological aspects of the illness can create barriers or problems for the individual.

There is no doubt that sex is better if one feels relaxed and uninhibited. Although few actually experience faecal incontinence during a flare-up, this fear, together with those of urgency, noise, soiling and odour, can make the individual tense and unable to enjoy sex, but also embarrassed to communicate these concerns to a partner.

When one is feeling unwell or tired, sexual desire is one of the first emotions to suffer and can generate feelings of guilt that you are not fulfilling your role, are letting your partner down and making them feel rejected. This issue can be even more difficult for male sufferers as their psyche is inextricably linked to their ability to achieve erection and orgasm.

One-third of females with IBD report dyspareunia and additional physical effects of IBD, such as perianal disease or rectovaginal fistulae. This may affect the individual's ability to have intercourse or to enjoy it comfortably and without embarrassment.

It is important too not to forget the partner, who may be afraid to even touch, let alone penetrate a loved one for fear of causing pain or damage.

It helps for nursing or medical professionals to address these issues with the couple, giving them the opportunity to express and discuss their personal fears and concerns, perhaps even just letting the couple know it is all right for them to have intercourse and offering them sensitive and practical advice as required. For example, taking anti-diarrhoea medication prior to intercourse will slow the bowel and lessen the fear of incontinence, and a change in position and use of a proprietary lubricant when making love may help women suffering from dyspareunia.

If the patient is within a new personal relationship he/she may want advice as to how and when to talk about the illness:

> I don't go out with men because I'm embarrassed, I don't want to tell them my problems as I don't think they'll understand, so I just steer clear.

Although IBD poses a dilemma for sufferers, most actually report nothing but interest and acceptance when they are able to disclose it.

Sex Following Surgery

For those patients whose disease has necessitated surgery and stoma formation there may be additional concerns pertaining to altered body image, the visible scar and having a bag. The stoma care nurse is trained to provide support and to proffer advice, such as using a petite unobtrusive bag whilst having sex and perhaps wearing underwear which is sensual but which will conceal the appliance.

For male patients who have extensive rectal disease a proctectomy may be necessary, although whenever possible surgeons these days endeavour to preserve this area. One reason is that the sympathetic and parasympathetic nerve supplies lie in close proximity to the rectum, and surgery may therefore cause damage to these nerves resulting in impotence.

The possibility of sexual dysfunction must, in this situation, be discussed with the patient and his partner preoperatively and provision for storage of sperm be made available if they so desire. This sensitive issue should be addressed again a few weeks after surgery and if difficulties are being experienced referral to a sexual health counsellor or consultant can be arranged. There are aids and devices available to assist the individual to achieve and sustain erection, such as vacuum pumps or instruction to self-administer penile injections.

Patients who are homosexual may be particularly distressed if their rectum is badly diseased or if its removal is necessary. Sexual counselling should be offered to the individual and his partner. It is also important for the stoma care nurse to establish who is the 'receiver' in the relationship and to place emphasis on not using the stoma for sexual penetration.

IBD and Fertility

IBD should not adversely affect the ability to conceive or carry a pregnancy to term; in fact some women report feeling healthier than they have for years during pregnancy. However, male sperm count may be reduced in the presence of Crohn's disease, particularly if the sufferer's weight and nutritional status are low; this may similarly affect a woman's fertility.

Once symptoms are well controlled with medication and general fitness improves, fertility should return to normal. Patients taking azathioprine are advised to stop this whilst trying to conceive, but those taking 5 ASA medication to maintain remission should continue with this (Kamm, 1996). On the other hand, patients who are taking the oral contraceptive pill should be aware that it may not be fully absorbed if they are suffering from diarrhoea, and additional precautions are advised during such episodes.

The Association to Aid the Sexual and Personal Relationships of People with a Disability (SPOD) produce useful supportive literature and telephone advice pertaining to sexual issues.

Social Implications of IBD

The unpredictable nature of Crohn's and colitis is reported by patients as being one of the most frustrating and troublesome aspects of living with the disease. At times when they are without symptoms it is possible almost to forget one has it, but during an attack carrying out even basic daily tasks can prove nearly impossible.

It is difficult therefore for sufferers to make any future social plans because of the threat of accompanying tiredness, fear of incontinence, odour and access to lavatories that go with a flare-up. Patients frequently report having to cancel arrangements at very short notice.

A normally enjoyable event such as eating out can present a nightmare situation. As will be discussed later in this chapter, many find certain foods exacerbate their symptoms. It is advisable to avoid foods that are thought to do this 6–12 hours before an engagement and to take loperamide if required.

Patients may feel reassured to know they may obtain a key to disabled lavatories via RADAR, plus an accompanying booklet outlining their location throughout the country.

Effects on Role and Employment

The unpredictability of IBD may also adversely affect patients' ability to maintain their 'normal' roles. For example if a mother caring for a young child is confined to the bathroom with unrelenting diarrhoea, even taking the child to school can prove impossible which may also generate feelings of guilt and worthlessness.

As alluded to previously, young people often fall behind in their course work and education. Being streamed into a class with younger pupils and away from their friends can be devastating. An additional area of concern was identified by Mayberry and Mayberry (1993), who found that young patients, although achieving equivalent qualifications, failed to gain comparable employment to their peers.

In noting the anxiety expressed by many patients regarding employment prospects, Moody et al. (1992) conducted a study into the attitudes of employers, obtaining only a 27% response rate! Many replied that a decision would rest upon the pre-employment medical.

Accessibility to lavatories whilst at work and an understanding of IBD both from employers and colleagues will help to reduce anxiety.

For those who are self-employed, the financial implications whilst being physically unable to work generate stress which will in turn exacerbate the disease symptoms.

Individuals will exhibit extraordinary degrees of resourcefulness to continue as normal: one man who was experiencing 35+ bowel actions a day had constructed a makeshift lavatory in the back of his van to use whilst working.

Involvement of a medical social worker who can provide knowledge and advice regarding benefits for which patients are eligible will help to address these concerns.

Treatments for IBD

> I don't think you ever come to terms with it really … I think I was angry at first because you think 'why me?'. And they can't tell you what's caused it and there's nobody out there who can tell you you're ever going to get better.

The fact that there is no known cause or cure for IBD makes it a frustrating and unknown entity for its victims, who do not know what future course or level of severity the disease will adopt and must face the ever present fear that surgery possibly resulting in stoma formation may one day be necessary.

In situations of chronic illness, compliance with treatments can be difficult. Patients become despondent often feeling that nothing, most notably a cure, is achieved by whatever efforts. Fulfilling individuals' desire for information and actively involving them with their care will help to aid compliance.

The main treatment for IBD at present is medication administered to relieve symptoms, reduce inflammation and prolong periods of remission. Drug regimes may be complex with worrying side-effects (Brian and Ferguson, 1993b). It has been suggested that compliance would increase if patients were actively encouraged to monitor their own symptoms, adjust their medication according to symptom severity and understand the dangers of discontinuing treatment (Kelly, 1986; Probert, 1991).

Medical Treatments

The choice of medication to be administered will be determined by the acuteness of the episode, but the most common is 5 aminosalicylate (5 ASA) for mild exacerbation, with the addition of oral or intravenous steroids for a more acute episode.

Mild Exacerbation

- 5 ASA medication   – sulphasalazine (Salazopyrin)

- New 5 ASA   ┌─ olsalazine (Dipentum)
  preparations with   ─┤ mesalazine (Asacol)
  fewer side-effects   └─ slow-release mesalazine (Pentasol)

Acute Exacerbation

- Steroids   –   oral prednisolone
                      ↓
                 if unresponsive
                      ↓
                 intravenous administration
                      ↓
                 if unresponsive
                      ↓
                 add intravenous cyclosporin (Kamm, 1996)

→ Reduce steroids gradually over 2–4 weeks, to allow the body's natural steroids to return to a normal level.

→ Maintain remission with 5 ASA medication.

→ If relapses occur more than once a year → long-term 5 ASA advisable.

→ If frequent relapses → add azathioprine.

→ If relapses are frequent and severe → consider surgical intervention.

Treatment of Proctitis

● Suppositories   prednisolone ⎯⎡⎯ administered at bedtime for
   or enemas   mesalazine   ⎣⎯ optimum retention.

Patients require training by the nurse to administer rectal preparations, aiming for them to extend as far proximally as possible. In cases of severe proctitis causing excessive diarrhoea and rectal bleeding, enemas may not be retained, therefore oral or intravenous steroids may be necessary.

Patients often experience concerns about their medication, dosages and side-effects which may be answered by an experienced nurse in the hospital or community.

Nursing Care during Acute Exacerbation

If an acute exacerbation should fail to settle with oral medication and the patient becomes very unwell, he/she will require hospital admission in order to monitor his/her condition, treat the symptoms and stabilize the disease. Patients in this situation need complete rest and an empathetic approach to care, and are ideally nursed in a area of the ward affording privacy, quiet and access to the bathroom.

Fluid Replacement

Unrelenting diarrhoea experienced during an exacerbation with subsequent fluid and electrolyte loss will cause the patient to become dehydrated and will require intravenous replacement and monitoring of fluid balance. At the same time it is necessary also to monitor signs or symptoms of electrolyte imbalance, in particular hypokalaemia (observe for muscle weakness and cramps) and hypernatremia (tachycardia and pyrexia).

Anaemia

Prolonged bleeding may result in iron deficiency anaemia. Haemoglobin levels should therefore be assessed and blood or iron supplements administered if required.

Vital Signs

Temperature, pulse and blood pressure should be monitored closely for signs of colonic dilatation or perforation, as should the abdominal girth and abdominal tenderness.

Radiology

Daily abdominal X-ray results and patient management should be discussed as a team approach between the physician, surgeon, nurses, dietitian and pharmacist.

Nutrition

Although there have been associations between high sugar consumption and Crohn's disease (Nicholls, 1998), diet has not been proven to cause or cure IBD. Despite this, patients do report particular foods as aiding or exacerbating their symptoms and is an area about which they want advice (Cooke, 1991). Offending foods are, however, individual to the sufferer which therefore creates difficulty when proffering dietary guidelines.

Advice should generally pertain to that of a well-balanced diet, eliminating foods which the patient personally identifies as aggravating the situation and bearing in mind pointers such as that dairy products can worsen symptoms of diarrhoea. Constipation sufferers may benefit from increased fibre. Use of fibre which does not ferment, such as the proprietary product Celevac, might improve the embarrassing problem of flatulence. Patients who avoid foods to aid their symptoms may need assessment to ensure that their diet is adequate and balanced.

During an exacerbation of IBD patients can experience rapid and marked weight loss and malnutrition which can be psychologically distressing and add to their feelings of tiredness and disability.

Nutritional assessment by the nurse, dietitian or nutrition specialist nurse is essential in the patient's management, considering such aspects as body mass, weight loss, muscle strength, stamina and serum albumin levels. Dietary improvements should first be achieved within the patient's normal everyday foods, trying to ensure he/she has three meals per day with snacks such as cheese and crackers in between.

If this is not sufficient, supplements can be prescribed, worse cases perhaps requiring supplementary tube feeding. Only in severe malabsorption, or if bowel rest is needed, should intravenous nutrition be considered.

The roles of elemental or polymeric diets orally or nasogastrically are still being evaluated; they have been found to produce a similar effect to steroids when given to patients with Crohn's disease for 4 weeks, but can be unpleasant, expensive and often result in early relapse (Nicholls, 1998).

Complementary Therapy Treatments

Patients may seek complementary therapies such as acupuncture, hypnotism, reflexology and massage to relieve their symptoms or in the hope of initiating a cure. Although the benefits of these are unproven in actually treating IBD it is possible to recognize their positive effects in managing and reducing stress, which some blame as predisposing to or worsening a flare-up.

Previous studies suggest that psychological counselling and stress management help to reduce anxiety and improve quality of life (Milne et al., 1986; Smith et al., 1995). Encouraging patients to adopt a method of relaxation which could realistically be incorporated into their lifestyle may provide a coping mechanism for them and produce some feeling of control in the knowledge that they are doing something positive to help themselves and their disease symptoms.

Surgical Treatments

In an ideal situation the gastroenterologist and surgeon will adopt a team approach in collaborative care for the individual patient, additionally involving other multidisciplinary team members such as nurses, the stoma care specialist, dietitian, pharmacist, the GP and community staff.

When the individual's condition is closely monitored in this way, if and when surgical intervention becomes an issue, the patient is psychologically prepared with opportunities for discussion over a period of time. Thus he/she is well informed, aware of the possible surgical options available, has spoken with the stoma or pouch nurse specialist and has met a fellow patient who has him/herself experienced such an operation and can offer a personal account.

An individual's reaction to surgery cannot be predicted. Some fear having to live with a stoma and therefore try to avoid an operation at all costs, whereas others actively welcome any intervention that will provide a cure and give them back control of their lives.

When patients have lived with distressing, debilitating symptoms for months or years, surgery involving stoma or pouch formation is understandably easier to accept than for those who develop a sudden, acute onset of IBD necessitating immediate surgery. These patients require enormous support post-operatively, often finding it difficult to comprehend having required something so radical and mutilating.

Surgery for Ulcerative Colitis

There are four situations which may lead to the decision to operate, the most common being failure of the disease and its symptoms to respond to medical treatment, with long-term use of steroids not being without possible serious side-effects. Other predisposing factors would be detection of dysplasia, i.e. malignant changes within the bowel. Extra-intestinal manifestations are described in Figure 6.4 for which, with the exception of sclerosing cholangitis, surgery is generally of benefit. An operation may prevent growth retardation in children and see adolescents through the 'normal' developments of puberty.

For the majority of patients the operation will be elective, therefore as previously discussed it is hoped they will feel psychologically prepared. However, a choice of surgical procedures may be available, and the patient will require as much information as possible to enable him/her to come to an informed decision.

Total Colectomy

A total colectomy with formation of an ileostomy and preservation of the rectal stump remains a popular choice in that it enables the individual to regain health and strength before deciding whether to go ahead with further restorative surgery, whilst giving time to see how he/she copes with and adapts to living with a stoma.

For patients in whom a definitive diagnosis between ulcerative colitis and Crohn's disease has been indeterminate, further opportunity

Surgical treatments for ulcerative colitis

1.	Total colectomy with ileostomy formation and preservation of rectal stump
2.	Total colectomy with ileorectal anastomosis
3.	Pan-proctocolectomy with formation of permanent ileostomy
4.	Kock pouch formation
5.	Restorative proctocolectomy with formation of ileoanal reservoir

Figure 6.8: Surgical intervention options for ulcerative colitis.

for histological investigation is also permitted. For those who require emergency surgery during an acute exacerbation this procedure is the one of choice, with the surgeon either suturing or stapling the remaining rectum or, if friable, bringing it to the skin surface as a mucous fistula (Nicholls, 1998).

Total Colectomy with Ileorectal Anastomosis

In previous years removal of the whole colon with direct ileorectal anastomosis was commonplace. However, this often resulted in frequency of loose bowel movements, with the patient having lost the capacity to store faeces and with the additional risk of recurrent colitis or cancer developing in the residual rectum. It is recommended therefore that such patients undergo annual screening and biopsy.

For children and adolescents this procedure may provide disease-free years prior to decisions regarding further surgery once they reach adulthood.

Pan-proctocolectomy and Permanent Ileostomy

Patients whose rectum and/or anus are badly affected may require removal of these together with their whole colon, thus resulting in a permanent ileostomy. Despite the radical and final nature of this procedure, it offers the patient a guaranteed cure from ulcerative colitis with no future concerns about developing colorectal cancer and is welcomed by some who wish to be free of frequent hospital visits and further surgery, involving time away from work and their families.

Although continual advances in the development of stoma appliances have addressed many of the problems previously experienced by ostomists, such as skin soreness, leakage and odour, patients may take some time or have difficulty in coping with the change in their body image and function. They and their partner will require empathetic support and education from the nursing staff and stoma care specialist during this period of adjustment, including follow-up contact on their return to the community (Porrett and Joels, 1996).

It is important also that the possibility of nerve damage, which may cause sexual dysfunction following rectal excision, is discussed with the individual preoperatively. The perineal wound can be uncomfortable and troublesome to the patient, often taking weeks or even months to heal (Nicholls, 1996) and additionally there is no guarantee that the ileostomy will itself not produce problems such as obstruction, retraction or parastomal herniation.

Age may help to select the nature of surgery with pan-proctocolectomy favoured by some surgeons for older patients with ulcerative colitis.

Kock Pouch

For patients who have had their anus removed and do not adapt to having an ileostomy, a kock continent pouch may be an option offered by some consultants.

This involves formation of an internal reservoir using terminal ileum and construction of a nipple valve which is tunnelled through the abdominal wall to the skin surface, resembling in appearance a tiny 'umbilical size' stoma through which the patient passes a Madena catheter in order to drain the faeces. However, many patients experience prolapse of the nipple valve which necessitates refashioning, and this procedure has been largely surgically superseded by the restorative proctocolectomy/ileoanal pouch.

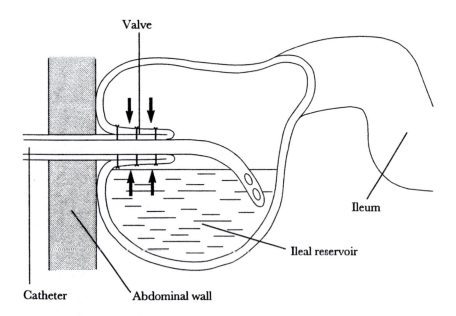

Fugure 6.9: Diagrammatic representation of a kock pouch.

Restorative Proctocolectomy

Restorative proctocolectomy was first described in 1986 by Sir Alan Parks as a sphincter-preserving operation and a means for patients to avoid a permanent ileostomy. Patients with ulcerative colitis may be suitable candidates for a pouch. Those with Crohn's are not, because of the risk of recurrent disease in the pouch lining.

The anus must be free from disease and tests are carried out which may include manometry, to ensure the sphincter muscle is adequate for continence.

When told about this operation patients may initially perceive it as an answer to their prayers, but it does have its share of potential problems. It is important that anyone considering pouch surgery has a realistic view and is made aware of the possible complications. The patient needs also to be motivated and psychologically prepared to cope with what are often difficult initial months following surgery.

Many surgeons perform this operation in two stages. The initial and major procedure involves excision of the colon and rectum to the anorectal junction, and an internal reservoir is constructed from loops of small bowel shaped into the form of an 'S', 'J' or 'W' thus providing some capacity to retain faeces. The base of the pouch is then hand sutured or stapled as an ileoanal anastomosis.

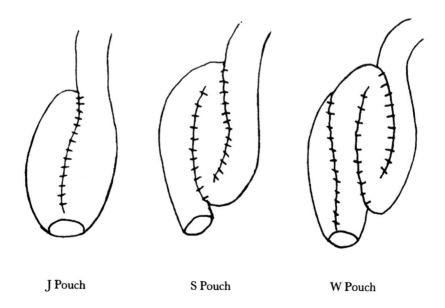

J Pouch   S Pouch   W Pouch

Figure 6.10: Diagrammatic representation of ileoanal pouch constructions.

A temporary loop ileostomy is generally fashioned to reduce the incidence of pelvic sepsis, and to allow time for pouch expansion and for the patient to recover prior to its activation. Reversal of the stoma takes place after approximately 8 weeks.

Output from the ileostomy is often quite excessive, so monitoring of fluid balance is essential, with administration of intravenous or oral electrolyte solution as necessary. Patients may also require medication to reduce bowel mobility, such as loperamide, which should be taken prior to meals.

Owing to the corrosive and irritant nature of the small bowel fluid it is essential that the patient has a well-fitting stoma appliance and is educated regarding care of the peristomal skin.

Informing patients beforehand of the estimated duration of their hospitalization will allow them to make personal and work arrangements. The first stay is likely to be 10–14 days, and for the reversal operation 5–7 days.

If patients are fully aware of what they can expect after their pouch is connected, unnecessary worry and panic situations can be avoided. They may initially be emptying the pouch 12–15 times per day and often experience soiling during sleep, when the sphincter muscles are relaxed. Dehydration and electrolyte imbalance can occur if loss is excessive and patients should therefore be aware of indicative symptoms, such as thirst, tiredness, lethargy and cramps, particularly in the limbs. This aspect will be monitored by the pouch or stoma care nurse specialist and electrolyte fluid or supplements recommended as necessary. It is also quite usual for patients to require loperamide or codeine phosphate medication during the initial postoperative weeks.

General dietary tips and guidelines are also useful, recommending foods that will reduce or thicken the output and avoiding those that may cause wind.

Passage of frequent loose stools will cause anal irritation and soreness. The patient should be advised that keeping the area clean by frequent douching using a bidet or shower and patting gently dry will help. This can be followed with sparing application of a barrier cream, or if the area is unbroken a peristomal protective wipe will act as a second skin.

Even a year after surgery bowel movements will average 3–6 a day and the efflux will continue to be loose. As patients report being unable to differentiate between faeces and flatus, frequent trips to the bathroom may be necessary!

The decision whether to have pouch surgery must rest with the individual once he/she has received information and counselling from the consultant and pouch or stoma care nurse.

In the UK, patient self-help groups have developed which can provide much needed mutual support and opportunity to learn from each other.

The patient should be aware of possible complications that can occur, perhaps resulting in pouch failure, such as pelvic sepsis due to anstomotic breakdown, poor pouch function and inflammation known as 'pouchitis' which has similar presenting symptoms to those of colitis.

Despite this, many find pouch formation gives them a feeling of 'normality' and after perhaps having lived with IBD for a number of years, will view five bowel actions a day as quite acceptable.

Surgery for Crohn's Disease

Unlike ulcerative colitis, surgery for Crohn's disease can never offer the patient a cure and is reserved primarily for complications of the disease such as enterocutaneous fistulae, which may require excision of the affected section of bowel, abscess which cannot be locally drained, intestinal obstruction, malignant changes or a failure of the disease to respond to medication.

Because of the danger of future recurrent disease necessitating further surgery and loss of precious bowel, resections tend to be conservative and limited to the affected segment. Patients who have a short bowel are likely to experience excessive diarrhoea with subsequent poor absorption, electrolyte imbalance and nutritional deficiency.

It should be noted that as the terminal ileum is responsible for absorption of vitamin B12, if this is removed patients will require 3-monthly injections of B12 for life in order to avoid development of megablastic anaemia.

Dependent upon the Crohn's site and extent, surgery may or may not involve stoma formation, although permanent colostomy may be necessary if the rectum or anus is badly affected and excision is necessary.

Conclusion

This chapter has presented an overview of inflammatory bowel disease and its current treatments, but more significantly for nurses has explored the physical, psychological and social implications for the individual and his/her family.

Effective communication and a multidisciplinary approach to care are essential, each member of the team contributing his/her own valuable skills. One may conclude that members of the nursing profession are ideally placed to play a key role in the coordination of this care.

Patients' needs for information and support have been identified and discussed, including an opportunity to talk, to be listened to sensitively and to receive education about the illness and its treatments, including information about medication and the possible side-effects.

Such self-empowerment and improvement within the patient/professional relationship can only lead to increased treatment compliance and enhance the patient's ability to cope.

References

Brian H, Ferguson A (1993a) Inflammatory bowel disease. Practice Nursing 15 June: 11–12.

Brian H, Ferguson A (1993b) Nursing needs in inflammatory bowel disease. Practice Nursing 20 June: 10.

Cooke DM (1991) Inflammatory bowel disease – primary health care management. Nurse Practitioner 16(8): 27–39.

Jewell DP, Chapman RGW, Mortensen N (1992) Ulcerative Colitis and Crohn's Disease – a Clinicians Guide. Edinburgh: Churchill Livingstone.

Joachim G, Milne B (1985) The effects of inflammatory bowel disease on lifestyle. Canadian Nurse 81(10): 38, 40.

Kamm MA (1996) Inflammatory Bowel Disease. London: Martin Dunitz.

Kelly M (1986) The subjective experience of chronic disease: some implications for the management of ulcerative colitis. Journal of Chronic Disease 39(8): 653–66.

Mayberry MK, Mayberry JF (1993) Practice nurses and chronic diseases of the gastrointestinal tract. British Journal of Nursing 2(3): 176–8.

Milne B, Joachim G, Niedhardt MD (1986) A stress management programme for inflammatory bowel disease patients. Journal of Advanced Nursing 11: 561–7.

Moody GA, Probert CSJ, Jayanthi V, Mayberry JF (1992) The attitude of employers to people with inflammatory bowel disease. Social Science and Medicine 34(4): 459–60.

Nicholls JR (1996) Chapter 6. In Myers C Stoma Care Nursing – a Patient Centred Approach. London: Edward Arnold, pp 90–122.

Nicholls, JR (1998) Chapter 8. In Phillips RKS Colorectal Surgery: A Companion to Specialist Surgical Practice. Philadelphia: WB Saunders, pp 141–78.

Porrett T, Joels J (1996) Chapter 18. In Myers C Stoma Care Nursing – a Patient Centred Approach. London: Edward Arnold, pp 283–94.

Probert CSJ (1991) Inflammatory bowel disease: patients' expectations in the 1990s. Journal of the Royal Society of Medicine 84(March): 131–2.

Pullan R (1996) Colonic mucus, smoking and ulcerative colitis. Annals of the Royal College of Surgeons of England 78: 85–91.

Pullen M (1997) Understanding ulcerative colitis. Practice Nursing 8(4): 24–7.

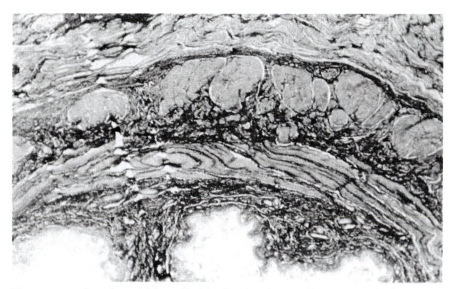

Transverse section of part of the wall of the foetal anal canal. The anal cushions are well developed. Deep to the submucosa lie the internal sphincter, the longitudinal muscle of the anal canal (more prominent in the foetus than adult) and the external anal sphincter. See page 78.

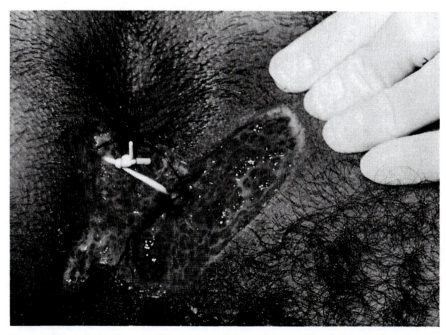

Trans-sphincteric fistulae with intersphincteric horseshoe and high ischiorectal extension. See page 88.

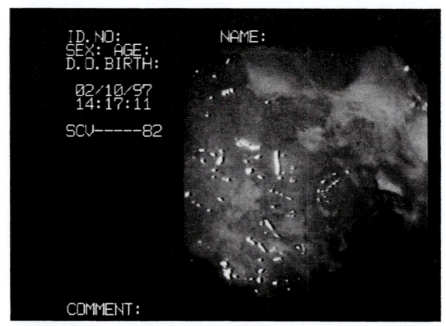

Ulcerative colitis. See page 121.

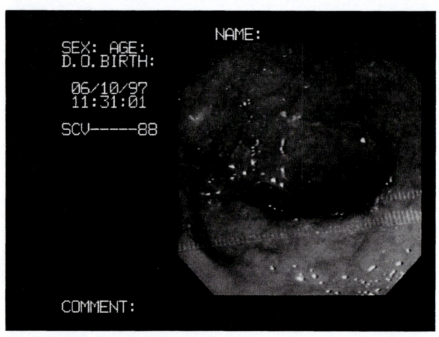

View of normal bowel mucosa. See page 121.

Scholmerich J, Sedlak P, Hoppe-Seyler P, Gerok W (1987) The information needs and fears of patients with inflammatory bowel disease. Hepato-gastroenterology 34:182–5.

Smith GD, Rogers D, Palmer KR (1995) Psychological morbidity in inflammatory bowel disease: a case for psychological counselling? Gut 36(4): April F268 (abstract from British Society of Gastroenterology spring meeting: BMJ publication).

Thompson NP (1995) Is measles a risk for inflammatory bowel disease? Lancet 345: 1071–3.

Useful Addresses

British Colostomy Association
15 Station Road
Reading
Berks RG1 1LG
UK
Tel: 01734 391537

British Digestive Foundation
3 St Andrew's Place
London NW1 4LB
UK

Ileostomy and Internal Pouch Support Group
Amblehurst House
PO Box. 23
Mansfield
Nottingham NG18 4TT
UK
Tel: 01623 28099

NACC
4 Beaumont House
Sutton Road
St Albans
Herts AL1 5HH
UK
Tel: 01727 844296

RADAR
25 Mortimer Street
London WIN 8AB
UK
Tel: 0171 637 5400

SPOD
The Association to Aid the Sexual and Personal Relationships of People with a Disability
286 Camden Road
London N7 0BJ
UK
Tel: 0171 607 8851

Chapter 7
Familial Adenomatous Polyposis

JUAN J. NOGUERAS MD, FACS, FASCRS, Head of Inherited Diseases Registry, Department of Colorectal Surgery, Cleveland Clinic Florida, Florida, USA

ELLEN McGANNON BSW, The David G Jagelman Inherited Colorectal Cancer Registries, Cleveland Clinic Foundation, Cleveland, Ohio, USA

Familial adenomatous polyposis (FAP) is an autosomal dominant disease characterized by multiple adenomatous polyps of the colon (Figure 7.1) and a variety of extracolonic manifestations. This condition was originally known as familial polyposis coli, but as awareness increased of a high incidence of adenomas arising in areas other than the colon, the name was changed to familial adenomatous polyposis. The estimated incidence of FAP ranges from 1 in 8000 to 1 in 29 000 births (Jagelman, 1990). The majority of cases are inherited, but up to 22% of patients with FAP have no retrievable family history, and are presumed to be spontaneous mutations (Rustin et al., 1990).

The last decade has seen dramatic advancements in our understanding of the molecular biology of this disease. The APC (adenomatous polyposis coli) gene is located on the long arm of chromosome 5 at 5q21–q22. Mutations of the APC gene account for the condition of FAP in addition to some cases of sporadic colorectal cancer (Nishisho et al., 1991). To date, over 250 different mutations have been identified, the majority of which occur in the 5' portion of the APC gene. These mutations are classified as point or frameshift mutations, and often result in a truncated protein. Recent research has focused on the phenotypic expressions of these various mutations (Nugent et al., 1994)

Historical Perspective

In 1882 Cripps reported the case of two family members with colonic polyposis, differentiating them from the polyposis seen in inflammatory bowel disease (Cripps, 1882). Handford (1890) described the adenoma to adenocarcinoma transition in a patient with polyposis. The disease was subsequently recognized as a genetic disorder, and the first FAP registry was established by Bussey and Lockhart-Mummery at St Mark's Hospital in London. The data accrued from long term follow-up of these families yielded valuable information on the disease process, and established the importance of organized registries (Dukes, 1952). In the past 20 years, numerous registries dedicated to FAP have flourished, including the Cleveland Clinic Familial Adenomatous Polyposis Registry, established by Dr David Jagelman in 1979.

In 1951, Gardner described a family with FAP with osteomas of the skull and mandible and multiple epidermoid cysts (Gardner, 1951). As he followed this family, other features developed, including supernumerary and impacted teeth, dentigerous cysts, and desmoid tumors of the abdomen (Gardner, 1969). Thereafter, this cluster of pathology was referred to as Gardner's syndrome. In 1959, Turcot described two cases of malignant CNS tumours in children with FAP, and this association became recognized as Turcot syndrome (Turcot et al., 1959). We now recognize that these conditions do not represent separate disease processes, but instead are different manifestations of the many extracolonic neoplasms associated with FAP.

The list of extracolonic manifestations is ever-expanding, and both benign and malignant lesions have been recognized (Table 7.1) (Jagelman, 1988).

Table 7.1: Benign and malignant extracolonic manifestations

Benign	Malignant
Endocrine adenoma	Duodenal carcinoma
Osteoma	Bile duct carcinoma
Epidermoid cyst	Pancreatic carcinoma
Hypertrophic retinal pigmentation	Desmoid tumour
Gastric fundic gland polyp	Carcinoma of the stomach
Duodenal adenoma	Adrenal carcinoma
Small bowel adenoma	Medulloblastoma
	Glioblastoma
	Thyroid carcinoma
	Small bowel carcinoma
	Carcinoid tumour of the ileum
	Osteogenic sarcoma
	Hepatoblastoma

Benign Extracolonic Manifestations

Osteoma

Osteomas in patients with FAP can be present in any bone; however, they occur more frequently in the jaw and skull bones. The osteomas are almost always benign, but there is one report of a family in which two members developed osteogenic sarcomas. Some of the jaw osteomas are non-palpable and can be detected only on radiographic examination. Utsunomiya demonstrated a high incidence of asymptomatic micro-osteomata in the mandibles of FAP patients who underwent screening Panorex X-ray examination (Utsunomiya and Nakamura, 1975). Because of the lack of specificity of these lesions for FAP, this radiographic test has not been useful as a screening modality for the disease.

Epidermoid Cysts

These cutaneous lesions are usually small, scattered throughout the body, and may be seen early in life in children with FAP. Leppard confirmed the histology of these lesions as epidermoid cysts (Leppard, 1974). They may precede the development of colonic polyps in some children, and thus may be helpful as a clinical marker of FAP.

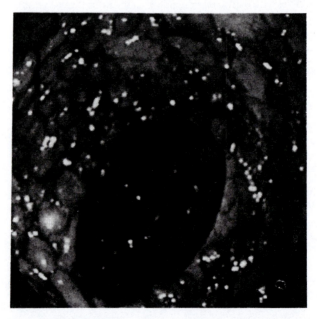

Figure 7.1: Typical colonoscopic appearance of multiple colonic polyps in patients with FAP.

Hypertrophic Retinal Pigmentation

Congenital hypertrophy of the retinal pigmented epithelium (CHRPE) is a manifestation of FAP which may be detected at an early age, even as young as 3 months (Jagelman, 1988). These lesions are detected with a dilated fundus examination by an experienced ophthalmic examiner. Pigmented retinal lesions are seen in the normal population, and are usually isolated, unilateral and flat. In the FAP patient population, specific criteria for defining a pigmented lesion as positive for CHRPE include a critical number of at least four pigmented lesions, with a bilateral distribution (Heyen et al., 1990). Using this criterion as a definition, CHRPE is found in 65% of families with FAP. When present in a family, it is found in all affected members within the family. Therefore, in kindred with the trait for CHRPE, a positive eye examination is predictive for the diagnosis of FAP. Because these lesions are present at an early age, the eye examination may help to confirm a diagnosis even before the onset of colonic polyps. Wide-angle survey fundus photography is useful to document precisely the number and location of these pigmented lesions. Because up to 34% of families do not carry the trait for CHRPE, ophthalmic examination cannot replace proctoscopic examination as a general screening tool for the entire population at risk.

Endocrine Adenomas

Adenomas of the adrenal, pituitary and parathyroid glands have been discovered as incidental findings in patients with FAP. Most of these adenomas are non-secreting and asymptomatic (Naylor and Gardner, 1981). The exact incidence of these lesions in the FAP population is unknown because the patients are asymptomatic and not generally screened for these lesions. There is a report of an adenocarcinoma of the adrenal gland in a 27-year-old woman with FAP (Painter and Jagelman, 1985).

Gastric and Duodenal Polyps

Gastric polyps in patients with FAP are usually fundic gland polyps with little premalignant potential (Figure 7.2) (Watanabe et al., 1978). Only a small percentage of gastric polyps are adenomatous, in contrast with duodenal polyps, which are typically adenomatous (Sarre et al., 1987a). The incidence of gastric cancer in patients with FAP differs between the western and eastern hemispheres. A survey of separate western hemisphere registries yielded a 0.6% incidence of gastric

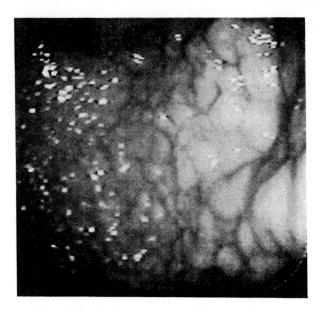

Figure 7.2: Fundic gland polyps seen during oesophagogastroduodenoscopy in FAP patients.

cancer compared with a 2.1% incidence reported by the Japanese Polyposis Center and a 4.2% incidence reported by the Korean Polyposis Registry (Jagelman, 1988; Utsunomiya et al., 1990; Park et al., 1992). This phenomenon may in part be due to the overall higher incidence of gastric adenomas in the general oriental population as compared with western countries, a fact which may reflect environmental, dietary or genetic factors.

The use of a side-viewing duodenoscope facilitates the inspection of the periampullary region, and increases the yield of positive examinations. Church et al. demonstrated an 88% prevalence of duodenal adenomas in FAP patients (Church et al., 1992). Moreover, endoscopically normal periampullary tissue revealed micro-adenomata in 50% of cases. The authors discuss the potential carcinogenic effect of bile on a genetically primed mucosa as a possible explanation for these observations. These genetic steps are still ill-defined, but recent data suggests that somatic APC mutations are uncommon, whereas K-*ras* mutations are relatively common during the adenoma-to-carcinoma sequence of periampullary tumorigenesis (Gallinger et al., 1995). Recent data suggest that this tumorigenic effect of bile on the duodenal mucosa may be pH sensitive, favouring a lower pH for adenoma formation, thereby suggesting a possible role for antacids as prophylactic treatment (Scates et al., 1995). Further work is necessary in this important area.

Malignant Extracolonic Manifestations

Arvanitis et al. examined the mortality records of 132 patients with a documented diagnosis of FAP utilizing data from the Cleveland Clinic Foundation FAP Registry (Arvanitis et al., 1990). The exact cause of death was not confirmed in 22 patients, but in the remaining 110 patients the cause of death was as follows: metastatic colorectal carcinoma 64 patients (58.2%), desmoid tumours 12 patients (10.9%), periampullary carcinoma 9 patients (8.2%), brain tumours 8 patients (7.3%), perioperative mortalities 5 patients (4.5%), adrenal carcinoma 1 patient (0.9%), and abdominal carcinomatosis 1 patient (0.9%). Ten patients died of causes not related to FAP. Of the 33 patients in the study who underwent prophylactic colectomy, the leading causes of death were desmoid tumours and periampullary malignancy.

In order to assess the long-term survival of patients with FAP following colectomy, Nugent et al. identified 222 patients who underwent total colectomy and ileorectal anastomosis at St Mark's Hospital in London (Nugent et al., 1993). Using life-table analysis, the FAP patients were compared with an age- and sex-matched group of the general population. The causes of death were identified and an odds ratio calculation determined the relative risk of dying compared with the general population. Of 222 patients, 53 deaths occurred during the follow-up period compared with 15.8 expected deaths. Therefore, the overall odds ratio calculation of the relative risk of dying for FAP patients following colectomy is 3.35. The causes of death in these 53 patients were: duodenal carcinoma 11 patients (21%), metastases unknown primary 8 (15%), rectal carcinoma 5 (9%), desmoids 5 (9%), perioperative complication 5 (9%). The overall survival of this group of patients was higher than the original St Mark's population of FAP patients who had neither screening nor prophylactic surgery, but the survival remains lower than the general non-FAP population by a greater than threefold factor.

Iwama et al. reported data from the Research Center for Polyposis and Intestinal Diseases in Tokyo, Japan on 1050 FAP patients (Iwama et al., 1993). Among all the patients, there were 11 cases of thyroid carcinoma (mean age 32.5 yrs), 23 cases of duodenal, periampullary, or small bowel carcinoma (mean age 43.7 yrs), 27 cases of gastric carcinoma (mean age 49.2 yrs) , and 71 desmoid tumours (mean age 32.2 yrs). The age of onset of thyroid carcinoma was statistically significantly younger when compared with onset of gastric and duodenal/small intestine carcinoma, but did not differ from desmoid tumours. The mortality/morbidity ratio was 0 for thyroid carcinoma,

0.11 for desmoid tumours, 0.48 for duodenal or small intestinal carcinoma, 0.44 for gastric carcinoma, and 0.66 for colorectal carcinoma.

Desmoids

Desmoid tumours arise from the musculoaponeurotic mesenchymal soft tissue and are composed of mature fibroblasts (Posner et al., 1989). They are locally invasive, non-metastasizing tumours relatively common in FAP when compared with the general population (Jones et al., 1986). The incidence of desmoid tumours in patients with FAP has been calculated to be approximately 8.9%, with a 3:1 female predominance (Tsukada et al., 1991). The patients with desmoids are relatively young (mean age 29.8 years), and in the majority of cases (86%) the desmoid tumours appear after colectomy (Figure 7.3). The majority of desmoid tumours in FAP patients are intra-abdominal mesenteric tumours, ususally large, and closely situated to vital mesenteric vessels, thereby precluding surgical resection (Figure 7.4).

Radiotherapy, which has had limited success in extra-abdominal desmoid tumours, has not achieved consistent results against intra-abdominal desmoid tumours in patients with FAP (Kitamura et al., 1991). Cytotoxic chemotherapy has produced some success, but reports are sporadic, anecdotal and lacking in adequate numbers for

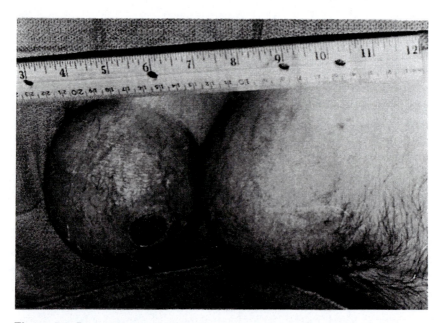

Figure 7.3: Desmoid tumours of the abdominal wall occurring at site of midline incision and parastomal location.

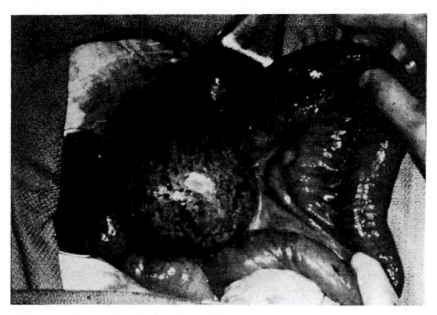

Figure 7.4: Desmoid tumour of the small bowel mesentery.

meaningful analysis (Kitamura et al., 1991; Lynch et al., 1994). Hormonal therapy is based on the observation that desmoid tumours are more common in women and are enlarged with pregnancy or oral contraceptives (McAdam and Goligher, 1970). Cytosolic receptors for oestradiol are present in 33–75% of desmoid tumours in FAP (Lim et al., 1986; Reitamo et al., 1986). *In vitro* studies of desmoid tumour cell cultures revealed a stimulatory effect of 17 ß-E2 on desmoid cell growth and collagen production in those FAP patients with positive oestrogen receptors in desmoid cells (Tonelli et al., 1994). Therapy with the anti-oestrogen agent tamoxifen has yielded some encouraging results, but reports are sporadic and limited in number (Kinzbrunner et al., 1983; Waddell et al., 1983). Non-steroidal anti-inflammatory drugs, such as sulindac, have yielded unexpected diminution of desmoid tumors, stimulating the establishment of ongoing clinical trials with this agent (Tsukada et al., 1992) A number of studies are currently under way evaluating each of these modalities alone and in combination for the optimal management of desmoid tumours in FAP patients.

Periampullary Carcinoma

Periampullary carcinoma represents the second most frequently diagnosed malignancy in FAP patients following colorectal carcinoma.

Periampullary carcinoma occurs in 2–3% of patients with FAP compared with the frequency of 0.02–0.05% observed in the general population (Jagelman et al., 1988). This represents a near hundredfold increase in risk. No significant risk has been found for gastric or non-duodenal small intestinal cancer in the western hemisphere.

The goal of an active surveillance programme is the prevention of malignant degeneration, and appropriate ablation of premalignant lesions. It is now recognized that prophylactic restorative proctocolectomy effectively eliminates the risk of colorectal carcinoma, and that periampullary malignancy represents a significant cause of death in these patients. Moreover, we do not have adequate information regarding the natural history and risk profile of periampullary cancer. Therefore, active screening of the periampullary region should be a part of the routine screening of these patients. There is still no data from large centres documenting a decrease in mortality from periampullary malignancy as a result of an active screening programme, but utilizing the adenoma-to-carcinoma sequence as our rationale, it is logical to pursue aggressive screening. We recommend UGI endoscopy with a side-viewing duodenoscopy every 1 to 5 years, depending on previous number of lesions, size, location and histology. Small duodenal lesions are removed endoscopically, random biopsies of endoscopically normal appearing periampullary mucosa are obtained, and large lesions are removed surgically. Pancreaticoduodenectomy is the preferred method for managing invasive cancers.

Other Malignancies

A variety of other malignancies have been reported in association with FAP (see Table 7.1), reflecting the generalized growth disorder of this condition. The true incidence of these other malignancies is not yet well defined.

Surgical Options

Once the diagnosis of FAP is established by the demonstration of multiple adenomatous polyps of the colon and the rectum, the timing of colectomy needs to be addressed. There are no hard-and-fast rules as to an optimal time for surgery other than the realization that it is a prophylactic colectomy for the prevention of colorectal cancer, therefore unnecessary delays are to be avoided. There are four surgical options: total proctocolectomy (TPC) with ileostomy, TPC with continent ileostomy, total abdominal colectomy (TAC) with ileorectal anastomosis (IRA), and restorative proctocolectomy (RPC) with ileoanal pouch (IAP).

TPC with ileostomy was the traditional surgical option, but it has been replaced by restorative procedures. Today, the primary indication for a TPC with ileostomy is a patient with a cancer of the lower third of the rectum or a failed sphincter-sparing operation.

Continent ileostomy is an appropriate choice for those patients with failed IAP, or those patients who desire conversion of a Brooke ileostomy after TPC. The advent of ileoanal pouch surgery has replaced continent ileostomies as a primary procedure in the majority of cases.

TAC with IRA is an acceptable option for young patients with few rectal polyps (Jagelman, 1991). There is no pelvic dissection, therefore there is no risk of autonomic nerve (sexual) dysfunction. The functional results are acceptable. The patient must be motivated and committed to close surveillance of the rectal segment because of the ever-present risk of rectal carcinoma. Overall, the risk of rectal carcinoma is relatively low. Bussey reported the St Mark's Hospital experience and found a cumulative risk of rectal cancer of 3.6% after 25 years (Bussey, 1975). The mortality from rectal cancer in this series was 0. This parallels the experience at the Cleveland Clinic in which 133 patients were evaluated (Sarre et al., 1987b). A total of 10 patients developed rectal cancer, and only 1 died of this complication. The actuarial survival free of rectal cancer was 88% at 20 years. Interestingly, more patients died of periampullary cancer than of rectal cancer in this series.

The final option of RPC with IAP is our preferred approach for the majority of patients. This operation offers the advantages of eradication of all disease at risk with acceptable functional results when performed by an experienced surgical team. The disadvantage of this option is the need for a pelvic dissection with all its attendant risks, the use of temporary diversion with loop ileostomy in many centres requiring a second operation for establishment of intestinal continuity, and the small risk of pouch-related complications, such as pouchitis.

Genotype–phenotype

The APC gene responsible for FAP has been identified, cloned, and more recently mapped in terms of different mutations. Attempts are under way to correlate the phenotypic expression of the disease, in terms of disease severity and extra-colonic manifestations, and the location of the mutations. Caspari et al. have summarized some of the recent work in this field, including their own research (Caspari et al., 1995). In patients with a mutation of a 5 base pair deletion at codon 1309, gastrointestinal (GI) symptoms and death from colorectal cancer appear 10 years earlier than in patients without this mutation. Conversely, mutations near the 5' end result in an attenuated form of the disease with relatively few polyps and later onset of symptoms. Mutations before exon 9 do not seem to produce CHRPE, whereas mutations from exon 9 up to codon 1387 seem to create ophthalmic lesions. Patients with mutations between codon 1445 and 1578 tend to have severe desmoids and no CHRPE.

Clearly, these correlations are but the tip of the iceberg. As our understanding of the molecular genetics of this disease broadens, so will our ability to predict for each patient which manifestation of the disease they are more likely to develop. Then, targeted surveillance programmes can be established, and perhaps prophylactic therapies will be improved.

Familial Adenomatous Polyposis Registries

Familial adenomatous polyposis is a family disease, affecting not only the patient and offspring, but potentially a large extended family as well as those family members not suffering from the disease. The foundation of family care in FAP is a complete family history that shows age of onset of polyps, colorectal cancer, other cancers, and extra-colonic manifestations. Most physicians are unable to devote time to collecting a complete family history documented by medical records to form the basis for estimates of individual risk and surveillance protocols. An FAP registry can perform these functions as well as coordinating patient care, providing education and facilitating research.

What is a Polyposis Registry?

It is an official record or list which follows patients and families with other inherited syndromes of colorectal cancer, such as hereditary non-polyposis colorectal cancer (HNPCC), juvenile polyposis, and Peutz-Jehger's syndrome. Registries vary in their orientation and the services they provide. Currently, there are 62 FAP registries representing 25 countries throughout the world. The first was established in London, at St Mark's Hospital, in 1925 and is an example of a registry in a major medical centre. Elsewhere in the United Kingdom, regional registries have been established where there is a uniform health care system with specialists who can provide direct patient care and the families are contained within a defined region. National registries are typical of smaller countries such as Sweden, Denmark and Holland where data collection is standardized, avoiding duplication of effort in tracing families. In North America registries tend to develop around a physician or team of physicians who work in a tertiary referral medical centre and who have a special interest in FAP and hereditary colorectal cancer syndromes. Patients may be referred because of the surgeon's technical ability or the unique services that the institution can offer. In this way, families are accumulated and a patient base is built. Patients may come from all over the country and make annual 'pilgrimages' to the registry for surveillance. An example of such a registry is at the Cleveland Clinic Foundation. Begun in 1979 by Dr David G. Jagelman, it has accumulated nearly 400 FAP families, and registers hereditary non-polyposis colorectal cancer (HNPCC), familial colorectal cancer, juvenile polyposis and Peutz-Jehger's families. The registry united with the Department of Medical Genetics in 1997.

Registry Team

A registry is an integrated team of physicians, nurses, geneticists, genetic counsellors, mental health professionals and data managers. The registry coordinator is the key person in this team, serving as a link between patients, their families and the registry. Over time a trusting relationship between coordinator and family develops. Duties of a coordinator include documenting and interviewing relatives to complete the family history; educating them about the disease, tests, surgical options and lifelong surveillance protocols; encouraging participation in study protocols; discussing issues regarding genetic testing; support over fear of tests and surgery; consulting over insurance issues, loss of employment or death of a loved one.

Role of a Registry

The main role of an inherited colorectal cancer registry is to prevent death from colorectal cancer. This is carried out by promoting knowledge of the risks and implications of a family history of colorectal cancer, by providing the best care to patients and families and by conducting important research.

Patient Care

Patient Identification

Every FAP patient and his/her family deserves to be included in a registry. However, in practice this is much harder to realize than in theory as 22% of newly diagnosed cases of FAP represent new mutations, the first family member to have this condition. Other factors confusing the pattern of inheritance include adoption and non-paternity. Break-up of families can make the business of supervising care more difficult. Patients may only know that a parent or immediate family members had colon cancer, diagnosed at a young age, and not know the hereditary aspects and ramifications of this condition.

Referrals to Registry

Patients are referred to the registry in many ways: by a gastroenterologist who is performing a colonoscopy or a surgeon who has removed a colon; by primary care physicians and nurses; by enterostomal therapists; by patients themselves, who have become more educated consumers. They may research the diagnosis on the Internet, through cancer and hereditary resource networks, the library or word of mouth. It is important to note that patients referred to the FAP registry are still under the care of their referring doctor. Registries do not want to assume care for their patients. Their role is an adjunctive one.

Pedigree Construction

The first step on referral to a registry is construction and documentation of the family history. This process begins with the registry coordinator meeting with the patient and family to record and document the family history. A complete family pedigree is begun and a family history questionnaire may be taken home to complete. This is an ongoing process as a family pedigree is always changing and is therefore never complete.

Consent for Participation

In the USA informed consent is obtained, and this involves confidentiality issues, the ability to contact other family members and the process of obtaining outside medical records. Prior to enrolment in the registry all patients and family members are asked to sign a consent to participation. Participation in the registry is voluntary. The registry coordinator will review the consent and answer any questions. The consent form should include: information on benefits, risks, treatment options; contact registry staff names and phone numbers; and costs. Specific items can include a request for a blood sample for banking and future research; confidentiality of records; discussion of screening and identification; and possible diagnosis and treatment.

Data Collection

Demographic and medical information about affected family members is necessary to document familial polyposis and other related conditions. Diagnostic and pathology reports, operative notes, and documentation of extra-colonic manifestations are collected for patients and family members. This documentation may be obtained from hospitals, physicians' offices and death certificates, and will confirm affected and at-risk status in a family enabling accurate evaluation of risk-screening recommendations. All data are entered into a database by data managers.

Genetic Testing

Patients who are interested in genetic testing can be referred to a clinical genetics or risk assessment programme. In the USA, through an Institutional Review Board (IRB) approved clinical programme a patient's appropriateness for testing is determined by a team of geneticists, genetic counsellors, physicians, nurses and mental health professionals. Genetic testing can be performed within the institution or referred to an outside laboratory. Results of the test are presented to the patient within the clinical programme by the geneticist and genetic counsellor and FAP physician who will provide a report of the results and risks, including preventive and screening recommendations.

Confidentiality

All registry data and genetic information including test results are maintained and kept in secured files within the registry.

Coordinating Medical Care

Patients with FAP may require multiple tests, treatments, minor surgical interventions and have appointments with multiple physicians for their surveillance examinations. Patients may have special needs when making their appointment. Patients who live out of state or at a distance from the medical centre where their surveillance exams are scheduled, may wish to have the tests performed on the same day. The registry coordinator can intervene to optimize appointments for patients and their families so that time away from home and work is minimized.

Encouraging Compliance

One of most important functions of the registry is to facilitate surveillance. Patients may have problems complying with protocols for a variety of reasons including health insurance issues, lack of knowledge, incorrect information or fear over tests and surgery. In the United States some patients may not have medical insurance and may not be eligible for federal programmes which can provide free medical care. Current managed-care providers may not cover testing or may not allow patients to go out of their health care network. Patients who are fearful of tests or surgery may need extra help in understanding the nature of the disease and necessity for surveillance, especially when they are not having any symptoms or discomfort. Patients may have incorrect information from family, friends or health care providers. Through intimate contact with patients and families, the registry coordinator can build a trusting relationship, allowing for honest feelings and fears to be discussed and dispelled. The insightful observations of the coordinator can steer patients to understand the importance of maintaining surveillance protocols for themselves and other family members.

Patient Advocate

The registry coordinator should always be an advocate for the patient. Patients have problems, which may be with insurance, employment, social or family stress, a need for a second opinion, or some other problem. The mismanagement of their problems can have a devastating effect on their medical care. To encourage lifelong surveillance, it is most effective for patients to know that they can rely on the coordinator as a resource. It helps when they understand that the registry coordinator will always have their welfare and their family's welfare in mind.

Education

Patients and their families should be taught the nature and implications of FAP. They need to be aware of how this condition will affect their life and their families. The rationale behind current surveillance protocols, surgical treatment options and genetic testing is explained to patients. Education should start at the first visit and be an ongoing process by the registry. Through booklets, newsletters and current articles from medical journals patients can keep up to date with new studies and treatments for FAP. Some patients are eager for detailed information, and the coordinator can help. To give informed consent, therefore, patients need to understand their disease process.

The registry should also be an educational resource for other health care workers and physicians. Promoting basic information about familial polyposis and the clinical implications will benefit patients. The registry should also encourage and foster the development of FAP registries and inherited colorectal cancer registries throughout the world.

Research

FAP registries with a large number of patients and families are an ideal place for conducting clinical and laboratory research. Studies can be done by one registry or by multiple registries working in collaboration. The registry becomes the foundation for these individual and multisite collaborative programmes. Upon enrolment families are educated about the important role that they will play in continuing research, allowing for a better understand of the issues surrounding inherited risk.

Organizations have been formed to facilitate such multi-centre research:

Leeds Castle Polyposis Group
Robin K.S. Phillips
The Polyposis Registry
St Mark's Hospital
Northwick Park, Watford Road
Harrow, Middx, HAI 3UJ
UK

Eurofap
Profesor J. Mohr
University Institute of Human Genetics
Panum Institute
Blefdamsvej 3b
DK-2200 Copenhagen N.
Denmark

The International Collaborative Group for the Study of HNPCC
Hans F. A. Vasen
The Netherlands Foundation for the Detection of Hereditary
    Tumours
Rijnsburgerweg 10, Big 50
2333 AA Leiden
The Netherlands

The Collaborative Group of the Americas on Inherited Colorectal
    Cancer
James M. Church MD
The David G. Jagelman Inherited Colorectal Cancer Registries
Medical Genetics T10
Cleveland Clinic Foundation
9500 Euclid Avenue
Cleveland, OH 44195
USA

References

Arvanitis ML, Jagelman DG, Fazio VW et al. (1990) Mortality in patients with famil-
    ial adenomatous polyposis. Diseases of the Colon and Rectum 33: 639–42.
Bussey HJR (1975) Familial polyposis coli. In Family Studies, Histopathology,
    Differential Diagnosis, and Results of Treatment. Baltimore: Johns Hopkins
    University Press, pp 65–6.
Caspari R, Olschwang S, Friedl W et al. (1995) Familial adenomatous polyposis:
    desmoid tumors and lack of opthalmic lesions (CHRPE) associated with APC
    mutations beyond codon 1444. Human Molecular Genetics 4: 337–40.
Church JM, McGannon E, Hull-Boiner S et al. (1992) Gastroduodenal polyps in
    patients with familial adenomatous polyposis. Diseases of the Colon and Rectum
    35: 1170–3.
Cripps WH (1882) Two cases of disseminated polypus of the rectum. Transactions of
    the Pathology Society of London 33: 165.
Dukes CE (1952) Familial intestinal polyposis. Annals of Eugenics London 17: 1.
Gallinger S, Vivona AA, Odze RD et al. (1995) Somatic APC and K-*ras* codon 12
    mutations in periampullary adenomas and carcinomas from familial adenoma-
    tous polyposis patients. Oncogene 10: 1875–8.
Gardner EJ (1951) A genetic and clinical study of intestinal polyposis: a predisposing
    factor for carcinoma of the colon and rectum. American Journal of Human
    Genetics 3: 167–76.
Gardner EJ (1969) Gardner's syndrome reevaluated after 20 years. Proceedings of
    the Utah Academy 46: 1–11.
Handford H (1890) Disseminated polypi of the large intestine becoming malignant.
    Transactions of the Pathology Society of London 41: 133.

Heyen F, Jagelman DG, Romania A et al. (1990) Predictive value of congenital hypertrophy of the retinal pigment epithelium as a clinical marker for familial adenomatous polyposis. Diseases of the Colon and Rectum 33: 1003–8.

Iwama T, Mishima Y, Utsunomiya J (1993) The impact of familial adenomatous polyposis on the tumorigenesis and mortality at several organs: its rational treatment. Annals of Surgery 217: 101–8.

Jagelman DG (1988) The expanding spectrum of familial adenomatous polyposis. Perspectives on Colon and Rectal Surgery 1: 30–50.

Jagelman DG (1990) Familial polyposis coli. In Fazio VW (Ed.) Current Therapy in Colon and Rectal Surgery. Philadelphia: BC Decker, pp 284–8.

Jagelman DG (1991) Choice of operation in familial adenomatous polyposis. World Journal of Surgery 15: 47–9.

Jagelman DG, DeCosse JJ, Bussey HJ (1988) Upper gastrointestinal cancer in familial adenomatous polyposis. Lancet 1: 1149–51.

Jones IT, Jagelman DG, Fazio VW et al. (1986) Desmoid tumors in familial polyposis coli. Annals of Surgery 204: 94–7.

Kinzbrunner B, Ritter S, Domingo J et al. (1983) Remission of rapidly growing desmoid tumors after tamoxifen therapy. Cancer 52: 2201–4.

Kitamura A, Kanagawa T, Yamada S et al. (1991) Effective chemotherapy for abdominal desmoid tumor in a patient with Gardner's syndrome: report of a case. Diseases of the Colon and Rectum 34: 822–6.

Leppard B (1974) Epidermoid cysts and polyposis coli. Proceedings of the Royal Society of Medicine 67: 1036–7.

Lim CL, Walker MJ, Mehta RR, Das Gupta TK (1986) Estrogen and anti-estrogen bonding sites in desmoid tumors. European Journal of Cancer and Clinical Oncology 22: 583–7.

Lynch HT, Fitzgibbons R Jr, Chong S et al. (1994) Use of doxorubicin and dacarbazine for the management of unresectable intra-abdominal desmoid tumors in Gardner's syndrome. Diseases of the Colon and Rectum 37: 260–7.

McAdam WAF, Goligher JC (1970) The occurrence of desmoids in patients with familial polyposis coli. British Journal of Surgery 57: 618–31.

Naylor EW, Gardner EJ (1981) Adrenal adenomas in a patient with Gardner's syndrome. Clinical Genetics 20: 67.

Nishisho I, Nakamura Y, Miyoshi Y et al. (1991) Mutations of chromosome 5q21 genes in FAP and colorectal cancer patients. Science 253: 665.

Nugent KP, Phillips RKS, Hodgson SV et al. (1994) Phenotypic expression in familial adenomatous polyposis: partial prediction by mutation analysis. Gut 35: 1622–3.

Nugent KP, Spigelman AD, Phillips RKS (1993) Life expectancy after colectomy and ileorectal anastomosis for familial adenomatous polyposis. Diseases of the Colon and Rectum 36: 1059–62.

Painter TA, Jagelman DG (1985) Adrenal adenomas and adrenal carcinoma in association with hereditary adenomatosis of the colon and rectum. Cancer 55: 2001.

Park J-G, Park KJ, Ahn Y-O et al. (1992) Risk of gastric cancer among Korean familial adenomatous polyposis patients: report of three cases. Diseases of the Colon and Rectum 35: 996–8.

Posner MC, Shiu MH, Newsome JL et al. (1989) The desmoid tumor: not a benign disease. Archives of Surgery 124: 191–6.

Reitamo JJ, Scheinin TM, Hayry P (1986) The desmoid tumors: new aspects in the cause, pathogenesis and treatment of the desmoid tumor. American Journal of Surgery 151: 230–7.

Rustin RB, Jagelman DG, McGannon E et al. (1990) Spontaneous mutation in familial adenomatous polyposis. Diseases of the Colon and Rectum 33: 52.

Sarre RG, Frost AG, Jagelman DG et al. (1987a) Gastric and duodenal polyps in familial adenomatous polyposis: a prospective study of the nature and prevalence of upper gastrointestinal polyps. Gut 28: 306.

Sarre RG, Jagelman DG, Beck DJ et al. (1987b) Colectomy with ileorectal anastomosis for familial adenomatous polyposis: the risk of rectal cancer. Surgery 101: 20–6.

Scates DK, Venitt S, Phillips RKS, Spigelman AD (1995) High pH reduces DNA damage caused by bile from patients with familial adenomatous polyposis: antacids may attenuate duodenal polyposis. Gut 36: 918–21.

Tonelli F, Valanzano R, Brandi ML (1994) Pharmacologic treatment of desmoid tumors in familial adenomatous polyposis: results of an in vitro study. Surgery 115: 473–9.

Tsukada K, Church JM, Jagelman DG et al. (1991) Systemic cytotoxic chemotherapy and radiation therapy for desmoid in familial adenomatous polyposis. Diseases of the Colon and Rectum 34: 1090–2.

Tsukada K, Church JM, Jagelman DG et al. (1992) Noncytotoxic drug therapy for intraabdominal desmoid tumor in patients with familial adenomatous polyposis. Diseases of the Colon and Rectum 35: 29–33.

Turcot J, Despres JP, St Pierre F (1959) Malignant tumors of the central nervous system associated with familial polyposis of the colon: report of two cases. Diseases of the Colon and Rectum 2: 465–8.

Utsunomiya J, Miki Y, Kuroki T et al. (1990) Phenotypic expressions of Japanese patients with familial adenomatous polyposis. In Herrera L (Ed.) Familial Adenomatous Polyposis. New York: Alan R Liss, pp 101–7.

Utsunomiya J, Nakamura T (1975) The occult adenomatous changes in the mandible in patients with familial polyposis coli. British Journal of Surgery 62: 45.

Waddell WR, Gerner RE, Reich MP (1983) Non-steroid anti-inflammatory drugs and tamoxifen for desmoid tumors and carcinoma of the stomach. Journal of Surgical Oncology 22: 192–211.

Watanabe H, Enjoji M, Yao T et al. (1978) Gastric lesions in familial adenomatosis coli: their incidence and histologic analysis. Human Pathology 9: 269–83.

Chapter 8
Faecal Stomas

SIOBHAN McCAHON BSC (Hons), RGN, Clinical Nurse Specialist
Stoma Care, Homerton Hospital, London, UK

Introduction

'Stoma' is a derivative of a Greek word meaning mouth or opening. It is constructed from a portion of large or small bowel, brought out of the abdomen and to the surface through a surgical incision, and varies in length according to its position and function. The normal colour of a healthy stoma is a pinkish red, which is comparable to the colour of the inside lining of the mouth.

Stomas can be divided into three categories (Devlin, 1985):

1. Input stomas – these are usually temporary and facilitate nutrients being put into the gut, e.g. gastrostomy, feeding jejunostomy.
2. Diverting stomas – these divert the contents of the gastrointestinal tract away from the diseased or damaged gut, e.g. loop ileostomy, loop colostomy.
3. Output stomas – these provide an outlet for the elimination of body waste, usually following excision of an excretory organ, i.e. bowel, e.g. colostomy or ileostomy

This chapter will encompass gastrointestinal diverting and output stomas. The nursing care that is entailed will be discussed from the preoperative period through to the long-term support required.

History of Stoma Care Nursing

Documentation of surgically fashioned stomas can be found as long ago as the early 1700s. Heister describes the damaged intestine of soldiers injured in battle whose bowel was brought to the abdominal wall forming an enterostomy (Richardson, 1973). However, no documentation of specific care to stoma patients can be found in nursing literature until Plumley (1939) in the *American Journal of Nursing*.

Development of Self-help Groups

Stoma patients had no access to specialized professional help until the second half of the twentieth century. Individuals relied on improvizational skill and advice from each other. In 1949 the first self-help group was set up by patients in Philadelphia, USA; this grew into the United Ostomy Association. In Europe progress was slow and it was not until 1956 that the Ileostomy Association of Great Britain and Ireland became the first European association followed by the other British self-help group, the Colostomy Welfare Group in 1966 (later renamed the British Colostomy Association).

Development of Stoma Care Nursing/Enterostomal Therapy Roles

In 1958 the first enterostomal therapist was enlisted in Cleveland, Ohio, USA to help with the rehabilitation of new stoma patients. Norma Gill was in fact not a nurse but an ileostomist who was employed by her surgeon Dr Rupert B. Turnbull after he recognized the need for stoma patients to be provided with a specialist service. Thus, Norma Gill became the first stoma therapist and went on to establish the first training course for enterostomal therapists in 1961.

Progress in Britain has been slower. Stoma care nursing was pioneered by Barbara Saunders, an experienced surgical ward sister at St Bartholomew's Hospital, London, who had developed an interest and expertise in stoma care. In 1969 she started a monthly clinic with a consultant surgeon and in 1971 was appointed a full-time stoma care nurse.

Research at the time from both sides of the Atlantic was highlighting a number of psychological and physical problems encountered by patients (Dyk and Sutherland, 1956; Orbach and Talent, 1965; Druss et al., 1968; Devlin et al., 1971). Although it was possible to care for a patient in a mechanistic way, dealing only with the physical problems, it was recognized that psychological and social trauma associated with the dysfunction and disfigurement which accompanies a stoma calls for a holistic and individualized approach to meet the patients' needs (Breckman, 1981).

In 1973 the first specialized training course for stoma care nurses began at St Bartholomew's Hospital and to this day on both sides of the Atlantic it is estimated that there are less than 20 of these courses in total.

Development of Appliances

Prior to the 1940s patients would use gauze pads, wadding, gamgees – anything they found that would contain the incontinent flow of faecal matter. The first ostomy appliance was reported in 1944 by Strauss and Strauss who described the Koenig bag. Koenig was an ileostomist who was an inventive chemistry student; he designed a bag for himself made of rubber which adhered to the skin using a latex solution. This bag became widely available, known as the 'black bag' and indeed is still used by some ostomists today.

Since then ostomy companies have invested considerable amounts of money in research and development to find the perfect bag. The advent of hydrocolloid adhesives in the 1970s helped to decrease the major skin problems which had been a frequent occurrence. Progress has continued to be rapid but the bag that will suit all skin types and stomas, yet be discreet and biodegradable, is still awaited.

Incidence of Stoma Formation

The total number of patients in the UK with stomas is not precisely known. In the 1980s the total number of stomas was estimated to be 120 000. It is approximated that in the last few years this figure has fallen to about 100 000; however, the number of temporary stomas is thought in fact to have tripled. This is due to the development of surgical techniques such as the ileoanal pouch and neo-sphincter operations. These procedures generally require a temporary stoma to be formed as part of the procedure. It is therefore felt that different types of stomas will continue to be formed well into the twenty-first century.

Types of Faecal Stomas

Figure 8.1 illustrates the positions on the abdomen where the stomas to be discussed are ideally sited.

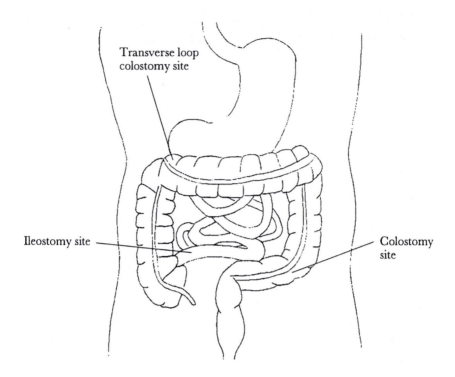

Figure 8.1: Preferred sites for stomas.

Colostomy

There are a number of different types of colostomies which will be formed for various reasons in different parts of the colon. The type of colostomy to be formed will be determined by the predisposing condition of the patient. For classification purposes the different types of colostomies have been divided into permanent and temporary colostomies.

Permanent/End Colostomy

The most common reasons for formation of a permanent colostomy are:

1. carcinoma of the lower third of the rectum;
2. extensive diverticular disease, including perforation;
3. sigmoid volvulus;
4. trauma, e.g. gunshot wounds or stabbing;
5. faecal incontinence;
6. carcinoma of the anus.

A permanent colostomy can also be referred to as a terminal or end colostomy and will generally be formed from the descending or sigmoid colon. Consequently most fluid reabsorption will have already occurred and the stool should be firm and well formed. It is important that the incision made in the skin is circular and large enough to allow the formed stools to be passed even when the abdominal muscles contract. The bowel is passed through the skin, turned over on itself and then sutured to the skin so that it will protrude by about 5 mm once postoperative oedema has diminished (Figure 8.2)

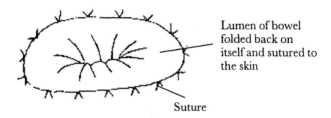

Lumen of bowel folded back on itself and sutured to the skin

Suture

Figure 8.2: Permanent colostomy.

Temporary Colostomy

The most common reasons for temporary stoma formation are:

1. carcinoma of the upper two-thirds of the rectum;
2. carcinoma of the sigmoid or descending colon;
3. diverticular disease and perforation;
4. Crohn's disease in the colon and rectum;
5. ischaemic bowel;
6. trauma, e.g. gunshot or stab wounds to the colon and upper rectum;
7. congenital abnormalities in children, e.g. Hirschsprung's disease.

There are several different options for the formation of a temporary colostomy:

1. loop colostomy – formed in the sigmoid or transverse colon;
2. double-barrelled colostomy – generally formed in the sigmoid colon;
3. Hartmann's procedure – formed out of the descending colon.

Loop colostomy: A loop of colon is brought to the surface through an incision in the left iliac fossa (sigmoid loop) or the upper abdomen/right upper quadrant (transverse loop). A plastic rod is placed under the loop to prevent the loop of bowel from retracting back into the abdomen; there is no need for this to be sutured in place. This rod will be removed after 5 days by an experienced nurse who turns the end of the rod so that it will not catch the stoma when it is gently pulled out. This is not a sterile procedure. An incision is made into the loop and the two ends folded back and sutured to the skin (Figure 8.3). This is a comparatively large stoma, therefore a larger aperture in the skin is required; consequently the risk of prolapse is far greater than if a smaller aperture was made.

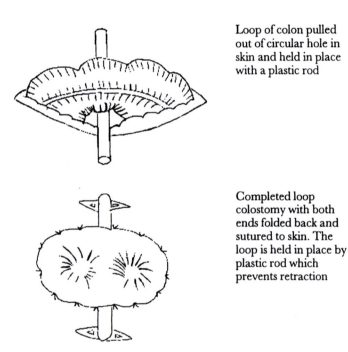

Loop of colon pulled out of circular hole in skin and held in place with a plastic rod

Completed loop colostomy with both ends folded back and sutured to skin. The loop is held in place by plastic rod which prevents retraction

Figure 8.3: Loop colostomy.

The output from a loop colostomy will vary depending on which part of the colon is used. A transverse loop will result in a semi-formed, often quite loose stool which may require a drainable pouch for management; this is due to the comparatively small amount of water reabsorption that has occurred. A sigmoid loop will result in more formed stools that permit a closed appliance to be used.

Double-barrelled: Two sections of descending or sigmoid colon will be brought to the surface through an incision in the left iliac fossa. The two lengths of bowel will be sutured together and then turned back on themselves before being sutured to the skin (Figure 8.4). This again results in a larger stoma with a large aperture incised in the skin being necessary. The output will consist of a formed stool and a closed appliance can be worn.

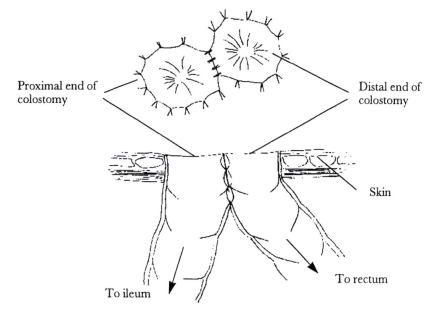

Figure 8.4: Double-barrelled colostomy.

Hartmann's procedure: This procedure is performed when it is considered too risky to anastamose together the two lengths of bowel. The proximal length of bowel consists of descending colon and is brought to the skin, as for an end colostomy. The distal length of bowel is oversewn and left inside the abdomen. The resulting colostomy is similar to an end colostomy in appearance and function; however, there remains the option to restore continuity at a later date.

Ileostomy

An ileostomy may be formed for one of the following reasons:

1. Crohn's disease;
2. ulcerative colitis;

3. familial adenomatous polyposis;
4. obstruction;
5. trauma, e.g. gunshot or stab wound.

Two different types of ileostomy exist: a loop ileostomy which is
intended as a temporary stoma and a terminal/end ileostomy which
will generally be a permanent stoma except if a mucous fistula has also
been formed allowing for restoration of continuity at a later date.

Temporary – Loop

A loop ileostomy has in recent years become the preferred procedure
over a transverse loop colostomy; and will be formed to temporarily
divert the faecal flow to allow an anastamosis to heal. A loop of terminal ileum will be brought to the surface in the right iliac fossa; the
circular hole in the skin will be smaller than for a colostomy owing to
the smaller diameter of the ileum. The loop of ileum will be pulled
through the skin and then the distal limb will be cut, folded back on
itself and sutured to the skin; this forms a flush non-functioning aperture. The proximal limb, while still partially attached to the distal limb,
is also folded back and sutured to the skin. This results in a spout about
2 cm long. To prevent the loop from retracting a plastic rod is sometimes used which will be removed after 3–5 days (Figure 8.5). The
spouted stoma is necessary in order for the skin to be protected from
the liquid corrosive output that contains digestive juices. A drainable

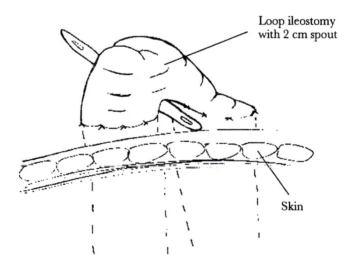

Loop ileostomy
with 2 cm spout

Skin

Figure 8.5: Loop ileostomy.

pouch must be worn and once established the ileostomy can be expected to produce 200–600 ml per day.

End Ileostomy

An end ileostomy will generally be a permanent procedure and will be formed from the terminal ileum unless this has previously been resected. A length of ileum will be pulled through the circular incision in the skin, folded back on itself and sutured to the skin in such a way that it will protrude by 2.5 cm on the top edge and 2 cm on the bottom edge (Figure 8.6). This ensures that the skin can be protected from the corrosive duodenal juices contained in the output. The output will be the same as for the loop ileostomy unless the stoma is formed from a more proximal section of bowel; in these circumstances the output will be greater.

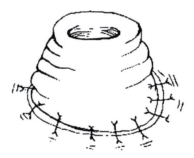

Figure 8.6: End ileostomy.

Jejunostomy

A jejunostomy will be formed only if the ileum and colon have previously been resected or are not viable. The formation and appearance of a jejunostomy will be as for an ileostomy. Due to the fact that it is formed higher in the gastrointestinal tract the output will be far greater (2000–4000 ml/day) and subsequent electrolyte imbalance will occur; electrolyte monitoring and correction is necessary on a regular basis. Deficiency in vitamin B12 may also occur due to the loss of the terminal ileum; levels must be monitored and supplements given if necessary.

Owing to the severe difficulties in management this is not a stoma of choice; it will tend to be a temporary procedure and often results in the patient having to remain in hospital to enable an adequate nutritional state to be maintained.

Preoperative Care

Psychological

Patients with a gastrointestinal complaint undergo a period of great uncertainty and anxiety while they are awaiting the results of the various tests that they have endured, still suffering the alarming and embarrassing symptoms that they originally sought help for. When the surgeon finally tells them of the need for surgery and stoma formation the patient may well find that he/she is unable to take in all the information at this time.

Patients may react in one of many ways, by being:

- stoical;
- shocked;
- in denial;
- blaming someone else;
- attempting to rationalize the information.

However patients react, it has been a well-documented fact that they will benefit from receiving more information, preferably on another date and in a relaxed and familiar environment, i.e. their home.

Much research has been published in the last 30 years to show that patients benefit from preoperative information. In fact, anxiety has been shown to increase in situations where people do not have sufficient information about what is happening to them (Elms and Leonard, 1966). The studies of Boore (1978) and Hayward (1975) are often quoted today as early studies which showed that providing preoperative information and discussion actually helped to alleviate anxiety. Kelly (1992) found that many patients emphasize a need to talk over health problems and obtain further information, especially in the time lapse between diagnosis and admission to hospital.

The preoperative meeting should occur with a stoma care nurse/enterostomal therapist who will endeavour to cover certain topics:

1. ascertain the patient's understanding of the disease, surgery and stoma;
2. illustrate descriptions of the pending surgery and stoma with annotated diagrams which the patient will find easier to comprehend;
3. allow time for the patient to ask questions;
4. describe what the stoma will look and feel like, i.e. the inside of the mouth;

5. show the patient an example of the type of appliance to be used postoperatively and on discharge, while giving reassurance that the ultimate choice will be his/her decision made with guidance from the stoma care nurse;
6. offer information booklets/videos to take away and look at;
7. offer to arrange for the patient to meet a person who already has a stoma and has adapted well;
8. if the rectum is to be excised ensure that the patient has been warned of the possibility of impotence or painful intercourse;
9. if the patient is agreeable encourage their partner to be present.

Marking of the Stoma Site

Time and consideration must be spent ensuring that the optimal site for the stoma has been marked. The following points should be considered:

- The patient must be able to see the stoma site.
- The stoma should be within the rectus abdominus sheath.
- Any bony prominences must be avoided.
- Skin creases or folds must be avoided.
- Any previous scars must be avoided.
- Ensure pendulous breasts are not obscuring vision of the stoma.
- The waistline of clothing should be avoided.
- Ensure there is enough flat skin around the site for adhering the bag to.
- Ensure that any prostheses do not cover the site.
- If the patient is wheelchair bound the stoma must be sited while he/she is in the wheelchair.

If the stoma is to be formed in an emergency, as many of these factors as possible should be considered while ensuring that any discomfort is kept to a minimum.

Postoperative Care

Psychological

In the first few postoperative days, physical recovery will take priority over the psychological recovery. Counselling is not appropriate until the physical pain and discomfort have subsided, the drains and infusions have been discontinued and the patient is able to mobilize.

The major abdominal surgery, diagnosis, possible sexual impairment, the loss of faecal continence and alteration in body image all contribute to the psychological difficulties a patient may have.

Devlin et al. (1971) suggested that the long-term psychological effects of having a stoma are underestimated, and psychologically disturbed patients may not be diagnosed. Although this evidence is over 25 years old it is felt that the psychological care that a patient needs in the postoperative period is still often neglected.

Model (1987) found that it can be helpful for a counsellor to be guided by the Kubler-Ross stages of grieving when considering the needs of a patient:

- denial and isolation;
- anger;
- bargaining;
- depression;
- acceptance.

It must be recognized that these stages take time to work through and it can take up to a year for patients to reach the acceptance stage; indeed some patients never successfully reach this stage.

Michael Kelly (1985) considered, from his own experience, that the psychological recovery needs to occur alongside the physical recovery if successful adaptation is to occur.

Altered Body Image

A major factor in the psychological recovery is that of adapting to an altered body image. Price (1990) described altered body image as 'Any significant alteration or body change occurring outside of normal, expected human development' – formation of stoma can quickly be seen to result in a major alteration in body image.

In order to understand the difficulty in accepting an altered body image it is important to understand how a normal body image develops. The development of a body image starts as a child and is a learned process that incorporates the following factors:

- cognitive development;
- the domestic environment;
- present and past perceptions;
- physiological functioning;
- the response of significant others (Salter, 1988).

The success with which a person adapts to an alteration in body image, such as the formation of a stoma, will depend on how developed these factors and therefore his/her body image are. The 'physiological functioning' of the body is totally changed with the formation of a stoma and the 'response of significant others' will be instrumental in ensuring that the body image is altered.

Hughes (1991) recognized that society places great value on having an attractive physical appearance; she saw that body image would affect not only how a person feels about him/herself, but also his/her ability to perform and interact with others. Previous studies (Devlin et al., 1971; Follick et al., 1984) have illustrated how ostomists have difficulty with social adjustment. Patients were particularly concerned about the reaction of others, were sensitive about their appearance, and fearful about leak and odours. It is imperative that patients are reassured that with advancements in appliance design, the appliance should not leak and odour should not be detectable unless the appliance is being changed.

At the same time as the altered body image comes a feeling of loss and Kelly (1985) describes these feelings as following a similar pattern to the bereavement stages described by Parkes (1972):

1. Realization –the bereaved person practises avoidance or denial of the loss followed by experiences of unreality.
2. Alarm – the individual exhibits anxiety, restlessness and fear, accompanied by feelings of insecurity.
3. Searching – this involves acute and episodic feelings of anxiety and panic and a preoccupation with the loss.
4. Internal loss – the individual has feelings of internal loss and mutilation. Some people experience morbid or atypical grief; if this happens the individual does not come to terms with the loss and cannot pass through to the other stages successfully.
5. A new social identity – the uncertainty and aimlessness of the early stages are resolved and the old ways of thinking and living are, at least partially, abandoned.

Practical Teaching

The practical teaching of stoma management needs to occur concurrently with the provision of psychological support. As patients develop practical skills they will develop in confidence both in themselves and in the appliance.

Follick et al. (1984) showed there to be a high correlation between technical expertise and the emotional, social and sexual adjustments. A later descriptive study (Kelly and Henry, 1992) also found that patients' main concerns centred around information about appliances and management of leakages and odours.

The focus of the postoperative teaching sessions should, therefore, be twofold:

1. To enable the patient/carer to develop the necessary practical stoma management skills to be able to care safely for the stoma in the home environment.
2. To educate the patient as to potential problems and to manage common stomal problems which can lead to leakage and odour.

The practical teaching of stoma management can seem overwhelming to the patient who may feel that he/she will not be able to achieve this goal. Dividing the ultimate goal into several tasks as in Figure 8.7 has several benefits:

- The patient is able to aim for many goals which can be quickly achieved giving a sense of success.
- The patient is likely to remain motivated as he/she can identify each goal as attainable.
- The level of independence that the patient has reached can be measured.

It is important that the patient understands that the procedure is not a sterile technique; the teaching should be kept as simple as possible and the use of accessories kept to a minimum. It is not necessary to use numerous skin preparations and warm water should be sufficient to clean the peristomal skin and the stoma; if soap is used it should be an unperfumed type which will reduce the risk of skin reactions.

It is essential to include the patient, his/her family and all caregivers at all stages of this teaching (Allison, 1996).

Irrigation

Irrigation is a method of cleaning the bowel by instilling lukewarm water via a colostomy every 24–48 hours. It enables the colostomist to be 'continent' again although is time consuming, and many patients find the idea distasteful. In the UK it is not very popular – about 1% of colostomists irrigate; however in the USA it is far more common.

Stoma care

Some simple steps to going home

Name -

Stoma type -

Date of surgery -

Discharge name of appliance -
              size of appliance -

Frequency of bag change -

When the patient has achieved all these steps he/she will be, in regard of stoma care, ready to go home.

	Please tick and date this column when patient has achieved the steps and feels confident about it.
11 Whole procedure without supervision.	
10 Whole procedure under supervision.	
9 Disposal of soiled bag/tissues.	
8 Reapply the new bag. (Identify the name and size of bag.)	
7 Cleanses skin, dries skin around stoma.	
6 Removes soiled bag.	
5 Prepares the new bag.	
4 Can identify all equipment needed to take to bathroom for bag change.	
3 Has observed stoma.	
2 Can empty bag with supervision and refasten clip.	
1 Able to fasten clip on bag.	

This must be updated by stoma care nurse specialist and ward staff on a daily basis.

Figure 8.7: Steps to achieving self-care.

Irrigation is not suitable for all patients: it has many disadvantages as well as advantages (Davis, 1996) and patients must be carefully selected and able to make an informed choice.

Advice Given to the Patient on Discharge

Encompassed within the teaching sessions should be advice about the stoma which could cause the uninformed patient alarm:

1. The stoma has no sensory nerves and therefore the patient cannot feel him/herself touching it.
2. Because of the thin mucosa and concentrated blood supply, contact bleeding will frequently occur when cleaning the stoma.
3. If the rectum is still intact, mucous and old cells may be passed rectally.
4. Constipation may occur in colostomists owing to the lack of voluntary muscle control; a high-fibre diet, plenty of fluids and laxatives may be necessary.
5. Diarrhoea may still occur; the consequences will be far more rapid, and constipating and bulking agents may be prescribed. Dietary advice will include starchy foods, such as white bread or rice and marshmallows.

Community Follow-up

Discharge from hospital can be a stressful and isolating time for the patient. Even the most proficient and informed patients will feel very alone and vulnerable when changing their appliance for the first time in their own home. The responsibilities of the stoma care nurse lie in supporting patients during this transition from hospital to home and continuing to provide support in the following months. It is only when patients are feeling physically stronger and have time to reflect that the psychological impact of what has happened hits them; this is often when patients begin to grieve for their former lifestyle and body part (Price, 1990).

Porrett and Joels (1996) recognized the importance of assessing the patient's bathroom facilities and his/her technique on a first home visit, as well as ensuring that the patient has received supplies and has remembered how to obtain them in future.

Assisting the family to understand the grief stages that the patient is passing through is important; recognizing at which times patients are known to feel vulnerable is also beneficial. Wade (1989) identified that

10 weeks postoperatively is often a psychological 'low point', and a home visit or clinic appointment at this time can be an invaluable opportunity to provide psychological support.

Effects of Different Cultures on Stoma Patients

Culture is seen to be an amalgamation of several different factors including ethnicity, religion, socioeconomic group, sexuality and sexual orientation, gender, colour, family and profession. The culture of a patient will affect the needs of a patient in relation to both general nursing care and specific stoma care.

Communication

It is important to allow every patient as much time as is needed to express grief, and to recognize whether the behaviour of the patient is due to his/her cultural way of expressing feelings or due to the grief process he/she is passing through. It is an acknowledged fact that the further east one travels around the globe the greater the emphasis on non-verbal communication. This fact can be illustrated by looking at different races from around the world, e.g. a Chinese wife may sit in the room of her terminally ill husband, not touching or speaking to him. Her actions of tidying the room and gradually removing the flowers (the signs of life) say everything necessary. An Islamic man in times of sickness may wish to be totally alone; however, the Jewish culture will tend to revolve around large family discussions before decisions can be made. Communication patterns within Europe and the USA vary greatly again; the British will have 'a stiff upper lip', the Italians are very emotional and the Americans will be very eloquent at expressing their viewpoint.

Self-esteem

As a result of religious beliefs, some Islamic races believe that a stoma renders a patient unclean; such individuals may be banned from eating in company or having intercourse and may even be divorced or ostracized from their community because of the shame they have brought to their family and society. Careful consideration of an individual patient's needs, education and discussion with their religious leaders prior to surgery can help to reduce this cultural problem. In some cultures placing the stoma above the umbilicus will render the patient clean again, in other religions exceptions may be made for the patient once the religious elders understand the need for surgery.

Additionally, the female patient who cannot speak English, and brings along her son to interpret, is put in a position where inappropriate questions need to be asked through her son, thus lowering her self-esteem. In many areas an advocate or professional interpreter can be arranged to translate either as a third person in the consultation room or on a three-way telephone.

Language

Finally, the language that health professionals use can be a problem when medical rather than lay terminology is used. If a patient looks up the word 'incontinent' in the *Pocket Oxford Dictionary* they may well understand that the doctor has told them they will be promiscuous after their surgery – the dictionary states that incontinent means 'lacking self-restraint (esp. sexual desire)'. It has been estimated that up to 80% of information given by a doctor may be lost due to a lack of understanding of the terminology; this may also be a problem for English-speaking patients with poor medical understanding.

Management of Stomal Problems

Prolapse

A prolapsed stoma occurs when the bowel falls out through the abdominal wall resulting in a larger stoma than initially intended. Prolapse of the stoma is most likely to occur if a loop stoma has been formed. The most susceptible type of stoma is the transverse-loop colostomy where a larger hole has been cut in the skin to allow the loop of colon to be pulled through without strangulation occurring. Lifting, heavy exertion or an enlarged liver increasing the intra-abdominal pressure may cause the bowel to prolapse out of the abdomen (Figure 8.8). The prolapse can be reduced manually, but it frequently recurs as soon as the patient moves around, and surgical intervention may be the only permanent solution.

It is important that the patient with a prolapsed stoma receives adequate support. The psychological effects of having a large amount of bowel outside the body are great, and fear can be a major problem. Practical care will centre around the need to keep the stoma clean and the skin healthy to reduce the risk of leakages. Most important will be the choice of appliance, which must be large enough to contain all the prolapse and the stool with ease. If the prolapse is pressing against the

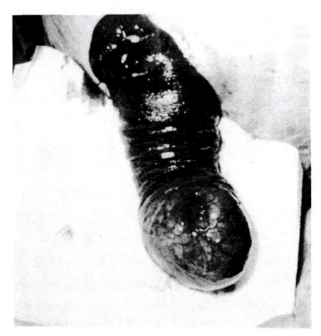

Figure 8.8: Prolapsed loop colostomy. See colour section.

sides of the appliance, pressure damage may occur on the bowel surface; if the appliance has been cut to fit too snugly around the stoma, the appliance flange may cut into the base of the prolapsing stoma.

Necrosis

Necrosis of the stoma is when the lumen of the bowel becomes black and dies due to poor perfusion and subsequent oxygen deprivation. It generally occurs within 24–48 hours postoperatively; for this reason it is important that the perfusion of the stoma be checked every 4 hours and the postoperative appliance must allow for direct viewing to occur. Necrosis will occur if the blood supply to the stoma is restricted, resulting in a compromised level of tissue oxygenation. Initially the stoma will become a dark red/plum colour over the surface, and then the stoma will rapidly turn black and necrotic (Figure 8.9). The blood supply to the stoma may be reduced for several reasons:

- the blood supply to the stoma has been cut during surgery;
- the opening in the skin is too small, resulting in the oedematous stoma becoming strangled;
- the bowel is under tension, due to distension, obesity or surgical technique.

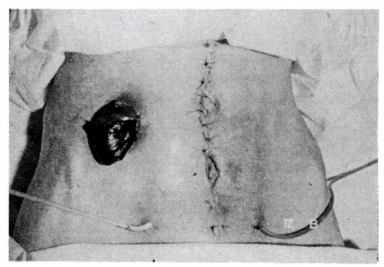

Figure 8.9: Necrotic stoma. See colour section.

If the necrosis is superficial the stoma will still be able to function and the necrotic tissue will 'slough off' with time. There have been some positive reports of local application of vasodilatory patches to prevent the necrosis from increasing; however, this is not yet a proven treatment. If the whole stoma becomes necrotic, peritonitis may occur and surgical intervention will be necessary.

Retraction

Retraction is when the stoma falls back into the abdominal cavity and does not protrude above the level of the skin. It may occur due to the bowel being under tension or once necrotic tissue has 'sloughed off'; this will generally occur within a month of surgery. Retraction may also occur long term as a result of weight gain, the abdomen increasing in size and the bowel being under greater tension. The resulting stoma will be below the surface of the skin and therefore leakages can be a major problem.

Appliance selection for the patient with a retracted stoma is important. The patient needs to sit, stand and lean over to allow for a careful assessment of the dips, creases and depth of retraction of the stoma.

The use of seals, convex inserts or appliances with built-in convexity will make the stoma protrude more, and therefore prevent the output from seeping under the adhesive. Belts may also improve the seal by pulling the appliance closer to the abdomen. Surgical intervention may be the only satisfactory solution for this condition.

Stenosis

Stenosis of a stoma is when the diameter has decreased to such an extent that the patient is at risk of an obstruction occurring (Figure 8.10). It will generally occur as a result of scar tissue around the stoma. The patient will be advised to ensure that soft fruits are peeled, vegetables high in cellulose are avoided, and nuts and sweetcorn avoided as these could all cause an obstruction. In severe cases all food may need to be pureed.

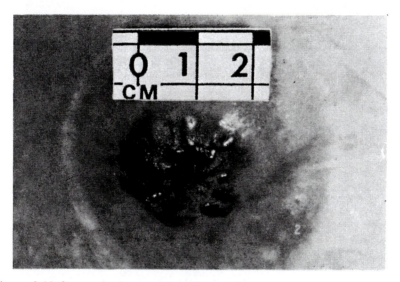

Figure 8.10: Stenosed colostomy. See colour section.

The patient can be taught to use a dilator on a daily basis to attempt to stretch the stoma; if this is not possible then surgical intervention is the only option.

Herniation

A parastomal hernia is when the abdominal muscle is not strong enough and the bowel pushes against the abdomen causing a spherical bulge around the stoma. Parastomal hernias may occur if the stoma is not sited in the rectus abdominus muscle, if the cut in the muscle is too large or if the abdominal muscles are very slack (Figure 8.11). The swelling which forms around the stoma can be alarming for the patient and much reassurance is necessary. Patient education is important, and heavy lifting and stretching should be avoided.

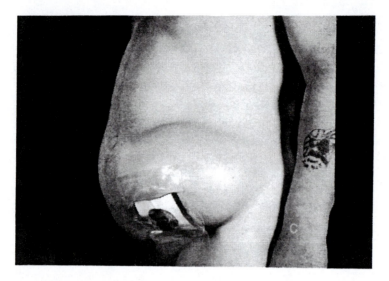

Figure 8.11: Parastomal hernia.

A surgical support belt can be made for patient comfort and the appliance needs to have a flexible flange to allow for it to be moulded around the hernia. Surgical correction may be necessary, though finding an alternative site for the stoma can be problematic, especially if many scars are present. If the stoma is resited it is important to advise the patient to continue to wear a support when physically active. Irrigation of a colostomy is not possible if a hernia is present.

Granulomas

Over-granulation of the bowel may occur especially if the appliance fits too tightly and continuous rubbing of the mucosa occurs. This over-granulation results in a granuloma. The patient may become alarmed at the bleeding which results when the stoma is cleaned and leakages can become a problem if the appliance then adheres to blood-stained skin. Cauterization of the granuloma will generally remove or decrease it in size, but granulation will frequently recur. Patient reassurance and education is important and the appliance must not rub against the stoma.

Conclusion

It can be concluded that the different types of stomas and nursing care comprise a vast subject. The specialist stoma care nurse/enterostomal therapist has the skills to educate and support the patient in the long recovery period and for continued management of the stoma. However, it is important that all health professionals have an understanding of the different types of stomas and the management of the ostomy patient; this chapter has endeavoured to provide the necessary information.

References

Allison M (1996) Discharge planning. In Myers C (Ed.) Stoma Care Nursing – A Patient-centred Approach: London: Arnold.

Boore J (1978) Prescription to Recovery: London: RCN.

Breckman B (1981) Stoma Care: A Guide for Nurses, Doctors and other Health Care Professionals. Beaconsfield: Beaconsfield Books.

Davis K (1996) Irrigation techniques: In Myers C (Ed.) Stoma Care Nursing – A Patient-centred Approach: London: Arnold.

Devlin HB (1985) Stoma Care Today: Oxford: Medical Education Sources.

Devlin HB, Plant JA, Griffin M (1971) The aftermath of surgery for anorectal cancer. British Medical Journal 14(August): 413–18.

Druss RG, O'Connor JF, Stern LO (1968) Psychologic response to colectomy, II: Adjustment to a permanent colostomy. Archives of General Psychiatry 20: 419–27.

Dyk RB, Sutherland AM (1956) Adaptation of the spouse and other family to the colostomy patient. Cancer 9: 123–38.

Elms RR, Leonard RC (1966) Effects of nursing approaches during admission. Nursing Research 15: 39–48.

Follick MJ, Smith TW, Turk DC (1984) Psychosocial adjustment following ostomy. Health Psychology 3(6): 505–17.

Hayward J (1975) Information: A Prescription Against Pain. London: RCN.

Hughes A (1991) Life with a stoma. Nursing Times 87(25): 67–8.

Kelly M (1985) Loss and grief reactions as responses to surgery. Journal of Advanced Nursing 10: 517–25.

Kelly M (1992) Self, identity and radical surgery. Sociology of Health and Illness 14: 390–415.

Kelly M, Henry T (1992) A thirst for practical knowledge. Professional Nurse 7(6): 350–1, 354–6.

Model GA (1987) Pre-operative and post-operative counselling. Nursing 21: 800–2.

Orbach CE, Talent N (1965) Modification of perceived body image and of body concepts (following colostomy). Archives of General Psychiatry 12(2): 126–35.

Parkes CM (1972) Bereavement Studies of Grief in Adult Life. London: Tavistock.

Plumley S (1939) Care of ileostomy. American Journal of Nursing 39: 275.

Pocket Oxford Dictionary (1990) Oxford: Clarendon Press.

Porrett T, Joels J (1996) Continuing care in the community. In Myers C (Ed.) Stoma Care Nursing: A Patient-centred Approach: London: Arnold.

Price B (1990) Body Image: Nursing Concepts and Care. London: Prentice-Hall.

Richardson RG (1973) The Abominable Stoma: A Historical Survey of the Artificial Anus. Maidenhead, Berks: Abbott Laboratories.

Salter M (1988) Altered Body Image: The Nurse's Role. London: Scutari Press.

Strauss AA, Strauss SF (1944) Surgical treatment of ulcerative colitis. Surgical Clinics of North America 24: 211–24.

Wade B (1989) A Stoma is for Life. Harrow, UK: Scutari Press.

Chapter 9
Diverticular Disease

MARC E. SHER MD, Assistant Clinical Professor of Surgery, Albert
Einstein College of Medicine, Long Island Jewish Medical Center,
New Hyde Park, New York, USA

LESLIE CHENEY RN, BSN, CGRN, Endoscopy Manager,
Department of Endoscopy, Cleveland Clinic Florida, Florida, USA

JULIA RICCIARDI RN, CGRN, Medical Nurse Clinician,
Department of Gastroenterology, Cleveland Clinic Florida,
Florida, USA

Introduction

Diverticular disease of the colon encompasses both diverticulosis and
diverticulitis, but its name only implies an out-pouching of the colonic
wall. Diverticulosis refers to an abnormal state in which non-inflamed
diverticula are present with or without symptoms, i.e. bleeding.
Diverticulitis results from inflamed diverticula, which may progress to
perforation with pericolonic infection (phlegmon), pelvic abscess formation, free perforation with generalized or feculent peritonitis, fistula
formation, or obstruction. Diverticulitis rarely presents with bleeding.

Before 1940, diverticular disease of the colon was rarely recognized
as a problem; reports estimated an incidence of only 5 to 10% (Spriggs
and Marxer, 1925). Recently, diverticular disease and its clinical consequences have become increasingly prevalent, paralleling western
patterns of living and eating, the aging population, and economic and
industrial development. In the United Kingdom, the United States,
and Australia prevalence has risen from 5%–50% (Almy and Howell,
1980). Diverticular disease also increases with age, occurring in 10%
of patients in their forties and rising to more than two-thirds of persons
in their eighties (Schoetz, 1993).

Most patients with diverticular disease of the colon are asymptomatic and complications such as haemorrhage or infection occur in only 10–30% of affected individuals. Moreover, only about 30% of these patients may require operative therapy (Telford, 1993). Thus, as our society ages and progresses, diverticular disease will remain a major public health concern and will continue to challenge physicians and nurses caring for these individuals.

Pathophysiology

Most diverticula of the colon are false diverticula composed of only mucosa and submucosa that have herniated through the muscularis externa at points of weakness, such as where the mesenteric blood vessels penetrate. Most colonic diverticula are found in the sigmoid colon although they may be pan-colonic (Figure 9.1).

Diverticular disease has been described as a disease of western industrialized civilization and as a consequence of refined food products where the intake of fibre has decreased. Diverticular disease is also unusual in Japan, where although industrialized, the population continues to eat a high-fibre diet including more raw fish and less red meat. First-generation Japanese born in Hawaii whose diet has been

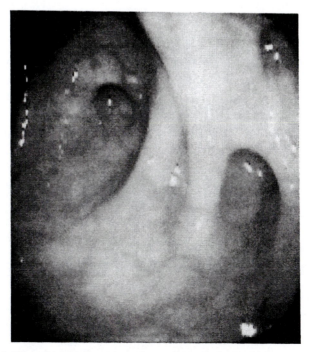

Figure 9.1: Diverticulosis (large intestine endoscopic finding).

westernized have an increased frequency of diverticular disease compared with native Japanese (Stemmermann, 1970).

Painter and associates hypothesized that diverticulosis is acquired based on segmentation, decreased wall tension, and forceful contraction of the colon containing small amounts of stool, as would occur with a low-fibre diet (Painter et al., 1965). The lumen may be totally occluded via contraction and segmentation, thus high pressures generated would permit herniation at weak points. Hypermotility has also been suggested to be a contributory factor. Nevertheless, the pathophysiologic changes common to all causes of diverticulosis of the colon have yet to be fully elucidated. Another hypothetical cause of acute diverticulitis is the inspissation of stool in the neck of the diverticulum with resultant bacterial proliferation and lymphangitis in the colonic wall and colonic mesentery leading to complications such as microperforation with peritonitis.

Epidemiology and Aetiology

The frequency of diverticular disease of the colon correlates mostly with advancing age. The rapidity of the increase in prevalence in western nations, Japanese immigrants, and in urban South African blacks points to environmental causative factors. In 1980, the introduction of milled wheat flour resulted in a lower intake of crude cereal grains, and an increased consumption of white flour, refined sugars and meats. These dietary changes have been linked to the increased prevalence of diverticular disease in England from 1910 onward (Almy and Howell, 1980). It is interesting that the death rate from diverticulitis in England and Wales increased steadily from 1923 to 1963 except between 1939 and 1945 when the British diet was implemented, focusing on a higher intake of whole grains, fruits and vegetables (Painter and Burkitt, 1971). Between 1909 and 1975, the total crude fibre content of the American diet declined by 28%, whilst the incidence of diverticular disease rose over tenfold (Heller and Hackler, 1978). Thus, fibre has become a major target in the preventative health care era of the 1990s.

Clinical Features

Typically, patients with acute diverticulitis present with a gradual onset of left lower quadrant pain, associated with a low-grade fever. Altered bowel habits, either constipation or diarrhoea, are common. Non-specific urinary tract symptoms such as frequency or urgency indicate the inflamed colon is adjacent to and irritating the bladder.

Pneumaturia or faecaluria are the hallmark of a colovesical fistula, the most common fistula of diverticular disease.

In addition to fever and tachycardia, physical examination usually reveals tenderness over the involved segment of colon. Because the sigmoid colon is the most common site, left lower quadrant or suprapubic tenderness is usually elicited. A lower abdominal mass or fullness may be palpated. Leukocytosis with a left shift is frequently encountered but not always. Urine analysis may reveal pyuria or haematuria.

Diagnosis and Investigation

An accurate diagnostic assessment is critical to decide where the patient fits in the clinical spectrum of inflammatory complications associated with diverticular disease. Some patients may be treated as outpatients and some require emergency surgery.

Frequent re-evaluation of patients afflicted with diverticular disease is the most important step to a successful outcome which should include abdominal examination, reassessment of vitals and a complete white blood cell count. A computer-assisted tomography (CT) scan is the best non-invasive study to diagnose diverticulitis and its complications. It also adds the advantage of percutaneous drainage, if necessary. Lower endoscopy is contraindicated in an acute attack for risk of perforation. A water-soluble contrast enema may be helpful to delineate the extent of disease, fistula, obstruction, perforation and also to confirm the diagnosis in difficult cases (Wexner and Dailey, 1986) (Figure 9.2).

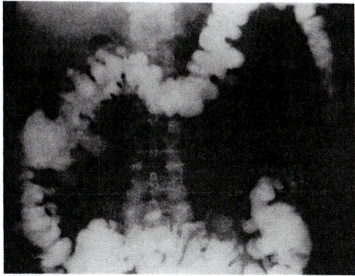

Figure 9.2: A barium study revealing multiple diverticula in the large intestine.

Indications for Surgery

The indications for surgery are the following:

- complications of diverticular disease: fistula; obstruction; haemorrhage; abscess; sepsis;
- recurrent attacks (two or more documented episodes confirmed by CT scan);
- persistent phlegmon or mass;
- stricture;
- persistent urinary symptoms associated with diverticular disease;
- unresponsive to conservative therapy or progression of symptoms after 48 hours;
- less than 40 years of age with an attack requiring hospitalization (one episode);
- unable to exclude carcinoma;
- unresponsive to percutaneous drainage;
- complications of diverticular disease associated with immunosuppressive states such as renal transplant patients and patients on steroids.

Complications

Complications of diverticular disease include:

1. haemorrhage;
2. acute diverticulitis;
3. abscess;
4. fistula;
5. perforation with peritonitis;
6. obstruction.

Haemorrhage

In over 70% of patients with diverticular haemorrhage, the bleeding stops spontaneously. Of those who stop, 75% do not rebleed. For the 25% who have recurrent bleeding, a segmental colectomy should be performed, as most will have subsequent haemorrhage. Massive bleeding is not uncommon with diverticulosis and tends to be right sided in origin (Welch et al., 1978).

Acute Diverticulitis

Acute diverticulitis can result from obstruction of the neck of the diverticulum, abrasion of a thin-walled diverticulum, a micro-perforation of a diverticulum or as a result of increased pressure leading to an invasive infection within the colon wall. The process can result in a self-limiting infection without symptoms, or can progress to a clinically significant infection requiring hospitalization and surgical intervention. If the infection progresses, other complications can occur. Most patients with acute diverticulitis severe enough to warrant hospitalization should be treated with intravenous fluids, bowel rest and broad-spectrum antibiotics. Signs and symptoms of complicated diverticulitis include fever, tachycardia, leukocytosis, pain and localized tenderness with voluntary guarding, and occasionally a mass. Patients who do not improve within 48 hours are usually stricken with complications of the disease process and require further investigation and therapy. Only 20% of patients with acute diverticulitis have complications with their first episode. This rises to 60% with recurrent episodes, therefore recommendation for elective surgery after more than one episode is encouraged (Telford, 1993).

A CT scan is the preferred test to diagnose a perforation or abscess. Also, percutaneous drainage can be performed to allow for the infection to subside and to continue with a segmental colectomy with primary anastomosis as a one-stage procedure without performing a colostomy. If drainage is not feasible or an abscess is not identified, surgical therapy is advised (Stable et al., 1990).

Segmental colectomy should be performed with the distal extent of resection extending to the rectosigmoid junction and proximal extent to normal pliable bowel even if diverticula remain more proximal. This reduces recurrence rates to less than 10% (Roberts et al., 1995).

Contraindications to primary anastomosis are: free perforation with generalized peritonitis, obstruction with an unprepped bowel, septic shock, ureteral injury, or other medical conditions that make a prolonged operation inadvisable. A large phlegmon may make primary anastomosis risky and a Hartmann procedure would be the procedure of choice. A Hartmann procedure includes resection of the involved segment with a diverting end, descending colostomy and a closed rectal (Hartmann) stump (Figure 9.3). A protecting loop ileostomy with primary anastomosis is another option in selected healthy patients.

Most patients with acute diverticulitis improve with intravenous fluids, bowel rest and antibiotics. Emergency surgery, therefore, is avoided. Intravenous and/or oral antibiotics should be continued for 7 days and feeding should be resumed when the tenderness has resolved and colonic transit has normalized, usually after 3 days. Complications such as abscess, fistula, free perforation or obstruction

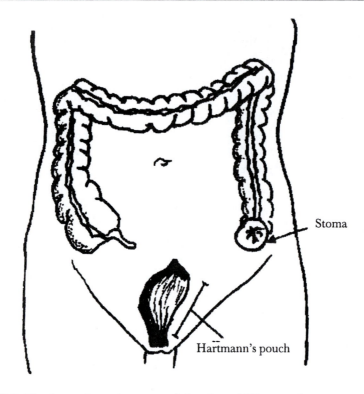

Figure 9.3: The descending colostomy and closed rectal (Hartmann) stump.

dictate operation before discharge. An uncomplicated attack of acute diverticulitis that quickly resolves allows the patient to be followed up as an outpatient. A second episode of diverticulitis, severe first episode of diverticulitis or acute diverticulitis in patients less than 40 years old should prompt surgical correction during the same admission as further episodes are associated with higher morbidity usually requiring a temporary colostomy (Ouriel and Schwartz, 1983). Also, elective resection is advised in immunosuppressed patients with only one prior attack such as renal transplant patients or patients on steroids.

Abscess

The most common complication of acute diverticulitis is the development of an abscess or a phlegmon. These abscesses can be located in the mesentery, abdomen, pelvis, retroperitoneum or scrotum. Often a tender mass is palpated on either abdominal or pelvic/rectal exam. Various degrees of sepsis may accompany a diverticular abscess. An abscess limited to the colon or mesentery is classified as Hinchey I disease. An abscess extending into the pelvis is Hinchey II disease (Hinchey et al., 1978).

Peritonitis

Rupture of a contained abscess or free perforation of a diverticulum into the peritoneal cavity may result in either purulent generalized peritonitis (Hinchey III disease) or faecal peritonitis (Hinchey IV disease). Most of these patients present with an acute abdomen and some degree of septic shock. The overall mortality rate is 6–18% for Hinchey III disease and at least 35% for Hinchey IV disease (Auguste et al., 1986).

Fistula

Fistulae occur in 2% of patients with diverticulitis but are present in 20% of patients who ultimately have surgery for diverticular disease (Woods et al., 1988). Internal fistulae arise as adjacent viscera adhere to the inflamed colon; 8% have multiple fistulae. Fistulae occur in men more often than women as the uterus serves as a protective barrier. Most females with colovaginal fistula or colovesical fistula have undergone a hysterectomy in the past. Most colocutaneous fistulae are iatrogenic secondary to an anastomotic leak. Colovesical fistulae account for 50–70% of all diverticular fistulae; pneumaturia is the most common symptom (Rao et al., 1987); colovaginal fistulae are the second most common. Patients usually complain of air or stool via the vagina more often with diarrhoea. A CT scan is the most sensitive test to diagnose a colovesical fistula; air is usually visible in a bladder that has no indwelling Foley catheter. Usually a one-stage operation with a sigmoid resection and primary closure of the bladder or vagina is possible to repair a colovaginal or colovesical fistula. A Foley catheter should be left in place for at least 5 days for drainage so that the bladder defect can heal.

Obstruction

Diverticular disease causes about 10% of large bowel obstructions. Partial obstruction is usually from oedema and spasm of the inflamed colon as a result of frequent or multiple attacks which can ultimately cause a stricture. It may be difficult to rule out cancer or colonic volvulus. All patients should have flexible sigmoidoscopy after the acute attack when it is safe, for fear of perforation. If a full bowel preparation is possible, patients with incomplete obstruction may undergo a one-stage resection. Patients with complete obstruction require resection and a diverting colostomy as an urgent procedure and the work-up should be delayed until the patient is more stable. A two-stage procedure is preferred rather than a three-stage procedure in almost all circumstances (Rothenberger and Wiltz, 1993).

Outpatient Therapy for Uncomplicated Diverticulitis

The decision to treat the patient with diverticulitis as an outpatient depends on the clinical impression of the physician, the severity of the disease process and the comorbid conditions the patient has. The experience of prior attacks and likelihood that the patient will respond to outpatient therapy are also important in the decision to treat as an outpatient. Patients should be able to tolerate a diet, be devoid of systemic symptoms and clearly lack peritoneal signs. Immunosuppressed patients or patients on steroids should not be treated as outpatients (Perkins et al., 1984). A complete blood count may be helpful to monitor the response to outpatient therapy with oral antibiotics.

Most of all, the patient must be reliable and/or have a reliable family, as worsening of symptoms or lack of improvement within 48 hours such as fever, increased abdominal pain or inability to tolerate a diet require hospitalization. After recovery from an initial episode of diverticulitis as an outpatient, the patient should undergo a colonoscopy or flexible sigmoidoscopy with barium enema to evaluate the entire colon and confirm the diagnosis.

Inpatient Therapy for Complicated Diverticulitis

Abscess

Complicated diverticulitis, i.e. abscess, fistula, obstruction or perforation, should be treated on an inpatient basis and individualized according to the Hinchey stages of disease. A small pericolic/mesenteric abscess (Hinchey I) (Hinchey et al., 1978) may resolve with intravenous antibiotics and bowel rest and not require urgent treatment. Large abscesses that do not resolve with medical therapy require percutaneous drainage or surgical therapy. Percutaneous drainage offers the patient stabilization and the avoidance of a temporary stoma (two-stage procedure). Some 70–90% of patients with unilocular collections are amenable to CT scan-guided percutaneous drainage. They may be successfully treated via this approach thus allowing a one-stage resection with primary anastomosis after 1 week of drainage with resolution of symptoms (Roberts et al., 1995).

Patients with abscesses not amenable to drainage or symptoms that persist after drainage require laparotomy. A Hartmann resection would be most appropriate which includes primary resection of the disease segment with an end stoma and a closed rectal remnant. Except for unusual circumstances, a three-stage procedure should not be performed as it is associated with increased morbidity (Auguste et al., 1986). If contamination is minimal and the bowel is pliable, an anastomosis may be performed in selective patients who are otherwise healthy. A covering-loop ileostomy will avoid return to the abdominal cavity with a difficult abdominal and pelvic dissection as part of the second-stage reversal of Hartmann procedure.

Perforation

Perforation of acute diverticulitis with purulent or feculent peritonitis is a surgical emergency requiring immediate resuscitation with intravenous fluids and intravenous broad-spectrum antibiotics, and an urgent operation. The degree of faecal contamination, length of time peritonitis was present and age of the patient usually determine perioperative mortality, which can approach 35%. The procedure of choice is a segmental resection with colostomy, i.e. Hartmann procedure. Resection of the perforated segment as a two-stage procedure has decreased mortality rates in these septic patients when compared with drainage of abscess alone with colostomy (Hackford et al., 1985; Auguste et al., 1986).

Fistula

Colovesical fistulae are the ones most commonly associated with diverticulitis, particularly if the uterus was previously removed. Other fistulae such as colovaginal, coloenteric and coloureteric are less common. The surgical principle should be to resect the diseased segment of colon with repair of the contiguous organ. In most cases, a primary resection with anastomosis can be undertaken if an adequate bowel preparation is achieved (Woods et al., 1988).

Obstruction

Patients with a large bowel obstruction presumably secondary to acute diverticulitis or chronic diverticular disease associated with a stricture should be resuscitated with intravenous hydration, antibiotics, nasogastric tube decompression, and undergo urgent surgery, usually a Hartmann procedure. The possibility of cancer must be strongly considered. If obstruction resolves quickly and bowel preparation is possible, a primary anastomosis may be performed. Nevertheless, the accepted standard operative procedure for a stricture resulting in a large bowel obstruction is a Hartmann procedure. Rarely, a very unstable patient may only tolerate a transverse-loop colostomy, which is more prudent and successful when a carcinoma is likely to be the aetiology of obstruction (Hackford, 1985).

Laparoscopic Approach

The laparoscopic approach for complicated diverticular disease is challenging; nevertheless it has shown promise in numerous series throughout the current literature (Sher et al., 1997). The study by Sher et al. (1997) showed that laparoscopic resections with primary intra-corporeal anastomoses for complicated diverticulitis were performed without additional morbidity when compared with a well-matched group of patients undergoing the same procedure by laparotomy. These patients were also stratified by severity of disease, and the benefits of a laparoscopic approach were more apparent in Hinchey I patients, notably no perioperative morbidity. They also documented a decreased length of stay (5 days) in both Hinchey stages I and II disease treated laparoscopically compared with the open approach. It is noteworthy that none of the patients in the laparoscopic group required a nasogastric tube. Perioperative morbidity was no different from the open group; moreover, as they ascend the learning curve, the morbidity reduced to less than that of the open approach. Other authors have noted similar findings, documenting a decrease in incidence of ileus, a decreased length of stay and a decreased morbidity (Bruce et al., 1996; Lieberman et al., 1996). Thus, the laparoscopic approach is a viable option for patients with complicated diverticular disease, specifically for patients with Hinchey stage I and II disease (Sher et al., 1997). Future data from prospective randomized trials will dictate the best approach, but the principles of excising the diseased segment with a tension-free anastomosis to the top of the rectum, not more proximal, are of particular importance and should not be compromised regardless of the approach.

Nursing Considerations

Owing to the increase of diverticular disease and its related complications in western society, nurses need to be aware that this disease poses a significant health problem. Because the nurse is an integral part of the care of the patient, knowledge of the pathophysiology, aetiology and clinical features of this disease should be acquired. Gaining such knowledge can occur through reading educational books, attending educational programmes in the hospital and the community and working closely with knowledgeable physicians.

The care of the patient incorporates a team of professionals. Planning the appropriate care requires the sharing of information and mutual support. The nurse's responsibility includes assessing the patient thoroughly. The assessment should include a medical/surgical history, medication, allergies, diet, history of the patient's chief complaint and physical examination. During the course of this process, as the nurse communicates with the patient, the nurse develops a rapport with the individual. The nurse should be able to evaluate the patient's level of education and understanding, psychosocial health status, coping mechanisms and expectations of care. This information will help the team decide on the course of evaluation and treatment. It also allows the team to better educate the patient on his/her level of comprehension. By utilizing the information set out in this chapter, the nurse will be prepared to care effectively for the patient with diverticular disease.

Patient Assessment

Patients with suspected diverticular disease should have their health history reviewed carefully during the nursing assessment. The nurse should begin by taking a health history of gastrointestinal disorders including diverticulosis, diverticulitis, previous evaluation and treatment and/or any hospitalizations for diverticular disease. Information should be elicited regarding endoscopic, radiologic or surgical procedures and their outcomes. Abdominal pain should be assessed indicating severity, location, duration, quality such as cramping, dull ache or sharp shooting and any other associated symptoms such as nausea, vomiting, flatulence and defecation. When discussing bowel habits with a patient, the nurse should differentiate between normal versus a change in bowel habits. It should be noted when the change occurred or if it was associated with diarrhoea or constipation. The description of bowel movements should include shape, size, colour, consistency, frequency, rectal bleeding and any associated symptoms such as fever, pain, flatulence and abdominal bloating. Additional assessment should include recent occurrence of fever and/or chills as well as a dietary history. This history should include a typical daily diet and daily fibre and fluid intake (Table 9.1).

Table 9.1: Fibre content of some foods

Fruits, grains, vegetables	Serving size	Fibre content
Banana	1	2 g
Apple	1	3 g
Pineapple	1/2cup	1 g
Cantaloupe	1/4	1 g
Strawberries	1 cup	3 g
Peach	1	2 g
Raspberries	1 cup	6 g
Acorn squash	3/4 cup	4 g
Peas	1/2 cup	4 g
Black-eyed peas	1/2 cup	4 g
Broccoli	1/2 cup	1 g
Brussels sprouts	1/2 cup	3 g
Lettuce	1 cup	1 g
Bagel	1	2 g
Wholewheat bread	1 slice	2 g
White bread	1 slice	1 g
Fibre One cereal	1/3 cup	12 g
Oatmeal	2/3 cup	3 g
White rice	1 cup	1 g
Brown rice	1 cup	3 g
Macaroni, spaghetti	1 cup	1 g

Abdominal Physical Examination

When performing an abdominal physical examination, four components should be included. Initially a visual inspection of the abdomen
should be done. From the right side of the bed, the contour of the
abdomen should be noted and observation made for peristalsis.
Increased peristaltic waves may indicate intestinal obstruction (Bates,
1983). Second, auscultation is useful in evaluating bowel motility and
abdominal complaints. Auscultation should be done before percussion
and palpation as these techniques may alter the bowel sounds.
Auscultation should be performed using a stethoscope noting the
bowel sound, frequency and character. Hyperactive bowel sounds may
indicate intestinal obstruction and high-pitched 'tinkling sounds' may
suggest intestinal fluid and air under tension in a dilated bowel
(Thelan et al., 1990). Absence of bowel sounds may indicate an ileus.
The third and fourth components of the abdominal assessment are
percussion and palpation. When performing percussion, tympanic
sounds may be found under circumstances where it is significant

enough to cause partial obstruction. When palpating an abdomen, note any tender thickened area of the sigmoid colon in the left lower quadrant. Also note any distention due to gas. These features may be indicative of diverticulitis.

Nursing Diagnoses

As stated earlier, nursing is an integral part of the care of the patient. Nurses must realize and keep in mind that there are problems a patient may experience that can be treated independently. These problems are more of a human response than a cellular response (Carpenito, 1983). Nursing diagnoses focus on these types of responses and help nurses implement their theoretical knowledge in the actual hands-on care of the patient (Carpenito, 1983). The following is a list of potential nursing diagnoses that may pertain to patients with diverticular disease.

Alteration in comfort:
- pain related to diverticular disease.

Alteration in bowel elimination:
- constipation related to low-fibre diet;
- diarrhoea alternating with constipation related to diverticular disease;
- anxiety related to concern about the possibility of complications and malignancy.

Knowledge deficit:
- symptoms of diverticulosis;
- symptoms of diverticulitis;
- lack of understanding of the relation between diet and diverticulosis. (Carpenito, 1984)

Dietary Advice

It is believed that the absence of roughage from the diet accounts for the high incidence of diverticular disease in developed or industrialized countries particularly the United States, United Kingdom and Australia (US Department of Health and Human Services, 1996). Because this condition was rare in the nineteenth century, a change in dietary habits was thought to be the incriminating factor (Corman, 1993). Studies have shown that in the past 100 years, the greatest change in people's diet has been the reduction in the amount of cereal and fibre (Corman, 1993). A diet enriched with fibre may reduce symptoms of diverticulosis and prevent complications such as diverticulitis. Fibre is a term used to describe the indigestible portion of plant foods. The most useful classification of dietary fibre is soluble and insoluble fractions. Most foods contain both in varying proportions. Purified (e.g. pectin or guar) or partially purified (e.g. wheat or bran) preparations are produced to serve specific functions such as bulk additives to cereal products, as thickeners in jams, ice cream and salad dressing, or as therapeutic agents (Jeejeebhoy, 1988).

Soluble fibre increases the viscosity of solutions thereby forming a gel. This type of fibre stays in the stomach and helps to slow food absorption. Soluble fibre is used to aid in the treatment of high cholesterol, diabetes and diarrhoea. It is found in cereals such as barley and oats, peas, dried beans, potatoes, apples and oranges (Jeejeebhoy, 1988). Insoluble fibres retain water, thereby producing softer, bulkier stools. This decreases the pressure on the colon wall, which in turn can help relieve pain and associated symptoms of diverticular disease. It also helps to promote better regularity. Insoluble fibres are found in many fruits, vegetables and whole-grain foods, such as wheat and rye bread, brown rice and pasta (Jeejeebhoy, 1988). A high-fibre diet should include 25–50 grams of fibre a day (Robinson et al., 1993) (see Table 9.1). Initially, people who typically consume low-fibre diets may experience flatulence, bloating and diarrhoea. To avoid this undesirable effect, the fibre should be increased gradually over a period of 6 to 8 weeks. While increasing fibre consumption, it is important to increase fluid intake at the same time. At least eight to ten glasses of fluid should be consumed daily. People who experience difficulty increasing fibre may benefit from over-the-counter fibre supplements such as Citrucel (Fybogel).

Health Education

An essential part of nursing care is health education. Nurses should strive to educate patients to the fullest regarding the disease. As with any disease it is important to provide patients with the knowledge and tools to best adapt to the residual effects of the illness. Providing patients with written material as well as verbal discussion should help to achieve this goal. Written material for diverticular disease should include information on definitions, symptoms, complications, diagnostic testing, treatment and dietary advice (Table 9.2). To aid in complying with a high-fibre diet it may be helpful to refer the patient to a nutritionist.

Table 9.2: Practical suggestions for increasing dietary fibre

Bread	Choose wholewheat, rye, pumpernickel multi-grain
Cereals	Select those with wholegrain ingredients or bran – wheat, oats, corn, rice
Crackers	Wholewheat or rye, or rice crackers made from brown rice
Rolls and muffins	Choose wholewheat, bran or oat bran
Pasta	Try wholegrain, or at least add a fibrous vegetable if serving with pasta
Rice	Substitute brown for white
Fruits and vegetables	When possible, eat fruits and vegetables with the skin or peel left on
Legumes	Increase consumption of kidney beans, split peas, lentils, chickpeas
Baking	When white flour is called for, substitute wholewheat for part or all of the flour

Source: Modified from: MacDonald HB, Howard M (1990) Eat Well, Live Well: The Canadian Dietetic Association's Guide to Healthy Eating.

Conclusion

The prevalence of diverticular disease is rising with the modernization and senescence of our society. Hospitalization with medical and surgical treatment has become more common in the ultimate management of diverticular disease. This has adversely contributed to the rocketing health care costs and crisis in the USA, Europe and throughout the continuously industrializing world today. This common treatable disease deserves more attention than it has received. Prevention with alterations in diet should be emphasized. In addition, identifying and treating patients who may benefit from surgical therapy early in the course of the disease will minimize the morbidity and mortality rate. Educating doctors and nurses and other health care professionals as to the natural history of diverticular disease will also decrease the morbidity and mortality associated with common colorectal disorders. There is, therefore, a need for health care professionals to participate actively in educational programmes in hospitals and in the community. The information provided should give patients an understanding of the importance of a high-fibre diet, as a result of which patients may report normal bowel patterns without constipation, diarrhoea or abdominal pain. There should also be an understanding of the symptoms of diverticulosis and its complications. In addition, the patient should express knowledge of the importance of following a high-fibre diet. Prevention and education will undoubtedly have a beneficial impact in the management and outcome of this prevalent disorder.

References

Almy JP, Howell DA (1980) Diverticular disease of the colon. New England Journal of Medicine 302: 324–31.

Auguste L, Borrero E, Wise L (1986) Surgical management of perforated colonic Diverticulitis. Archives of Surgery 151: 269–71.

Bates B (1983) A Guide to Physical Examination. Philadelphia: JB Lippincott.

Bruce CJ, Coller JA, Murray JJ, Schoetz DJ Jr, Roberts PL, Rusin LC (1996) Laparoscopic resection for divertcular disease. Diseases of the Colon and Rectum 39: 51–6.

Carpenito LJ (1983). Nursing Diagnosis Application to Clinical Practice. Philadelphia: JB Lippincott.

Carpenito LJ (1984) Handbook of Nursing Diagnosis. Philadelphia: JB Lippincott.

Corman, ML (1993) Colon and Rectal Surgery. Philadelphia: JB Lippincott.

Hackford AW, Schoetz DJ Jr, Coller JA, Veidenheimer MC (1985) Surgical management of complicated diverticulitis. The clinic experience 1967 to 1982. Diseases of the Colon and Rectum 28: 317–21.

Heller SN, Hackler LR (1978) Changes in crude fiber content of the American Diet. American Journal of Clinical Nutrition 32: 1510.

Hinchey EJ, Schaal PGH, Richards GK (1978) Treatment of perforated disease of the colon. Advances in Surgery 12: 85–109.

Jeejeebhoy K (1988) Current Therapy in Nutrition. Toronto: BC Decker.

Lieberman MA, Phillips EH, Carroll BJ, Fasslas M, Rosenthal R (1996) Laparoscopic colectomy vs traditional colectomy for diverticulitis. Surgical Endoscopy 10: 15–18.

MacDonald HB, Howard M (1990) Eat Well, Live Well: The Canadian Dietetic Association's Guide to Healthy Eating. Toronto: Macmillan of Canada.

Ouriel K, Schwartz SI (1983) Diverticular disease in the young patient. Surgery, Gynecology and Obstetrics 156:1–5.

Painter NS, Burkitt, DP (1971) Diverticular disease of the colon: a deficiency disease of western civilization. British Medical Journal 2: 450–4.

Painter NS, Truelove SC, Ardan GM et al. (1965) Segmentation and the localization of intraluminal pressures in the human colon with special reference to the pathognesis of colonic diverticular disease. Gastroenterology 49:169–77.

Perkins, JD, Shield CF III, Charge FE et al. (1984) Acute diverticulitis: comparison of treatment immunocompromised and non-immunocompromised patients. American Journal of Surgery 148: 745–8.

Rao PN, Knox R, Barnard RJ, Schafield PF (1987) Management of colovesical fistula. British Journal of Surgery 74: 362–3.

Roberts P, Abel M, Rosen L et al. (1995) Practice parameters for sigmoid diverticulitis. Supporting documentation, ASCRS Standard Task Force. Diseases of the Colon and Rectum 38: 127–32.

Robinson CH, Weigley ES, Mueller DH (1993) Basic Nutrition and Diet Therapy.

New York: Macmillan.

Rothenberger DH, Wiltz O (1993) Surgery for complicated diverticulitis. In Wolf BG (Guest Ed.) Surgical Clinics of North America. Philadelphia: WB Saunders.

Schoetz DJ (1993) Uncomplicated diverticulitis. In Wolf BG (Guest Ed) Surgical Clinics of North America. Philadephia: WB Saunders.

Sher ME, Agachan F, Bortul M, Nogueras JJ, Weiss EG, Wexner SD (1997) Laparoscopic surgery for diverticulitis. Surgical Endoscopy 11: 264–7.

Shils ME, Olson JA, Shike M (1994) Modern Nutrition in Health and Disease, 8th edn. Malvern: Lea & Feiberger.

Sorensen K, Luckman J (1979) Basic Nursing: A Psychophysiologic Approach. Philadelphia: WB Saunders.

Spriggs EI, Marxer OA (1925). Intestinal diverticular disease. Quarterly Journal of Medicine 19: 1.

Stable BE, Puccio E, Van Sonnenberg E, Neff CC (1990) Preoperative percutaneous drainage of diverticular abscess. American Journal of Surgery 159: 99.

Stemmermann GN (1970) Patterns of disease among Japanese living in Hawaii. Archives of Environmental Health 20: 266–73.

Telford GL (1993) Diverticular disease. In Greenfield L (Ed.) Surgery, Scientific Principles and Practice. Philadelphia: JB Lippincott.

Thelan LA, Davie JK, Under LD (1990) Texbook of Critical Care Nursing Diagnosis and Management. St Louis: Mosby.

US Department of Health and Human Services (1996) Diverticulosis and Diverticulitis, NIH Publication No. 97-1163. Washington, DC: US Department of Health and Human Services.

Welch CF, Athanasoulis CA, Galdabini JJ (1978) Hemorrhage from the large bowel with special reference to angiodysplasia and diverticular disease. World Journal of Surgery 2: 73.

Wexner SD, Dailey TH (1986). The initial management of left lower quadrant peritonitis. Diseases of the Colon and Rectum 29: 635–8.

Woods RJ, Lavery IC, Fazio VW et al. (1988) Internal fistulas in diverticular disease Diseases of the Colon and Rectum 31: 591–6.

Yamada T, Alpers DH, Owyang C, Powell DW, Sylverstein FE (1995) Textbook of Gastroenterology, Vol. 2. Philadelphia: JB Lippincott.

Chapter 10
Constipation

ELINOR TEAHON RGN, Staff Nurse, Halley Ward, Homerton
Hospital, London, UK

What is Constipation?

Constipation is not a disease in itself, but a symptom that may
indicate that a variety of pathological factors may be present. It
presents as the infrequent or incomplete passage of hard, dry stools.
There may not be any urge to defecate and pain is often experienced
in the anus, perineum or abdomen, which can be accompanied by
abdominal bloating. Other general symptoms include a bad taste in
the mouth, nausea, headache and malaise. Some patients are only able
to defecate by inserting a finger into the rectum (digitating) (Norton,
1996).

There are many different definitions of constipation, none of which
seems to be universally accepted, and it is worth noting that very often
patients and doctors will have different opinions as well. Most doctors
will classify simple constipation objectively as passing two or fewer
stools a week, whereas patients will often report being constipated
when they experience the more subjective symptoms such as difficult
or incomplete evacuation, pain, hard, dry stools, straining, nausea and
bloating – even if they are opening their bowels every day (Pfeifer and
Wexner, 1996). There is a common belief amongst the general public
and the medical/nursing profession alike that if individuals do not
have their bowels open daily they are constipated. Many people do not
have their bowels open daily but instead have their bowels open every
two to three days, passing a large soft formed stool with ease. This is
not constipation but their normal bowel habit. Constipation should be
considered as the passing of multiple small, hard stools with difficulty.

For a diagnosis of chronic constipation that would require further investigation into the underlying cause the most popular definition is two or more of the following criteria for at least 12 months:

- straining at defecation at least 25% of the time;
- lumpy or hard stools at least 25% of the time;
- a sensation of incomplete defecation at least 25% of the time;
- less than two bowel motions a week. (Pfeifer and Wexner, 1996)

- Infrequent/incomplete passage of stool
- No urge to open bowels
- Stools that are difficult to pass
- Digitation necessary to open bowels
- Pain in abdomen, perineum or anus
- Rectal prolapse
- Haemorrhoids
- Abdominal bloating
- Bad taste in mouth
- Headache
- Nausea
- Malaise

Figure 10.1: Symptoms of constipation.

The Normal Defecation Process

There are three sphincters involved in the normal defecation process. The first is a weak sphincter at the junction of the sigmoid colon and the rectum which keeps the rectum empty for most of the time. Further down, just inside the anus is the internal anal sphincter which is a circular structure of smooth muscle, and immediately outside that is the external anal sphincter constructed from striated muscle fibres and controlled by the somatic nervous system.

Approximately 600 ml of faecal matter enters the colon from the small bowel every day, and after absorption of fluid the rectum will receive around 150–200 ml of this (Norton, 1996). The defecation process is commenced when a mass movement forces faeces into the rectum through the first sphincter. The autonomic nervous system is triggered by sensory nerve fibres in the full rectum sending signals to the sacral part of the spinal cord which, via a reflex arc known as the defecation reflex, signals back to the descending colon, sigmoid colon, rectum and anus to commence strong peristaltic actions and the internal anal sphincter relaxes. The rectoanal inhibitory reflex is believed to play an important part in continence and the physiology of defecation (Martinelli, 1997). When the internal sphincter relaxes, pressure decreases in the upper part of the anal canal and the rectal content comes into contact with nerve terminals in the anal canal, telling the brain that the rectum is full.

Efferent (motor) neurones initiate other actions via the somatic nervous system which include taking a deep breath and closing the glottis, and contracting the abdominal muscles. This forces down on the faeces in the colon whilst causing the pelvic floor muscle to pull out and up on the anus therefore moving the faeces downward. The external anal sphincter can then be relaxed and defecation can occur. Except in babies and other cases such as spinal cord damage or some severe learning difficulties, the external anal sphincter is controlled at will by the individual. If it is not convenient at the time the urge is felt, defecation can be delayed by increasing the contraction of the external anal sphincter until the urge passes, usually a matter of a few minutes. The defecation reflex will not return until more faeces pass into the rectum, often several hours later. A mass movement can sometimes be initiated by taking a deep breath and contracting the abdominal muscles, which forces faeces into the rectum thereby creating a new defecation reflex. However, these self-initiated reflexes are never as effective as naturally occurring ones and so individuals who continually suppress their natural urge to defecate usually become severely constipated.

Causes of Constipation

Extra-colonic Constipation

Extra-colonic constipation is often referred to as simple constipation because it results from factors outside the colorectal area and usually responds well to simple treatment and does not require further investigation. For this reason it is sensible to exclude all the causes of simple constipation before extensive and often unpleasant investigations are commenced.

The most common cause of extra-colonic constipation is the modern lifestyle. The majority of fibre that naturally occurs in unprocessed foods has been refined out over the years in preference for highly processed convenience foods. Physical exercise has also declined with labour-saving machines taking over household tasks and

Lifestyle:
- Refined diet and low fluid intake
- Lack of exercise

Pharmacological:
- Laxative abuse
- Anticholinergics
- Antidepressants
- Opiates

Metabolic:
- Diabetes
- Hypothyroidism
- Menstrual cycle
- Pregnancy

Neurological:
- Muscular sclerosis
- Paraplegia
- Parkinson's disease
- Cerebral vascular accident

Figure 10.2: Causes of extra-colonic constipation.

a huge increase in car ownership. Unfortunately our colons have not adapted as readily as our minds.

Fibre resists chemical digestion and absorbs water therefore providing bulk and moisture to the faeces. Peristalsis in the colon is controlled by pressure receptors in the colon wall which are influenced by the volume of faeces in the colon. If fibre intake has been high and the faeces are bulky, the transit time in the colon will be decreased by strong peristaltic action and larger softer stools will be expelled more easily. A diet that is low in fibre but high in protein and fats (the typical refined diet of the West) will produce faeces that are smaller and less able to retain water. Transit time in the colon is slower which allows the colon to absorb more water, resulting in small, hard and dry stools that require straining to expel. The amount of fluid that we take in is as important as the amount of fibre. A normal soft stool contains 70% water so the amount of fluid in our system not only affects the consistency, but also the size and the transit time of the stool produced. Exercise has a direct effect on colonic motility. Changes in position vary the pressure throughout the intestines and using the abdominal muscles creates a wave of pressure throughout the colon. The combination of these encourages peristalsis, thus decreasing transit time. When a decrease in abdominal muscle tone occurs (for instance after a period of prolonged bed rest), transit time is increased and straining becomes less effective.

These factors must be considered for all patients admitted to hospital. Their normal eating and drinking patterns are immediately disrupted through lack of availability or the inability to eat and drink owing to investigations or surgery. Exercise is normally limited because the patient feels unwell and privacy can be hard to maintain especially when assistance is needed to use the toilet or, even worse, the bedpan. Surgery, particularly abdominal or pelvic, makes defecation painful and the patient may be receiving opiate analgesics, compounding the problem (Charlwood, 1987).

Certain groups of drugs given for other conditions have a side-effect of constipation. These include anticholinergics, antidepressants, iron supplements, diuretics, some antacids and opiates (and their derivatives such as codeine). When administering these drugs, bowel function should be monitored and laxatives given if necessary. However, long-term laxative use can in itself cause constipation. Many people, mainly the elderly, become overly concerned with opening their bowels on a daily basis and will take a laxative every day to prevent constipation occurring. When the colon is artificially stimulated in this way it loses its natural ability to function. Laxative abuse can also lead to diarrhoea, dehydration either through excess fluid loss or the inability to absorb water, a deficiency in the fat soluble vitamins A, D, E and K and an increased risk of anaemia and osteoporosis in the elderly through absorption difficulties.

Certain psychiatric disorders have a marked effect on bowel function. The disturbance of neurotransmitters shown in clinical depression can alter the regulation of the body biochemically and slow down gastric and intestinal movements affecting both normal eating and elimination patterns. If this is coupled with the constipating effect of antidepressant medication the result can be severe constipation. In anorexia nervosa the basal metabolic rate is lowered and this, together with a greatly reduced dietary intake, leads to slow transit of small stools through the bowel.

Other conditions that slow down the metabolic rate through hormonal control and cause an increased risk of constipation are diabetes and hypothyroidism. The majority of constipation in young adults is suffered by women, usually in the second half of their menstrual cycle; it is also a very common side-effect of pregnancy. The

expanding uterus puts pressure on the colon; the increased proges-
terone level has a relaxing effect on smooth muscle including the
colon; nausea and cravings can result in dehydration; and light, low-
fibre diets and haemorrhoids and perineal repairs can cause extreme
pain on attempted defecation.

Neurological disorders cause constipation through a disordered
nerve supply. Parasympathetic stimuli are lost and voluntary control is
absent or greatly reduced. This results in reduced colonic motility
and/or an absent defecation reflex with little or no control over the
anal sphincters. The main disorders causing this are multiple sclerosis,
spinal cord injury, Parkinson's disease and cerebral vascular accidents.

Colonic Constipation

Colonic dysmotility:
- Slow transit constipation
- Constipation-predominant irritable bowel syndrome
- Carcinoma
- Diverticular disease

Disordered rectal evacuation:
- Rectal prolapse
- Rectocele
- Hirschsprung's disease
- Mega-colon or mega-rectum
- Anismus

Figure 10.3: Causes of colonic constipation.

Colonic constipation results from abnormalities within the bowel itself
and demands further investigation and treatment of the underlying
cause. This can be the result of slow transit times in the colon or difficulty in evacuation.

Irritable bowel syndrome is well known to present as diarrhoea or a
cycle of diarrhoea and constipation, but can present as constipation
alone. Owing to the excessive muscular activity it results in pellet-like
stools passed frequently rather than infrequent defecation.
Diverticular disease can increase transit time by abnormal muscle
contractions which at worst can result in total bowel obstruction.

Idiopathic slow transit constipation is, as its name suggests, a condition in which the transit time around the colon is increased allowing more
fluid to be absorbed from the faeces, resulting in small hard stools. There
is reduced peristalsis but the colon appears normal in size and shape.

Tumours may cause constipation in a number of ways. A tumour growing within the bowel will gradually form an obstruction by narrowing the lumen of the bowel, whereas a tumour growing elsewhere in the pelvis may obstruct the bowel by placing pressure on it or by shifting the colon out of its normal position. Blood supply to the colon may be impeded affecting motility, or peritoneal metastases may invade the colon causing obstruction. All carcinomas of the bowel will usually cause a change in bowel habit without necessarily causing an obstruction.

Adhesions and strictures from previous surgery can also cause constipation or even total obstruction. Adhesions are cobweb-type structures of scar tissue that can form around the bowel or peritoneum whereas a stricture is a thickening and narrowing of the lumen of the bowel, in this case caused by surgery, but stricture can be caused by carcinomas or inflammation as from ulcerative colitis or Crohn's disease.

Conditions which cause difficulty with evacuating faeces from the rectum can also be grouped under the term pelvic outlet obstruction. Faeces move correctly through the colon, but the rectum is unable to pass them out, resulting in a backlog which then enables the colon to absorb more fluid from the faeces, so the already dysfunctioning rectum or anus then has to deal with smaller, harder stools.

Adult Hirschsprung's disease is a very rare condition in which small parts of the rectum or colon are totally without a nerve supply and have inefficient motility. It is usually diagnosed a few days after birth when the meconium is not passed, but a fraction of the small group with this disease will not be diagnosed until early adulthood.

A rectocele results from an abnormally thin rectovaginal septum. All the nerves supplying the rectum and anus are intact, but when straining occurs the faeces create a bulge in the septum (the muscle wall between the rectum and vagina) instead of moving down and passing out of the body. This bulge protrudes into the vagina and can be manipulated back into place until straining occurs again. Some women apply pressure to the posterior vaginal wall whilst straining to prevent it occurring, whilst others find it necessary to digitate their anus to achieve a bowel movement. Although the defect in the rectovaginal septum may have been present for several years, it will not normally become symptomatic until the woman reaches her forties or fifties.

In some cases there is an inappropriate contraction of the external anal sphincter and pelvic floor muscles which does not allow faeces to pass through. The individual will strain excessively, totally unaware that he/she is actually contracting these muscles. This is known as paradoxical contraction or anismus.

A rectal prolapse will cause constipation because the prolapsed mucosa will interfere with the nerve signals which trigger the defecation reflex.

If any of the causes of constipation are left untreated for a prolonged period the result can be a mega-rectum or mega-colon. As the colon or rectum has been overstretched for some time it becomes enlarged with decreased elasticity and muscle tone, making the peristaltic actions ineffective and therefore the transit of faeces more and more difficult.

Investigations

Investigations to find the cause of constipation can be divided into two categories. Structural tests look for abnormalities of the anatomy of the bowel, whilst functional tests look for abnormalities in the physiology of the bowel. However, the primary and most important investigation must be a detailed history of the problem. If this is done properly then the cause can often be identified and rectified with no invasive procedures whatsoever.

A history should include details of the normal bowel habit, how it has changed and over what time-scale, any recent lifestyle changes or changes in diet, a full pharmacological history and details of any other

---

- History
- Anal examination

Structural investigations:
- abdominal X-ray
- sigmoidoscopy
- colonoscopy
- barium enema

Functional investigations:
- colonic transit studies
- defecating proctogram
- anorectal manometry
- electrophysiological studies

Figure 10.4: Investigations into the cause of constipation.

illness or syndrome that the patient may have. This should reveal any causes of extra-colonic constipation that may be resolved with a simple alteration to diet, lifestyle or medication, but it does not exclude any colonic causes which may need more urgent treatment (such as neoplasms), so details of weight loss, nausea and vomiting, previous bowel disorders or abdominal surgery are essential. The history should be accompanied by a digital examination of the anus (and vagina in women if a rectocele is suspected) which may reveal haemorrhoids, bleeding, hard dry faeces, watery faeces, pain, or any low masses. If anything is suspected other than an obvious extra-colonic cause, then more investigations must be undertaken, usually starting with the structural ones.

Structural Investigations

A plain abdominal X-ray is able to confirm that the bowel is loaded with faeces and will also often identify whether there is an obstruction present. Once this has been done it is usual to move on to perform an endoscopy. A sigmoidoscopy will enable detailed examination of the rectum and sigmoid colon and a colonoscopy will enable the practitioner to visualize as far as the caecum. These procedures will reveal any abnormalities in the lining of the rectum or colon, such as polyps, diverticuli or growths, or any changes to the size of the bowel such as mega-colon, and allow for biopsies to be taken at the time of the test. If the rectum is not loaded a sigmoidoscopy requires no physical preparation (in the case of a full rectum an enema may be given) whereas a colonoscopy will require full bowel cleansing over a two-day period. A barium enema gives a very clear picture of the structure of the colon. An enema of barium contrast is given to the patient and a series of X-rays taken over about an hour, during which time the patient's position is changed to enable the barium to reach all parts of the colon. This investigation also requires full bowel cleansing.

Functional Investigations

If nothing has been revealed in the structural investigations then an examination of the function of the colon, rectum and anus should be made. These are often highly technical procedures and require referral to a specialist centre.

Colonic transit studies reveal the time it takes for faeces to travel through the colon. The patient swallows radio-opaque markers which move through the bowels in the faeces. On the fifth and seventh days X-rays are taken which show where the markers have reached. A normal colon will have expelled 80% of markers on the fifth day and all of them by the seventh. This will show whether there is a slow-transit constipation or if the transit time is normal but there is a backlog at the rectum.

A defecating proctogram is useful when a pelvic outlet obstruction is suspected, particularly a rectocele. A thick barium paste is introduced into the rectum and X-rays are taken while the patient attempts to pass the paste. This will show the angle of the anal canal and the direct effect of contracting or relaxing the muscles and sphincters during attempted defecation.

Anorectal manometry measures the pressures within the anal canal. A small tube is inserted into the rectum which records the pressure created by the anal muscles contracting and relaxing. This is useful in diagnosing anismus or adult Hirschsprung's disease (although a rectal biopsy is required to confirm this).

The defecation reflex can be examined using electrophysiological studies. These can highlight nerve or muscle damage, particularly that caused by childbirth.

Treatment

Simple Constipation

The first-line treatment of simple constipation is to increase the fibre content of the diet accompanied by an increased fluid intake. Fibre should be sought from a variety of sources and intake should be spread throughout the day, not just taken at breakfast (Chiarelli and Markswell, 1992). Food manufacturers have improved their labelling of products vastly over the years and the fibre content of most foods is now easily identifiable on the label. It is widely agreed that 27–40 g of fibre a day is a sufficient amount for an adult. Fruit, vegetables, cereals, and nuts all contain varying amounts of fibre and at least one (preferably two) groups should be included at every meal. Wholemeal or wholegrain bread is better than white or brown, as are breakfast cereals with a high bran content. Wholemeal pasta and brown rice can easily be substituted for white and pulses can be 'hidden' in soups and casseroles if they are disliked. Potatoes are most fibrous when eaten with their skins on and vegetables should be lightly cooked to avoid breaking down valuable fibre.

If these dietary changes fail to produce an effect, the patient may require added bran in his/her foods. This must be done with caution (particularly in the elderly), starting slowly and then building up until the desired effect is reached. This allows the colon time to readapt to a more normal stool size and consistency and not to be suddenly over-loaded and unable to function.

A recommended starting point is two teaspoonfuls added to every meal and slowly increased after two weeks until the patient is able to defecate regularly without straining. Once the individual's require-ment is reached, he/she should continue to take the same amount to prevent constipation recurring (Painter, 1980).

As fibre keeps the stool soft by retaining water, adequate fluids must accompany any increase in fibre in the diet. The recommended daily intake is two litres and caffeine should be kept to a minimum. Few people manage to drink that amount every day, so it is worth examin-ing how much the patient drinks at present and then aim to increase that to two litres or more until a balance is reached. Asking someone who normally takes only one litre a day to double the amount is prob-ably quite unrealistic!

If possible, exercise should be increased. This does not have to be anything too vigorous: taking the stairs instead of the lift, walking some of the bus route, or a brisk walk in the evening should be sufficient to aid peristalsis.

At first laxatives may be needed to get things moving. This should always be viewed as a short-term measure to be tailed off once the increased fibre and fluids start to take effect. Stimulant laxatives act by irritating the colon and therefore increasing motility. Many of the old-fashioned laxatives commonly used by the elderly such as syrup of figs and castor oil fall into this group. Lubricants soften the stool and coat the lining of the bowel, which makes the passage of faeces easier.

Osmotic laxatives retain water in the bowel, as the name suggests, by osmosis, and bulking agents increase the bulk of the stool in much the same way as fibre. Bulking agents must be given with caution when being taken with a high-fibre diet and fluids must always be increased to avoid causing an obstruction of large dry and hard faeces.

Suppositories are beneficial as they often have an effect almost immediately which tends to relieve any acute perineal pain. They should be placed in the rectum (past the anus) next to the wall and retained for as long as possible to allow them to act, and this is best achieved if inserted blunt end first (Abd-El-Maeboud et al., 1991). If suppositories fail, then an enema should be tried. Although they are usually the most effective pharmacological means to relieve simple constipation, enemas are also the most distressing and embarrassing for the patient so are usually best left until other measures have failed.

If the patient has a history of long-term laxative use it can be difficult to convince him/her that this is why he/she is constipated now and it may be necessary to spend a lot of time reassuring such patients that it is beneficial to try other means to counteract their constipation. They may have a misconception about what constipation actually is, believing themselves to be constipated if they do not open their bowels every day. The laxatives should first be substituted with milder ones and then slowly withdrawn, allowing the colon plenty of time to readjust to normal.

It is also important to tell patients how to open their bowels. It should be emphasized that enough time must be allowed for the procedure and that there are right and wrong positions. Shortly after eating, particularly after breakfast, is often a good time as the gastrocolic reflex has stimulated waves of peristaltic action, and they should be encouraged to allow about 15 minutes if needed. Modern pedestal toilets do not make defecating any easier as the ideal position in which to open the bowels is squatting (the position that young children automatically adopt). This allows the anal canal to open fully and the pelvic floor is braced, supporting the anus. Both feet should be flat with knees apart and elbows placed on knees. A foot-stool can be used to raise the knees above the level of the hips (Chiarelli and Markswell, 1992).

Colonic Constipation

Patients suffering from colonic constipation do not respond well to increased fibre intake. Indeed, it can actually lead to worsening pain and bloating. Many patients will become resistant to oral laxatives and even enemas will have a limited effect (Storrie, 1997). This small group of patients is left with two treatment options: biofeedback and surgery.

Biofeedback is an effective treatment for retraining the nerves and muscles in evacuation disorders, and is based on B.F. Skinner's operant conditioning. The patient is given information or feedback about an aspect of his/her biological state, in this case the rectum and anus, and is reinforced for altering that state (Atkinson et al., 1990). A balloon is placed in the rectum which produces the feeling of needing to defecate and electrodes are placed near the external anal sphincter. These are then linked to a display screen and the patient is able to see the effects of attempts to contract and relax the sphincter. He/she is encouraged to perform relaxation exercises before attempted defecation and is taught to use the abdominal muscles effectively. The training takes place over a number of sessions and is often accompanied by counselling and behavioural therapy, such as setting a routine time every day to practise the exercises in the toilet. Ongoing support is crucial to this treatment as results may take weeks to take effect, and it is carried out at specialist centres involving a multidisciplinary team of biofeedback specialist nurse, psychologist, physiotherapist, continence nurse specialist and clinical scientist (Storrie, 1997).

Surgical intervention is the last resort in the management of colonic constipation. Patients will usually have had problems for many years and will not have responded to conservative treatments. It is not an effective treatment for anismus, but in the case of combined slow-transit constipation with anismus it can be successful when used after a period of biofeedback training (Pfeifer and Wexner, 1996).

Bowel resections for slow-transit constipation include subtotal colectomy with either ileorectal anastamosis, ileosigmoid anastamosis or caecorectal anastamosis. However, in their study Pfeifer et al. (1996) found that subtotal colectomy with ileorectal anastamosis had the highest success rate at 90%. This approach carries the same success rate when performed for idiopathic mega-bowel. Occasionally a proctocolectomy with formation of an ileoanal pouch can be performed but this is drastic action with a moderate success rate so it is usually performed after previous surgery has failed. The other alternative is to raise an ileostomy (Pfeifer and Wexner, 1996).

In the treatment of Hirschsprung's disease anorectal myectomy, rectal myectomy or anal sphincterotomy is used (i.e. the diseased part of the muscle is removed), or a bypass of the segment may be performed. In a small number of cases extensive colonic resection may be required (Moriarty and Irving, 1993).

Rectoceles require surgical repair of the rectovaginal septum and respond better when this is done transrectally then transvaginally.

Nursing Management of Simple Constipation

Assessment

1. Assess patients' knowledge of constipation:
- does the patient regard constipation as not opening the bowels every day even if the stools are soft and easy to pass?

2. Assess previous bowel function:
- Does the patient often suffer from constipation?
- How often does the patient normally open his/her bowels?
- Does the patient usually have to strain to open his/her bowels?

- Is there a particular time of day that the patient opens his/her bowels?
- Does the patient use a laxative and if so how frequently?

3. Assess current bowel function:
- How often does the patient currently open his/her bowels?
- What is the appearance of the stools, i.e. are they harder and smaller than usual?
- Does the patient have to strain to open his/her bowels?
- Over what time-scale has the change occurred?

4. Assess cause of constipation:
- Has there been a recent change in diet?
- Has there been a reduction in fluid intake; does the patient appear dehydrated?
- Has there been a reduced activity level?
- Is the patient taking any medication that may cause constipation?
- Does the patient have a disorder that may predispose to constipation, e.g. sacral cord lesion?
- Is it painful for the patient to open his/her bowels and if so where is the pain?
- Is the patient able to maintain privacy and dignity when opening his/her bowels?
- Is the patient able to communicate the need to open his/her bowels?

Planning

The aim is for the patient to be able to pass soft stools when he/she feels the need to do so, with maximum privacy and dignity.

Implementation

- Record all bowel actions daily.
- Provide assurance and education regarding what constitutes a normal bowel habit, i.e. opening bowels from between two or three times a day to three times a week as long as the output is soft and easy to pass.
- Encourage patient to increase fibre in diet. Liaise with dietitian if necessary.
- Ensure adequate fluid intake, by intravenous route if necessary.
- Encourage patient to take gentle exercise as tolerated. Liaise with physiotherapist as required.

- Examine all current medication for constipating side-effects. Liaise with doctor to withdraw or replace constipating medication, or to add an accompanying laxative if this is not possible.
- Administer an appropriate laxative to relieve current constipation. Withdraw this as soon as a regular bowel pattern becomes re-established.
- Relieve pain associated with straining by giving prescribed analgesics with an accompanying laxative if necessary. If pain is associated with recent abdominal surgery teach patient to take deep breaths to increase intra-abdominal pressure, whilst gently supporting the wound. If pain is associated with haemorrhoids, give prescribed medication. Ensure that the patient is aware that delay in opening their bowels will make the pain worse not better.
- Encourage the patient to maintain his/her usual routine as far as possible, i.e. if the patient normally has breakfast and then opens his/her bowels, ensure that he/she is given the time and facilities to do this.
- Maintain as much privacy and dignity as possible. Use the bathroom whenever possible and ensure that the patient feels safe, comfortable and unhurried. Only use commodes or bedpans when the patient is unable to be moved from the bedside.
- If there is a communication difficulty attempt to overcome this by using written words or pictures.

Evaluation

- Has the patient re-established his/her normal bowel pattern?
- If the outcome is unsuccessful, re-assess and liaise with doctor regarding further investigations.

Constipation is a common complaint in the western world which can vary in severity and duration. It can be a socially isolating problem which patients may treat in private for many years before seeking medical help. The nurse is often the first person to be aware of the problem and in many cases the sensitive handling of the situation by the nurse can lead to a rapid improvement for patients. The effects and/or causes of constipation should never be trivialized and the informed nurse practitioner has much to offer patients in the form of advice and support.

References

Abd-El-Maeboud et al. (1991) Quoted in Norton C (1996) The causes and nursing management of constipation. British Journal of Nursing 5(20): 1252–8.

Atkinson R, Atkinson R, Smith E, Beni D, Hilgard E (1990) Introduction to Psychology, 10th edn. Florida: Harcourt Brace Jovanovich.

Charlwood J (1987) Problems of the Lower Bowel Causing Constipation. London: Baillière Tindall, pp 774–7.

Chiarelli P, Markswell S (1992) Let's Get Things Moving – Overcoming Constipation. NSW, Australia: Gore & Osment Publications.

Martinelli E (1997) Computerised analysis of the rectoanal inhibitory reflex in impaired recto anal function. Techniques in Coloproctology 1: 64–7.

Moriarty K, Irving M (1993) ABC of Colorectal Diseases. London: BMJ Publishing Group.

Norton C (1996) The causes and nursing management of constipation. British Journal of Nursing 5 (20): 1252–8.

Painter N (1980) Constipation. The Practitioner 224: 387–91.

Pfeifer J, Wexner S (1996) Surgery for constipation. Postgraduate Doctor Surgery 5(4): 94–8.

Pfeifer J, Agachan F, Wexner S (1996) Surgery for constipation – a review paper. Diseases of the Colon and Rectum 39: 444–60.

Storrie J (1997) Biofeedback: a first-line treatment for idiopathic constipation. British Journal of Nursing 6(3): 152–8.

Chapter 11
Irritable Bowel Syndrome

PAULA TAYLOR RGN Colorectal Nurse Practitioner, St Mary's
Hospital NHS Trust, London, UK

Introduction

Irritable bowel syndrome (or IBS for short) affects millions of people
around the world in different ways, to different degrees and for
different reasons. It is thought a third of the population will at some
time or other experience IBS, and about one in ten people will suffer
symptoms bad enough for them to go to see their general practitioner.
Females tend to outnumber males by about 2:1 and symptoms
normally present in early adult life (15–40 years old). IBS is more
common in the developed countries of the West than in the East. This
has led to IBS being labelled as a 'disease of civilization' due to
increased consumption of more refined and 'junk' food with less
manual work and exercise; however, medical care in the West is much
more accessible than in the East and this could simply be the reason
for this apparent difference.

What Actually is IBS and Why does it Occur?

No one knows the answer to this question, but studies are going on
around the world to try to resolve this. IBS is a functional bowel disorder in which the intestinal muscle appears to react abnormally to
outside influences such as stress, infection and some foods. Faeces
normally move along the bowel with smooth, rhythmical contractions
of the muscles in the gut wall where they squeeze then relax in order to
propel the faeces along to be expelled from the anus (peristalsis).

With IBS sufferers these contractions become irregular for some
reason and can either be too strong or too weak. This could be due to a

malfunction in the peristaltic action or a problem with the way in which the nerves controlling bowel sensations work, giving IBS patients enhanced sensation and perception of their bowel functions making the gut more sensitive to certain foods, medication and stress; or perhaps it could be a combination of these two theories.

Researchers at Columbia University, New York, suspect IBS stems from an abnormality in the enteric nervous system (a branch of the autonomic nervous system that controls the digestive tract) and with the development of this system at the embryonic stage. This congenital abnormality, they say, can then be exacerbated by psychological stress. Dr Gershon and colleagues have identified the critical role played by the neurotransmitter serotonin in the motility of the digestive tract. His studies have shown that IBS sufferers respond differently to hormones released by the upper part of the gut. The researchers hope their work will eventually translate into more highly targeted drug therapies (Gershon, 1995).

Why is IBS Difficult to Diagnose and Treat?

IBS is a very complex problem to deal with for many reasons:

1. the variety of symptoms with which it presents itself;
2. the symptoms mimic other diseases of the bowel which therefore must be excluded;
3. IBS can be so different to treat from one patient to the next, with one intervention helping one patient and the same intervention making the next patient worse or having little effect;
4. the medical profession's lack of knowledge on the subject;
5. investigation results will appear normal.

Because of the complexity it takes time, understanding and knowledge on the part of the health professional to find a cause for the patient's symptoms and to plan appropriate care for each individual, looking not just at the symptoms but the patient as a whole to consider physical, psychological, emotional and social issues.

Medical help offered can vary from telling the patient it's all in the mind and he/she will have to live with it, to prescribing medication and telling the patient that this will make him/her better, to taking a careful thorough history and referring the patient to the appropriate health professional or for complementary therapies.

Studies looking at nurses' perceptions of IBS and patients with IBS showed nurses hold negative attitudes towards these patients. Sue

Letson carried out the study, using 254 qualified nurses from 18 London hospitals. The vast majority of nurses agreed with statements that IBS patients are demanding, unable to cope with life, lazy and crave attention and waste the doctor's time. Only half believed they would recognize the symptoms and felt they had a good understanding of the disorder. Half of the sample believed that doctors and other health professionals had a poor understanding of IBS. Letson concludes that such attitudes can surely only be detrimental to the treatment of those patients with IBS (Letson and Dancey, 1996).

What Symptoms Commonly Occur with IBS?

'Syndrome' is a medical word meaning a collection of symptoms that tend to occur together. The most common symptoms with IBS include abdominal spasm, pain and bloating, diarrhoea, constipation or both alternating, painful noisy wind, feeling of incomplete evacuation, a sharp pain felt low down inside the rectum, urgency or faecal incontinence and mucus from the back passage. The symptoms can vary greatly from patient to patient.

Manning et al. (1978) devised diagnostic criteria for IBS to differentiate it from other gastrointestinal disease. The six symptoms they describe are:

1. relief of abdominal pain with defecation;
2. looser stools with the onset of pain;
3. more frequent bowel movements at the onset of pain;
4. abdominal bloating or distension;
5. feeling of incomplete evacuation;
6. passage of mucus per rectum.

Generally, the more Manning criteria present the more likely it is the patient has IBS. The criteria state that the symptoms must have been present for 3 months in order to make the diagnosis. The grouping of these symptoms only occurs in IBS, whereas other conditions will produce only one or two of them.

The abdominal pain usually occurs in the left iliac fossa but can occur anywhere in the abdomen. The pain can range from a dull ache to pain so severe that the patient cannot cope with day-to-day activities. It tends to come in waves causing a crampy feeling and is typically relieved by passing flatus or a motion but for some patients the pain intensity may be more closely related to particular times of the day or to their menstrual cycle. Bloating of the abdomen is very common with IBS patients and sometimes it can remain even if the pain has been relieved by passing flatus. This can be very distressing for people trying to buy clothes to fit and feel comfortable in.

Patients with IBS may predominantly suffer with either diarrhoea or constipation or have an alternating combination of these. There may be a period of constipation or normal stool followed by a sudden attack of diarrhoea; usually the same quantity is excreted as normal, though it is more frequent and 'sloppy' rather than watery like an infective diarrhoea. Patients usually complain that their bowels are worse in the morning and can then settle throughout the day even though they feel they have to be constantly on the alert as to where the nearest toilets are.

Patients who complain of constipation but have frequent bowel movements usually feel their bowels have not been emptied completely, which can create further anxiety.

Patients often say they feel they are producing excess flatus; however, it is usually the case that the gas is just unable to escape, so building up inside the intestine, stretching the bowel and causing discomfort. Allowing the air to be expelled will help the discomfort even though this event is very embarrassing for the patient.

Mucus may be passed in the stools or passed on its own. This can cause itching around the anus as it comes into contact with the peri-anal skin.

Other gastrointestinal symptoms have also been seen in some IBS patients; examples include nausea, vomiting, heartburn and dyspepsia.

Non-gastrointestinal symptoms include dysmenorrhoea, dyspareunia, urinary frequency, loin pain, back and thigh pain, headaches, insomnia and psychiatric symptoms, especially depression.

Many patients with IBS symptoms will try to deal with these themselves by seeking advice from pharmacists and reading about self-help strategies in IBS books. Patients who do present to their doctor tend to have more serious or prolonged symptoms by the time they visit the surgery.

How is IBS Diagnosed?

A diagnosis of IBS will vary from person to person depending on the duration of the symptoms, the patient's age and clinical presentation. A careful detailed history is the first, most essential part of assessing these patients. A battery of tests is not always the right way to manage them. Unfortunately one specific test does not diagnose IBS: a diagnosis can only be made by a process of elimination when all tests show a normal healthy bowel.

Patients may have one or more of the investigations listed below in order to exclude other bowel disorders such as inflammatory bowel disease, diverticular disease, slow-transit constipation or bowel cancer.

- stool specimen for occult blood and for ova and parasites;
- blood test for anaemia and malabsorption;
- rigid sigmoidoscopy;
- flexible sigmoidoscopy;
- colonoscopy;
- double-contrast barium enema X-ray;
- barium meal
- defecating proctogram with transit studies and anorectal manometry;
- hydrogen breath test for lactose intolerance.

During the investigative and diagnostic stage it is vital to maintain the patient's respect, dignity and understanding. Nurses need to appreciate patients' anxieties as fear of malignancy is often in their mind. The investigations should be explained clearly so they understand the reason for them. Patients need to be informed how soon they will get the results and when they will be seen in the follow-up clinic.

It is important to enquire whether the patient can tell you what, if anything, may have started the symptoms of IBS. This may be an attack of gastroenteritis (which can make the bowel more sensitive); a time of stress, e.g. financial worries, divorce, exam nerves etc.; certain foods; a course of antibiotics (which can alter the balance of good bacteria in the gut); regular use of laxatives (which can irritate the bowel); or in some cases there does not appear to be any particular reason for the onset of symptoms.

After a full history has been taken from the patient a general examination, abdominal and rectal examination should be performed in the GP's surgery.

If the GP suspects IBS he/she will commonly prescribe an antispasmodic tablet and/or a bulking agent then review the patient within 4 to 6 weeks. If the symptoms have not improved GPs will tend to refer the patient to a hospital specialist.

As more is understood about IBS more doctors are keeping the amount of investigations to a minimum. Most of the tests are uncomfortable and can be embarrassing for patients and all to no avail. Today, for people under the age of 40 years old who have no family history of cancer or bowel disease, many doctors will now diagnose and treat IBS without investigation or will do a routine rigid sigmoidoscopy in clinic. People over the age of 40 may need at least a flexible sigmoidoscopy (as the left side of the colon is where the majority of serious bowel disease occurs); however, if a patient of this age has a family history of bowel disease the gold standard is to have a colonoscopy with a series of biopsies.

With patients who complain in particular of diarrhoea with excess mucus, inflammatory bowel disease needs to be excluded as this predominantly is diagnosed in the same age-group as IBS. The appropriate investigation in this case would be a colonoscopy with a full series of biopsies from terminal ileum to rectum (Crohn's disease can often start in the terminal ileum whereas ulcerative colitis usually starts in the rectum). In general, IBS sufferers are in good health apart from their IBS symptoms and do not pass blood per rectum, whereas inflammatory bowel disease sufferers will usually have blood per rectum, mucus and loose stool and are often unwell in an acute episode. An example where an IBS sufferer may have some rectal bleeding will be if in the presence of haemorrhoids from constipation; this bleeding will typically be bright red in colour, occur after defecation and seen on the toilet paper. A proctoscopy can be done to confirm this diagnosis.

Infective diarrhoea also needs to ruled out, though this can usually be done by checking whether the patient has a fever or if other family members are affected and asking the patient whether he/she has travelled abroad recently. Otherwise a stool specimen can be taken.

A double-contrast barium enema may be ordered in patients over the age of 40 who complain of hard, small, pellet-shaped motions with abdominal pain. This will exclude diverticular disease and cancer. A barium enema is not advisable in female patients under the age of 40 because of the large amount of radiation used, which can affect their reproductive organs.

A barium meal may be organized to exclude gastric and small bowel disease. This is usually only performed when the lower and upper bowel appear normal but the patient continues to have diarrhoea as the main symptom.

A defecating proctogram with transit studies may be organized for patients complaining predominantly of constipation whereby they do not pass a motion for many days and when they get the urge to go they are unable to do so. This will exclude such conditions as slow-transit contipation, intussusception and rectocele formation. Anal manometry may also be done with these symptoms to check that the patient's internal and external sphincters are functioning correctly.

A hydrogen breath test may be needed to exclude lactose intolerance.

This will be ordered if the patient feels the symptoms are related to food eaten, especially milk and milk products.

Patients who are told that their symptoms are likely to be due to IBS and that their test results are normal should be fully informed about the syndrome, how it can affect them, how to help themselves and what symptoms they should return to their GP with, as it can occur that a patient with long-term IBS subsequently develops cancer or another bowel disease.

Nurses can educate patients with IBS by informing them which bowel symptoms need to be reported to their GP which are not typically related to IBS. These include blood on or appearing mixed in the motion; a dark brown or black stool; severe pain in the abdomen that will not go away; vomiting (especially coffee-ground in appearance); losing weight when not trying to, with a poor appetite.

How can Nurses Support Patients Diagnosed with IBS?

With the nature of IBS symptoms being so diverse it is essential to manage the patient holistically. As the Greek philosopher Plato once said, 'The cure of the part should not be attempted without treatment of the whole'.

There is no one good general treatment for IBS. Different things work for different people and unfortunately the only way to know exactly what works for an individual is by trial and error. This takes time, commitment and perseverance. Often patients are referred back to the GP from the hospital with normal results and a probable diagnosis of IBS, and the patients try antispasmodics, bulking agents, analgesia or antidiarrhoeal drugs. In general the emphasis on care and long-term management of these patients does seem to come back to the primary care setting.

The difficulty with IBS patients is that they do need time to explain their symptoms and to explore why they may occur and this time is rarely available in the clinic setting, with most patients allocated just 5 or 10 minutes. Research done in Sweden showed that IBS sufferers given eight sessions of simple supportive listening and advice about lifestyle had fewer symptoms and disability, both physical and psychological, 3 months after being seen than a similar group who received no such help (Arn et al., 1989).

A specialist nurse in coloproctology or a nurse who is interested in learning about the problems facing IBS sufferers and how to help them (for example a practice nurse in the surgery setting) would be ideal to inform, guide and support newly diagnosed IBS patients until such time as they can manage the symptoms for themselves.

There are certain points that nurses need to discuss with IBS patients:

- There needs to be a careful explanation of what IBS actually is, that it is not cancer and it does not mean sufferers are more likely to get bowel cancer.
- They need to understand that it is a real medical condition, the causes of which are only now just beginning to be understood with research going on to try to find some answers.
- They need reassurance that despite what some people will say it is not all in the mind and there are things that can be done to help them.
- They need to be aware of the reality of the problem – that at present there is no cure – but reassured that the long-term observation of these patients shows that IBS does seem to improve as patients get older.
- Nurses should ensure patients have access to information to read about the syndrome, how they can help themselves and be kept updated on new findings.
- Patients should be informed about the IBS Network, how to contact them and what the benefits are of doing this. Also there is much information for IBS sufferers by accessing the relevant pages on the Internet.
- It is important that close family understand the problem so they can appreciate that even though the medical tests are normal there is a real condition that needs to be dealt with. Nurses can make sure family members are involved if this is acceptable to the patient with IBS.

What can IBS Patients do to Help their Symptoms?

Abdominal Bloating, Discomfort and Excess Flatus

This is probably the symptom most commonly reported by IBS patients, who feel as if they have excess gas which they cannot expel which in turn causes great discomfort and embarrassment. Studies have shown that people with IBS produce the same amount of gas as people without IBS. This discomfort is usually relieved by passing flatus or a motion.

Patients can be advised to avoid eating certain foods which are known to create more wind or to at least try having a smaller portion of those foods. Foods suggested are listed below (this is by no means an exhaustive list and some of the foods may be fine for some people; again it is a case of trial and error):

- artichoke;
- banana (under-ripe);
- beans (all types including baked beans);
- broccoli;
- Brussels sprouts;
- cabbage;
- cauliflower;
- cold potato salad;
- cucumber;
- curry;
- eggs;
- fizzy drinks;
- lentils;
- mushrooms;
- onions;
- pasta (if cooked, cooled then re-heated);
- radish;
- sweetcorn.

- General advice to avoid build-up of wind is to advise patients to eat slowly and chew each mouthful well before swallowing. Also more wind can accumulate if talking whilst eating or chewing gum.
- There are some products that can be bought from health food shops which can help some people to break down the wind so that there is less discomfort, for example Windeeze and Windcheaters. Also 'Ido Air', made by Nature's Best, is a natural enzyme which helps to stop the production of excess wind. It is best taken with or just before meals as it acts on complex carbohydrates, helping them to break down to simple sugars that can be comfortably absorbed without causing wind. It can be taken just before going out to eat to avoid embarrassing bloating and wind.
- Some people may find it helps to suck peppermints or take peppermint essence in warm water and drink it slowly after meals.
- Cinnamon or nutmeg added to warm water or milk can help soothe a bloated feeling in the abdomen.
- Charcoal tablets or biscuits can be bought from health food shops. These can help to break up flatus and reduce any odour.

Constipation

When patients say they are constipated they need to explain exactly the problem, i.e. is the motion hard, or difficult to pass or are they passing a normal stool but less frequently than usual for them. Bowel habits can alter from time to time for different reasons so this is why a detailed history needs to be taken to determine the real problem.

If the constipation is related to the other IBS symptoms then some of the following may help:

- Advise the IBS patient with constipation to increase the amount of fibre in the diet by eating fresh fruit, raw or lightly cooked vegetables, wholemeal bread and pasta. However, fibre needs to be introduced into the diet gradually, especially if patients suffer from abdominal bloating, to give the bowel a chance to adapt. The wheat and bran fibre products (i.e. the non-soluble fibre) should be avoided initially as these can make the problem worse owing to their harsh nature. If the patient finds it difficult to increase the amount of fibre within the diet initially, he/she should be advised to try a bulking agent, for example Fybogel, which will help to bulk the stool, which can then push more effectively against the bowel wall so that complete expulsion will take place. It is always important when advising patients on increasing their fibre intake to also increase the amount of fluid they drink as the extra fibre will need to be 'soaked up' to help it move along the bowel effectively, i.e. they should aim for approximately 10 cups of fluid a day. Some foods, such as melon, soups, ice cream and oranges, contain a lot of fluid and can be suggested if the patient finds it difficult to drink this amount.
- The nurse should ensure the patient is aware that it is not a good idea to ignore the urge to defecate, because the motion will go back up into the rectum to the colon where further absorption of water will take place, making the motion even harder and more difficult to pass.
- Difficulty in passing a motion can sometimes be due to the position a patient adopts on the toilet. Squatting is said to be the optimum position for easy evacuation but when sitting on a toilet it can help if the patient is advised to lean slightly forward from the waist and to use a small stool under the feet to press on to. If both hands are then placed on the abdomen the patient should feel the muscles pushing against the hands, thus knowing that the correct muscles are being used.
- Biofeedback therapy has been effective for some people with IBS, however, it needs to be carried out in unison with counselling, coor-

dination exercises and health education for it to have its full effect (this technique is described in more detail later in the chapter).

- Linseed and liquorice are a natural way to help prevent constipation and are available from health food shops; they can be used in cooking or sprinkled on to food.
- A deep hot bath can help ease the pain or a hot water bottle over the abdominal area can be effective for bloating.
- Regular, light daily exercise can help the motility of the bowel.
- Massage of the abdomen may help, using large stroking movements up the right side and across under the rib cage and down the left side of the abdomen. This is the direction of peristalsis and can sometimes help to get things moving or at least help relieve some trapped flatus. The patient should be advised to repeat each circular movement several times in the same spot before moving on, and always to move in the same direction as the movement of the gut. The patient should experience some relief within about 10 minutes. The use of oils to aid the massage may feel relaxing and soothing.

Diarrhoea

As with constipation the patient needs to be asked exactly what is meant by diarrhoea. Is the motion watery or just loose, is the patient passing a motion more regularly throughout the day, is there a problem with getting to the toilet in time, etc.? It is also important to establish how long the diarrhoea has been going on as bowel habits can vary from time to time for no apparent reason.

It is more common for IBS patients to suffer with diarrhoea than with constipation. It can put people off leaving their home, as they always have to be aware of the nearest toilet in case they cannot get to the toilet in time after getting the urge to pass a motion.

Diarrhoea in the IBS patient seems to occur when the muscles in the bowel are overactive and there are more squeeze than relax impulses, therefore the food passes along much quicker and the colon has much less time to do its job of absorbing water back into the system. Morning tends to be the worst time for IBS, with symptoms gradually settling throughout the day.

- High-fibre eating and a bulking agent such as Fybogel can help some people with diarrhoea as it binds the loose stools together. It is worth trying but if things do not improve within a week this needs to be reviewed.
- Antidiarrhoeal tablets are usually effective, for example codeine

phosphate or Imodium. These work by slowing the motility of the gut so allowing the colon more time to absorb water back into the system from the food residue.

- With diarrhoea-related IBS it is worth investigating the patient to see if there is a food intolerance (see below).
- The patient should be advised to avoid fatty and fried foods as they will pass through the bowel too quickly, exacerbating the diarrhoea
- Patients should try to avoid too much salad, curried and spicy foods and also citrus fruits.
- The nurse should inform the patient about the IBS Network (or similar charity in the USA), which will supply patients with a 'can't wait' card to get quick access to toilets in public areas.

What Medication is Commonly Prescribed for IBS Patients?

Some of the drugs prescribed by doctors may help with the symptoms but it may only be short-term relief that is gained, and a more permanent answer may need to be sought. Medication may not get to the root of the problem and patients need to be made aware of this.

The main groups of drugs prescribed are antispasmodics, anticholinergics, bulk laxatives, antidiarrhoeal tablets, benzodiazepines and antidepressants.

Antispasmodics

The pain associated with IBS is thought to be due to spasm in the bowel and if this tends to be the most troublesome symptom to the patient antispasmodics are worth trying. They work by either slowing down intestinal movement or by exerting a direct relaxant effect on intestinal muscle:

1. Dicyclomine (Merbentyl) appears to work in both ways, relieving stomach cramps and colicky abdominal pain with few unwanted side-effects.
2. Mebeverine hydrochloride (Colofac) and alverine citrate (Spasmonal, Relaxyl) claim 80% effectiveness in their trials; however, studies using a placebo group have been inconclusive. Both mebeverine and alverine have few side-effects as they act only on the digestive tract and are generally tolerated better than the anticholinergics (described below) although there is no evidence that they are any more effective.

3. Peppermint oil (Colpermin, Mintec) is a non-anticholinergic smooth muscle relaxant which also has antispasmodic effects. It may be tried as an alternative to, or in combination with, another antispasmodic if an inadequate response is obtained with the latter. It can sometimes take several weeks to produce a response. It can help to suppress colonic spasm and relieve the discomfort of trapped wind, and the flatulence expelled tends to smell more acceptable (like peppermint). Recommended dosage is two capsules up to three times a day. Adverse effects are minor, e.g. irritation of the mouth if the capsule is not swallowed whole, and occasional dyspepsia.

Anticholinergics

Anticholinergic agents work by decreasing the abnormal sensitivity of cholinergic receptors in the smooth muscle of the gut. Examples include hyoscine butylbromide (Buscopan) and propantheline bromide (Pro-Banthine) which are used quite widely but the evidence shows little real effect. Patients should be warned about possible adverse effects such as a dry mouth, blurred vision and difficulty in micturating. These drugs should be avoided in people with glaucoma and patients with a history of prostatic or cardiac disease as they can cause dysrhythmias. They can also tend to constipate so they are best avoided in the group of IBS patients who suffer predominantly from constipation. They are best used on an 'as required' basis in order to prevent dependence.

Bulk laxatives

These may be of use to patients who suffer mainly from constipation-related IBS. One study showed a significant improvement with 82% resolution of symptoms (Prior and Whorwell, 1987). They work by softening the stool by retaining water, and can also help some people with diarrhoea by making the bowel function more regular by binding the stool; however, they can also make the patient feel much worse. It is always important to advise sufferers to increase the amount they drink when taking a bulk laxative such as Fybogel.

Commonly prescribed laxatives for constipation, e.g. Duphalac (lactulose) can cause more colonic spasm and pain and are therefore best avoided with IBS sufferers. Its side-effects are flatulence, stomach cramps and nausea; however, this drug is often prescribed for IBS patients with constipation. Senokot (senna) is a stimulant laxative which will increase the activity in the colon and hence cause more pain. These products should certainly be avoided long term in IBS sufferers.

Antidiarrhoeal drugs

These drugs, e.g. loperamide (Imodium), help to slow the motility of the bowel to reduce the frequency of defecation so that the patient can exert a degree of control to reduce urgency and incontinence. The dose can be adjusted to the patient's need to the lowest that will produce a satisfactory response. Long-term use should be safely monitored by the patient's doctor.

Benzodiazepines

These drugs can sometimes produce relief from IBS symptoms although the effect may often be short term with a high risk of dependence. They also may effect the patient's ability to deal with an underlying problem which may be exacerbating the symptoms. Lorazepam and diazepam (Valium) are examples. Their side-effects can include drowsiness, changes in vision and confusion. When IBS symptoms are accompanied by anxiety or panic attacks a short course may be useful, or when a particularly traumatic event has temporarily made symptoms worse, but generally they are best avoided.

(Passiflora is a natural tranquillizer, is readily available in the form of tablets taken before going to bed and is not habit-forming.)

Antidepressant drugs

These are sometimes prescribed if the patient's IBS is associated with depression. They are thought to have a direct action on the gut so that they modify gut sensation, leading to altered brain perception about what is occurring in the gut. Examples include imipramine (Tofranil), dothiepin (Prothiaden) and fluoxetine (Prozac).

A combination of the medicines described above will often give relief in the short term but IBS is more often than not a long-term disorder, so drugs cannot really be the permanent answer. Sometimes the solution may lie in what is eaten, or how patients live and cope with their lives. Once bulk laxatives have produced a soft stool for a period of two weeks then this state should ideally be maintained by a high-fibre diet. Similarly with antispasmodics, when they reduce the pain the patient should be encouraged to look at what is causing any tension and how it could be dealt with positively. Some medication for IBS is now available without prescription, including:

- alverine citrate (Relaxyl);
- Boots IBS relief (this contains 135 mg mebeverine hydrochloride);
- Colofac IBS (this contains 135 mg mebeverine hydrochloride);
- Colpermin and Mintec (0.2 ml peppermint oil).

It is important for patients trying 'over the counter' treatment to read the literature in the packet to make sure the medication is suitable for them, or they should discuss the product with a health professional. If the symptoms continue or do not improve, they should be advised to see their doctor.

What Effects can IBS have on the Individual's Life?

In June 1996 the results of an IBS postal survey were published in *Gut Reaction* newsletter from the IBS Network. This was conducted nationwide amongst people who had enquired about IBS. There were 827 questionnaires returned and analysed. The results are as follows:

- 75% claim that IBS has a negative effect on their lives and over half of these said their symptoms caused them to cancel social engagements;
- 55% find their symptoms embarrassing;
- 79% have to watch what they eat;
- 29% found using public transport a problem;
- 62% said their worst symptom was abdominal pain. Other symptoms in order of severity were flatulence, bloating, diarrhoea, constipation and nausea;
- 29% said IBS had a negative effect on their relationships and affected their sexual life;
- a third of those who said it had a negative effect on their relationships also complained that their partners were unsympathetic and some found it too embarrassing to talk about it with them;
- 39% of those in full-time employment had taken time off work as a result of their symptoms. Of theses 43% claimed not to have given IBS as a reason for missing work;
- 71% of those taking time off work thought that IBS had a negative effect on their career and over half of these said that they were frightened to go to work because of the pain;

- 21% claimed their colleagues were unsympathetic to their symptoms;
- 63% felt stress was the main cause of their symptoms (rising to 72% amongst 15- to 44-year-olds). Over half agreed that they had stressful lives and admitted to suffering from other stress-related conditions such as indigestion, headaches, hay fever and asthma;
- three in 10 sufferers experienced their symptoms for more than 5 years before a diagnosis was made and 37% for between 1 and 5 years.

Are there any Foods which should be Avoided by the IBS Patient?

Unfortunately there is no 'ideal' diet for people suffering from IBS. Foods which suit one person will not suit another. This is because people will suffer different symptoms but the condition is still termed IBS and one person's symptoms could be due to a food intolerance or be the result of stress or a medical problem. This is why the newly diagnosed IBS patient needs a thorough history taken and assessment made of symptoms, diet and lifestyle so that real help may be offered. The underlying cause needs to be found to be able to treat the problem effectively.

One of the first things most people with IBS are told to do is to increase the amount of fibre in their diet as it is thought IBS may be the result of a lack of fibre in the diet but research shows this generally not to be the case. Some patients with constipation-predominant IBS find increasing the amount of fibre in their diet will help their symptoms but the majority find that excess bran makes their symptoms much worse. In one study more than 70% of patients gained relief from their symptoms when placed on a simple bland diet of plain fish, lamb, and a few vegetables (Allun-Jones et al., 1982).

Some foods do contain chemicals which appear to upset the lining of the bowel and therefore bring on the symptoms of IBS. Wheat seems to be a common problem for IBS sufferers. It is found in many products such as flour, biscuits and pasta, so lists of ingredients need to be read to check for this. Health food shops sell products that specifically do not contain wheat; these are manufactured for people with coeliac disease and are gluten-free.

The other common food problem appears to be related to milk and milk products. This is due to the lactose sugar found in milk, which is broken down in the gut by an enzyme called lactase. Unfortunately not everyone produces enough lactase so lactose cannot be broken down fully, or not at all. This can give symptoms of diarrhoea and discomfort.

It is a good idea to advise the IBS patient to try to cut out all the foods which are known to have caused problems commonly in other IBS sufferers for approximately 2 to 3 weeks. Examples are listed below:

Avoid these foods:	*Foods to try instead:*
Wheatbran and wheat-based cereals	Fresh fruit and vegetables
Milk and milk products	Skimmed or soya milk
Fatty or fried foods	White meat or lean red meat
Brown bread	White, wholemeal or soda bread
Spicy foods	Cottage cheese or low-fat cheese
Citrus fruits	All plain fish
High-yeast-containing foods	Seafood
Processed foods	Natural yoghurt
Baked beans	Pulses, chick peas and lentils
Onions	White or wholemeal rice or pasta
Fizzy drinks	Spring, still water
Tea and coffee	Herbal teas
Alcohol	Unsweetened fruit juice

General advice to give to IBS patients regarding food:

- Eat regularly each day instead of having one large meal which makes the bowel overwork.
- Avoid drinking liquid with meals as this can enhance abdominal distension.
- Avoid going without breakfast as this could mean that the bowel is missing the important gastrocolic reflex triggered by the first meal in the day.
- Eat slowly and chew well.
- Eat in a relaxed atmosphere and stop eating when feeling full.
- Eat fresh foods where possible, ensuring a balanced diet, low in animal fat, salt and sugar and high in fresh fruit and vegetables (preferably organic).
- Wash fruit and vegetables, meat, fish and rice well with cold water.

Can a Food Intolerance Give Rise to IBS Symptoms?

A food intolerance is described when there appears to be an adverse reaction to a food. This is different from a food allergy where there is an immune reaction. Some people with IBS have specific food intolerances to wheat, beef, onions, spices, coffee, milk and/or fatty foods.

Ideally patients should be referred to a dietitian who can help safely guide them to eliminate the foods likely to be contributing to the symptoms of their IBS. The dietitian will ensure essential vitamins and minerals are not left out of the diet, which would make the patient feel unwell.

A common elimination diet is started by eating only rice, lamb and pears (as these foods rarely cause problems) for at least 2 weeks (some patients trying this diet have reported worsening of symptoms before improvement). If the symptoms seem to settle down then the patient should start introducing different foods into the diet one by one, keeping a food and symptom diary of what foods are eaten, when and what symptoms were experienced each day if any, how stressful the day was, what medication was taken and where she is in the menstrual cycle (if appropriate). Once a food has been identified the dietitian will decide whether it affects the balance of the patient's diet and whether he/she needs a vitamin or mineral supplement. (There are now simple blood tests that can be done to show what foods, if any, the patient is intolerant of.)

Dr John Hunter, from Addenbrookes Hospital, believes food intolerance may be the cause of IBS and has suggested two ways in which this may work. First as a direct effect of chemicals found in food, e.g. caffeine, tyramine and histamine (the latter two both found in cheese), monosodium glutamate and various additives such as tartrazine. Enzymes produced in the gut and the liver will break these chemicals down so they are then harmless. In IBS Dr Hunter believes that perhaps for genetic reasons sufferers produce fewer protective enzymes than other people, leaving them vulnerable to their toxic effects. Research has shown that many people with food-intolerance diarrhoea do not produce enough lactase, i.e. lactose intolerance (Hunter, 1991).

Second, as a result of an imbalance of the different bacteria in the gut. Research shows that some IBS sufferers have abnormal balances of these bacteria and Dr Hunter believes this may cause certain foods to be converted into toxic chemicals in the colon to produce the IBS symptoms. Dr Hunter, through his research, has found that the most commonly eaten foods are usually the problem, with 60% of patients affected by wheat, 44% by milk and corn, 39% by cheese, 33% by coffee and 24% by citrus fruits.

Unlike true allergies, food intolerance sufferers often find that after avoiding a food for some months, it no longer upsets them when they come to eat it again as long as it is in moderation. Dr Hunter's exclusion diets have now been published.

The 'Hay system' is a theory with no scientific support which involves the patient not eating carbohydrates and proteins at the same meal. The idea for this diet came from Dr William Howard Hay some 50 years ago. Some sufferers of IBS have claimed it has benefited them. It is a wholefood diet where vegetables, salads and fruits provide the main part of the diet with no processed foods eaten at all (Hay, 1934).

In summary, dietary manipulation often proves to be important in the attempt to alleviate the symptoms of IBS, though it is not usually the complete answer.

What is the Relationship Between IBS and *Candida albicans?*

Candida albicans is a fungus which lives on and in our bodies. It is normally found in the bowel and mouth from infancy and so long as it stays in these areas where the body's defence system can keep it under control everything is fine. Some medications can upset the delicate balance of bacteria in the gut, e.g. antibiotics, contraceptive pills, steroids, tranquillizers, etc. Also some researchers argue that mercury leaking from dental fillings can interfere with the immune system and kill friendly bacteria in the bowel allowing overgrowth of candida and other yeasts.

It is thought that as the candida takes over the bowel it becomes an overactive fermentation tank causing a lot of gas, abdominal bloating and alteration of bowel habit, as well as weakening the immune system. It has been suggested by Trickett (1990) that if candida may be the reason for the symptoms of IBS it can be confirmed by the patient taking Brewer's yeast for 3 to 4 days. If soon after doing this the patient has developed an itchy rectum, bloated or uncomfortable abdomen, diarrhoea, rashes or insomnia it is likely that this is the problem.

To kill off candida the patient needs to cut out or restrict:

- bread and any refined carbohydrates;

- food and drink containing high levels of sugar;
- refined cereal products such as breakfast cereals, biscuits;
- sweets, chocolate, ice cream;
- alcohol;
- yeast-containing foods, e.g. cheese and vinegar;
- yeast and meat extracts, e.g. Marmite, Bovril, stock cubes;
- some tinned and packet soups;
- citrus fruits;
- vitamin preparations containing yeast, particularly Brewer's yeast.

Instead advise that they eat:

- lots of vegetables (preferably organic as no pesticides are used) and salads;
- garlic;
- fish, meat and poultry;
- seafood;
- plain live yoghurt;
- cottage cheese;
- lentils, peas and beans;
- rice;
- soda bread.

When restricting food intake it is always sensible to seek a dietitian's advice to avoid any vitamin and mineral deficiencies (this can be organized by the GP in the primary care setting, or by the doctor in the clinic if being treated by a hospital specialist).

Garlic is reported to have safe anti-fungal properties. Patients with candida overgrowth causing IBS should be advised to try three cloves a day ideally; these should be crushed to release allicin, taken with yoghurt and swallowed like a medicine and then washed down with plenty of water. If it is difficult for the patient to take this much, capsules of garlic can be taken instead but the packaging must state that it contains allicin for it to be effective ('Kyolic' is available in health food shops). As candida overgrowth can affect the immune system patients should be advised to take fresh linseed oil daily because it is rich in essential fatty acids which are vital for a healthy immune system. Apart from changing the diet as above it is advisable for the patient to reduce or stop smoking, take regular exercise and make time to relax every day.

Can Stress Affect IBS Symptoms?

Many IBS sufferers will say their symptoms are made worse by periods of stress or anxiety in their lives and researchers have tried to find links between IBS and a person's psychological state. They claim IBS patients have higher rates of psychiatric problems such as anxiety and depression, but these studies are of patients who have had IBS for many years so it may be the result of living with the IBS that causes the stress.

When people experience stress quite often the bowel is affected to some degree, from 'butterflies' to severe abdominal cramps and diarrhoea. With stress, adrenaline is released into the bloodstream in order to give increased energy levels to deal with the stressful situation through a 'flight or fight' response. If both these responses are ignored the muscles tend to stay in a state of tension and the nerves in the digestive tract start to behave in a disorderly way, which in turn causes pain, loss of appetite and digestive upsets which can lead to more anxiety. The food is then not fully absorbed and subsequently bloating and discomfort are experienced which can create more tension build-up.

Stress in itself is not necessarily a bad thing. However, if it is unrelenting and unmanaged it will inevitably take its toll on an individual's health.

One-third of patients who have had an attack of gastroenteritis go on to develop symptoms typical of IBS. Over time an increasing percentage lose their symptoms. The higher psychometric scores (results based on patient questionnaires relating to personality, anxiety and bowel symptoms) in patients with gastroenteritis who have subsequently developed IBS support the hypothesis that psychological factors are important in IBS (Gwee and Read, 1996).

How can IBS Sufferers Reduce their Stress Levels?

Relaxation can help stress. The nurse should discuss with the IBS patient possible ways of relaxing which are suitable and manageable for them. Examples may include:

- Making time each day to do something enjoyable such as having a long soak in a hot bath, reading a novel, watching a favourite programme on television or listening to some relaxing music.
- Getting involved in some type of regular activity such as walking the dog, swimming or a sporting pursuit.
- Patients should be encouraged to write down situations which they

know bother them most, then make a note if the bowel becomes more irritable at such times. The patient should try to imagine being in these situations and visualize him/herself as pleasantly relaxed, lowering the shoulders, breathing deeply and evenly and relaxing tense muscles until he/she is able to think of that situation without so much anxiety or with none at all.

- Saying no to unreasonable requests and delegating tasks at work and at home.
- Patients should be helped to find a way to sort out their daily priorities and then plan action positively but also realistically.
- It should be explained that it is important to eat slowly, taking time to enjoy the food and digest it.
- Relaxation tapes and videos are now widely available.
- Deep or diaphragmatic breathing can help to relax the body. The IBS sufferer can try the following exercise:

1. Locate a quiet warm and comfortable place where approximately 15 minutes can be set aside without the patient being disturbed.
2. Release any tight clothing.
3. Lie on the back with feet slightly apart, or sit in a comfortable chair.
4. Close the eyes and put one hand on the abdomen and the other on the chest area and breathe in and out through the nose slowly, steadily and deeply so that the breathing, its rhythm and rate can be felt with the hand.
5. Pull in the abdominal muscles when breathing out and become more aware of the abdominal wall pushing out.
6. Place the hands by the sides and continue to breathe, focusing on the rise and fall of the abdomen.

- Progressive muscle relaxation is a technique used to release tensions and stress. The aim is to progressively tense and relax each set of muscles to achieve a state of full relaxation. This can make a patient aware of how a tense muscle feels in order to feel the muscles relaxing. This can be done in conjunction with the deep breathing exercise so that when the patient tenses the muscles he/she takes a deep breath in and then breathes out slowly through the mouth as the muscle is relaxed. The patient needs to be completely focused on this for it to have some benefit. With this method it is advised that the patient starts by tensing and relaxing the foot muscles, holding the breathe to maintain the tension, then relaxing the muscle while breathing out. This should be repeated, focusing on the different parts of the body. This is a good exercise to try if a patient finds it difficult to sleep at night.

- Yoga aims to harmonize the mind, body and emotions and should help to improve muscle tone, increase suppleness, and improve breathing and blood circulation. It involves adopting postures, using stretching movements, breathing exercises and relaxation techniques. The whole body is systematically exercised and the aim is to leave one feeling revitalized and calm by restoring balance and removing energy blocks and chronic tensions. The best advice is for the patient to try going to a local yoga class; courses are often held under the auspices of the local council or there are plenty of books and videos available in bookshops.

What is Biofeedback Therapy and How can it Help IBS Patients?

Biofeedback can give IBS patients information about what is happening to their body. It is a technique which allows the patient to watch how the anal muscles are functioning, which can highlight any problems.

Biofeedback therapy is pain free and has no side-effects. The treatment will entail a series of approximately five sessions every 2 to 3 weeks, each session lasting between 30 and 60 minutes. Patients are given time to discuss things in life that cause them to become stressed. Advice is also given concerning diet and medication. The aim is to restore the patient's normal colonic function with correct defecatory muscle control (Schwarz et al., 1986).

The therapist will insert a balloon into the back passage and inflate it with a small amount of air; this mimics a bowel motion and hence the patient will feel the need to defecate. Electrodes linked to a computer are placed on to the buttocks either side of the back passage. A display screen will show the patient a graph which is affected by the squeeze and relaxation of the anal muscles. When the patient tries to expel the balloon the computer will tell which muscles are being used. The patient can see the graphs and by making a conscious effort to change the display can make alterations; this learning can help in daily life without the display.

Patients may need to be taught to sit correctly on the toilet, leaning forward with the feet slightly raised; how to relax before defecation; how to widen their waists for effective propulsion and how to relax rather than squeeze the muscles of their back passage. The exercises can be practised at home in between visits to the hospital.

Biofeedback may take some months before any improvement is seen and then it may only be a slight improvement; but most people tend to find they do learn a great deal from the therapist to improve their bowel function generally.

Can Exercise Help IBS Patients Manage their Symptoms?

Research has proved that most people with IBS show a definite improvement with regular exercise. Spollett (1989) stated from his research that physical exercise can help with abdominal distension and constipation and can also therapeutically reduce anxiety. It can make people feel more lively and energetic, which in turn can help with relaxation and lower stress levels that have built up. It is important that the exercise is enjoyable. Exercise at safe levels can help reduce symptoms of mild anxiety and mild depression and can help improve self-esteem and confidence. It is also beneficial for general good health.

To gain real benefit, once the patient has chosen a suitable activity he/she should aim to do it for about 15 to 20 minutes at least two or three times a week. Exercise needs to be thought of as a natural, essential part of life, just like eating or sleeping.

Getting started can be the difficult part. A companion is a good idea as the two keep one another motivated. The IBS patients should be advised to arrange time in his/her diary as lack of time can be an easy excuse. Realistic goals should be set so even if the patient feels too busy one week, just trying to fit a little extra walking into the day – for example by using stairs instead of a lift – will help. Patients should start slowly and build up; if they experience any pain or get very tired they should stop and rest for a while. If they have significant medical history it is worth discussing increased exercise with their GP before commencing.

Physical activity does not have to be intensive to improve the day-to-day quality of life. Walking, gardening and even housework can all help if they are done on a regular basis. The current official guidelines recommend 30 minutes 5 days a week, e.g. a brisk walk, swimming, cycling.

Patients should be given some useful tips to follow before vigorous activity, such as warming up first with gentle running on the spot and stretching to avoid muscle or joint injury, and wearing loose comfortable clothing and good supportive training shoes. Other advice is given below:

- The local library will have information about courses run by the local authority or a leisure centre if the commitment of a course seems too much.

- Swimming is a good all-round exercise which can do little harm.
- Working out at a gymnasium may appeal to some people, though it is always sensible to complete a simple fitness test beforehand with an instructor who can give guidance on what individuals should be aiming for.
- Aerobics with a trained instructor is another option, or a reputable video may be bought which can be played at home to exercise at one's own pace.

Can Complementary Therapies be Effective in IBS?

Sceptics say complementary therapies are still unproven. Research into their effectiveness is very limited compared with research into conventional treatments. People with IBS may get to the stage where they have tried different diets, different medication and tried ways to reduce stress but still have no relief from their symptoms and are keen to try anything. The effects of complementary therapies are often discovered through word of mouth or by reading health and women's magazines.

The therapies that have been reported to work well for IBS are homeopathy, hypnotherapy, aromatherapy, acupuncture, herbal medicine and reflexology.

Homeopathy

Homeopathy has been used now for around 200 years. It is the medical practice of treating 'like with like', jolting self-healing powers into action. It sees the symptoms of an illness as the body's reaction against the illness as it attempts to overcome it, and will seek to stimulate and not suppress this reaction (as with conventional treatment). It is a natural therapy which stimulates the body's own natural healing forces.

Nobody is completely sure how it works but it seems to be that the more dilute the remedy, the more effective it is. Remedies come as tablets, granules, powders or liquids and can be taken by mouth or as creams or drops. They are made from plant, mineral and animal extracts.

The choice of which remedy is appropriate depends on the individual's reaction to illness mentally and emotionally rather than on the signs and symptoms presented. The idea is always to treat the person holistically.

Remedies are safe and non-addictive with no unwanted side-effects. Individual response is varied but usually there is some feeling of well-being within a week even though a degree of the symptoms may remain. When the patient notices an improvement he/she should increase the interval between the doses; if improvement continues then treatment should be stopped, and restarted if there is a recurrence of symptoms. It is recommended that the most appropriate remedy should not be repeated more than four times. Patients should be reassured that it is safe to take prescribed drugs at the same time as taking homeopathic medication; however, it is best to advise patients to discuss this with their GP and there should be communication between the GP and the homeopathic doctor. Sometimes symptoms are aggravated initially but this usually means the body is responding well and the patient should try to persevere until the aggravation passes (the patient will need to be fully informed of likely effects). The nurse should ensure the patient is aware of the British Homeopathy Association (or the US equivalent).

Examples of homeopathic therapies that may help with the symptoms of IBS are:

- Natrum sol for loose stool and abdominal cramps;
- Podophyllum for watery yellow stools;
- Sulphur for diarrhoea associated with excess wind;
- Carbo veg for people with bloating and distension relieved by passing wind;
- Lycopodium can be taken for sensation of fullness in the abdomen after eating even a small amount, and noisy abdominal rumblings;
- Nux vomica or aesculus are worth trying for patients who have the sensation of not completely evacuating the motion with a residual burning sensation once the bowels have acted;
- Belladonna can be effective for abdominal distension;
- Argent nit is used for symptoms of flatulence and constipation alternating with diarrhoea, and if mucus is passed in the stool;
- Colocynth 6C can be tried if a patient experiences griping pains relieved by doubling up or pressing on the abdomen.

Hypnotherapy

The intention of hypnotherapy is deep relaxation but not unconsciousness. Once the patient is in a hypnotic state the therapist will make suggestions aimed at helping the person change the way he/she experiences or respond to something, using a slow soothing voice. Nobody is completely sure how it works but one theory is that the left, analytical side of the brain switches off, giving free rein to the right, creative side. The therapist will try to convince the patient that he/she is confident, capable and is becoming physically well, by putting these suggestions into the patient's subconscious. A course of this therapy can last about 45 minutes to an hour weekly for 10 to 12 weeks. The therapist may teach techniques of self-hypnosis or give a relaxation and confidence-boosting tape to the patient to listen to at home.

A study by Whorwell et al. (1984) demonstrated an overall 80% response rate to hypnosis in IBS. The technique he used was 'gut-directed hypnosis'. Patients are given a simple account of how the gut works so that during hypnosis they are asked to modify the way their gut works to a more normal function. The results were dramatic and definitive.

For it to be effective the patient has to be in a state of deep relaxation by using the breathing and muscle relaxation methods described above. Patients need to fix their attention on an object that is placed slightly above eye level so the eyes have to turn upwards. They then need to tell themselves that the eyelids are feeling heavier and heavier. The process needs to be repeated until the eyelids close. Patients should concentrate on their breathing and tell themselves that they are becoming more and more relaxed. When they are ready to finish they should tell themselves they will be out of trance by the count of five, so that they are safely out of the trance.

In a study on the effects of hypnosis looking at 33 patients, 20 experienced significant improvements and 11 reported improvement in all their symptoms (Walker et al., 1984).

Aromatherapy

This complemetary therapy is based on the supposed healing properties of essential oils, that is extracts of the flowers, fruit, seeds, leaves and bark of certain plants.

Some substances can be absorbed through the skin and inhaled substances can enter the bloodstream.

Many of the oils have been used for thousands of years and are safe, but a trained aromatherapist should always be consulted before using these oils as they may *not* be advisable for everyone, such as pregnant women, the very young, the frail and elderly and for those who have high blood pressure, epilepsy or a nervous disorder. Aromatherapy is often used with therapeutic massage and this can help relieve both physical and mental tension. The circulation of blood and lymph is stimulated, resulting in excretion of toxins from the body and return to the body of a balanced tone in the muscles. As the body starts to change and heal with regular massage, feelings of depression and irritability should be released.

All essential oils must be diluted in an appropriate carrier oil, for example sweet almond oil. The main routes of administration are via the skin and through smell. With massage, oil molecules are dissolved in the carrier oil which permeates the skin to reach fine blood vessels and thence cells and body fluids; with inhalation the cells of the olfactory system relay messages directly to the brain then the brain releases appropriate neurochemicals, i.e. sedative or stimulating, to have their effect.

Examples of essential oils used for symptoms of IBS include:

- Marjoram and rosemary with abdominal massage can help to alleviate constipation problems;
- Neroli is thought to be the best essential oil for diarrhoea caused by stress – this can be used in the bath, for massage or to inhale before a stressful event;
- Camomile, cypress, lavender, rosemary and peppermint all have antispasmodic properties which help with abdominal cramps and build up of flatus;
- Lavender has anti-inflammatory properties and is calming and soothing;
- Clary sage acts as a relaxant, and has anti-inflammatory, antispasmodic and calming effects.

It is important that patients with IBS who try these oils for themselves (as they are now widely available) know where to get more information about them, i.e. the Aromatherapy Organisations Council.

Acupuncture

Acupuncture is an ancient system of healing developed over thousands of years from the eastern countries. Needles are placed in appropriate places depending on the nature of the problem and then left in for either seconds or up to 30 minutes depending on the effect required. The warming of acupunture points, called moxibustion, through the use of smouldering herbs can be used as a supplement, and the needles can also be stimulated using a small electric current. This can give the patient a feeling of relaxation. Response will vary from person to person, but usually five treatments are needed weekly before effects are seen. Patients embarking on this form of complementary therapy would be advised to let their GP know they are doing this (acupuncture can be safely combined with drug therapy).

The aim of acupuncture is to treat the whole patient and restore the balance between the physical, emotional and spiritual aspects of the individual. Acupuncturists believe health is dependent on the balanced functioning of the body's motivating energy known as Qi (pronounced 'chi'). This Qi flows throughout the body but is concentrated in channels beneath the skin, known as meridians. The aim is to restore the balance between the equal and opposite qualities of Qi (the 'Yin' and the 'Yang'). Upsetting the balance and disturbing the flow of Qi can be due to emotional states such as stress, anxiety, anger, fear and grief; and also poor nutrition, infections and poisons.

The first visit to an acupuncturist involves a consultation to determine the nature of the problem. Symptoms, past medical history, family history, lifestyle, diet, sleep patterns and emotional feelings will be discussed. This helps both parties to look at the total picture.

The number of acupuncturists practising in the NHS in Great Britain is growing and some GPs are also learning the technique. The patient wanting to find a registered practitioner should be advised to contact the British Acupuncture Council, which works to maintain common standards to ensure the health and safety of the public at all times.

Herbal medicine

This is the use of plants or plant extracts in the treatment of disease. The herbs can be taken as tinctures, teas, inhalations or suppositories.

Examples that may help patients with IBS include:

- Valerian, melissa and scullcap help to relieve nervousness and anxiety by relaxing the mind and nervous system.
- Camomile has anti-inflammatory, sedative and tissue-healing effects on the gut.
- Viburnum opulus (cramp bark) can help alleviate spasticity of the colon.
- Peppermint and camomile tea can be drunk for relaxation and to reduce abdominal spasm.
- A tablespoon of fennel seeds heated in boiling water and drunk whilst hot can help with painful flatulence.
- 5 g of lavender may be infused in a litre of boiling water, left to cool and drunk between meals.

- Four leaves of fresh mint may be infused in a cup of boiling water.
- Cooking with herbs such as cumin, fennel, garlic, mint, thyme, rosemary and marjoram can help to aid digestion.
- Valerian acts as a relaxant and antispasmodic for the whole body (this is not recommended for regular consumption).
- Golden seal is a Native American remedy which works as an anti-spasmodic and also as a tonic to the bowel wall and helps to aid digestion.
- Wild yam and agrimony may help with spasm pain and if passing a lot of mucus from the back passage.
- Cinnamon or ginger can gently warm the bowel to soothe it.
- Bach flower is a herb containing different flowers, rock rose, clematis, impatiens, cherry and plum, it has a calming effect and is ideally taken if there are problems emotionally or a stressful time is imminent.

Reflexology

Reflexology is based on the idea that specific areas of the feet represent certain organs and areas of the body. Tension or disease in the body will be shown in the corresponding area on the foot called the 'reflex zone'. Through careful massage of this area by a trained reflexologist this tension can be relieved and the process of healing begun.

The reflexologist will feel the feet and hands, noting the position of tender reflex areas, and a case history is taken. Treatment consists of compressing and massaging the feet as a whole, paying particular attention to the tender areas to break down the crystalline deposits and free the energy flow. If there is some problem the patient will feel a pain or pricking sensation.

The patient should be told what he/she is likely to experience in the first few days after the treatment, e.g. sweating, increased urination and bowel movements. Explain that this is regarded as a good thing as it shows the treatment is working. There is no limit to the amount of treatments a patient should have.

Is there an Association for Patients with IBS in the UK?

The IBS Network is a registered charity based at the Northern General Hospital in Sheffield. It is a self-help organization for people with IBS. It was set up in 1991 by Susan Backhouse and Christine Dancy. It produces a quarterly journal called *Gut Reaction* which has information on the latest research into IBS, sufferers' experiences, members' experiences that they wish to share with other sufferers – particularly anything that has helped them, so that useful information can be shared. Also dietary advice is discussed and there are articles about alternative and complementary therapies. There are book reviews and experts in the field of IBS will write articles of interest. There is a small subscription fee for members.

Members receive a 'can't wait card' which can be shown to staff in shops, restaurants, etc. to access a toilet if the need is urgent. Members also have the opportunity to participate in research if they so wish. The Network operates a befriender and penpal scheme and coordinates local self-help groups.

There is also an IBS helpline run by the Medical Advisory Service, staffed by specialist nurses on weekday evening from 6 pm to 8 pm to answer queries and offer guidance (tel: 01543 492192).

Are there any Self-help Groups for IBS Patients?

Most people who are asked about the benefits of self-help groups will be overwhelmingly positive. Meeting and talking to others who have similar problems and feeling one is not alone with the problem can help. Some studies have shown that support groups can actually help reduce the severity and frequency of the symptoms.

Payne and Blanchard (1995) measured patients' symptoms, anxiety and depression after 2 months and again after a 3-month period. The patients were split into three groups: one group received cognitive psychotherapy, the second group formed a self-help group and the third group did neither. The cognitive therapy group came out best with a 67% reduction in symptoms; the self-help group achieved a reduction of 31%; and the third group 10%. The only problem with cognitive therapy is that it does cost money whereas the support group costs nothing except perhaps the travel fare.

If there is not a local group one can be set up, though it does take time and commitment but the benefits will be worth it.

- Its always advisable to let GPs in the area know that such a group is starting. They may offer to be the first guest speaker or else they may know of people who could participate.
- A gastroenterologist at the local hospital may agree to come and talk about what can be done, give advice on dealing with the problem and outline current research into the syndrome.
- Practitioners in alternative and complementary therapies are

usually keen to come and discuss the different therapies and give a demonstration.

- IBS topics can be discussed to increase patients' knowledge and share experiences and update them on research.
- It is a good idea to set up an information library of books, articles, tapes and videos, etc. that can be shared among the members of the group.
- Fund-raising activities for research can be organized among the members; at least then there is a feeling of actually doing something positive to help researchers find some answers.
- Ideally there should be a coordinator and a structure to the meetings and all members should have a role within the group.
- The IBS Network will send details of the local group out in the newsletter and put people in contact with others who have successfully set up a group. Local newspapers will often give free publicity, and local libraries and surgeries will help advertise the group.

Irritable bowel syndrome is undoubtedly a complex problem for any health professional to deal with and affects many people's lives. Sufferers need to be listened to and then guided appropriately so that they can learn how to manage their symptoms. This chapter demonstrates the multiple areas in which nurses can facilitate and support patients following a diagnosis of IBS.

References

Allun-Jones V, Shorthouse M, McLaughlan P (1982) Food intolerance: a major factor in the pathogenesis of IBS. Lancet 2: 1115–17.

Arn I, Theorell T, Uvnas-Moberg K, Jonsson (1989) Psychodrama group therapy for patients with functional gastrointestinal disorders – a controlled long-term follow up study [University of Stockholm, Sweden]. Psychotherapy 51 (3): 113–19.

Barnes J (1996) Helping people who have irritable bowel syndrome. Community Nurse 2: 30.

Bennett P, Wilkinson S (1985) A comparison of psychological and medical treatment of the IBS. British Journal of Clinical Psychology 24: 215–16.

Farthing M (1995) Irritable bowel, irritable body, or irritable brain? British Medical Journal 310: 171–5.

Gershon (1995) Journal of the College of Physicians and Surgeons of Columbia University 15(3).

Greener M (1996) The Which? Guide to Managing Stress. London: Consumer's Association.

Hogston R (1993) Nursing management of irritable bowel syndrome. British Journal of Advanced Nursing 2: 214–17.

Hunter JO (1991) Food allergy or enterometabolic disorder. Lancet 338: 495–6.

Letson S, Dancey CP (1996) Nurses' perceptions of irritable bowel syndrome (IBS) and sufferers of IBS. Journal of Advanced Nursing 23: 969–74.

Manning AP, Thomson WG, Heaton KW, Morris AF (1978) Towards a positive diagnosis of the IBS. British Medical Journal ii : 653–4.

Payne A, Blanchard E (1995) A controlled comparison of cognitive therapy and self-help support groups in the treatment of IBS. Journal of Consulting & Clinical Psychology 63: 779–86.

Schwarz SP, Blanchard EB, Neff DF (1986) Behavioral treatment of IBS: a 1-year follow-up study. Biofeedback and Self Regulation 2 (3): 189–98.

Spollett GR (1989) IBS: diagnosis and treatment. Nurse Practitioner 14(8): 32–44.

Reading List

IBS – A Complete Guide to Relief from Irritable Bowel Syndrome, by Christine Dancy and Susan Backhouse.

The Irritable Bowel Syndrome and Diverticulosis: a Self Help Plan, by Shirley Trickett (Thorsons).

Coping Successfully with your Irritable Bowel, by Rosemary Nicol (Sheldon Press).

The Troubled Gut, by Barbara Rowlands (Headline).

What You Really Need to Know About Irritable Bowel Syndrome – patient information video, by Norgine Limited.

Sounds Like IBS – audiotape with information and relaxation music, by Norgine Limited.

Let's Get Things Moving – Overcoming Constipation, by Pauline Chiarelli and Sue Markwell (Neen Health Books) .

Recipes for Health: IBS, by Jill Davies and Ann Page-Wood.

Irritable Bowel Syndrome – Special Diet Cookbook, by Ann Page-Wood and Jill Davies.

The Complete Guide to Food Allergy and Intolerance, by J. Brostoff and L. Gamblin (Bloomsbury).

Beat IBS through Diet, by Dr Alan Stewart (Vermilion).

Beat Candida – from Thrush to Chronic Fatigue, by Gill Jacobs (Vermilion).

The Allergy Diet, by Dr John Hunter (Vermilion).

Pocket Massage for Stress Relief (Dorling Kindersley).

Herbal Medicine for Sleep and Relaxation (Amberwood).

Step by Step Massage for Pain Relief (Gaia Books).

Banish Anxiety: a Common-Sense Plan for Gaining Control of your Life, by Dr Kenneth Hambly.

Stress: Proven Stress-Coping Strategies for Better Health, Leon Chaitow.

Classic Relaxation Programme, by Dr Hilary Jones (Deutsche Grammophon/ Polygram).

Relaxation; Sleep Better; Meditation; Body Relaxation Exercises; four tapes by Anthony Ross (produced by Relaxation Centre Cassettes, 7–11 Kensington High Street, London W8 5NP. Tel: 0171 938 3409).

Personal Hypnotherapy series: Deep Relaxation; Eliminate Stress; Sleep like a Log; by Paul McKenna Productions.

The Complete Family Guide to Alternative Medicine (Element).

Eating Right for a Bad Gut: The Complete Nutritional Guide, by James Scala (Hal/Dutton, USA).

IBS Handbook: Learning to Live With IBS, by Gerard Guillory (MTA Publishing, USA).

Relief from IBS, by Elaine Shimberg (Evans, USA).

Food Combining for Health, by Doris Grant and Jean Joice (Thorsons) (based on Dr William Howard Hay's book Health Via Food, Harrap, 1934).

Associations

British Digestive Foundation
3 St Andrew's Place,
London NW1 4LB
Tel: 0171 487 5332

Green Farm Nutrition Centre
Woodlands, London Road,
Battle, East Sussex TN33 0LP

British Society for Allergy
Environmental and Nutritional
Medicine, PO Box, Totton,
Southampton SO40 2ZA
Tel: 01703 812124

**The Institute of Individual
Wellbeing**
99 King's Road,
London SW3 4PA

British Acupuncture Council
Park House,
206–8 Latimer Road,
London W10 6RE
Tel: 0181 964 0222

**Aromatherapy Organisations
Council**
Tel: 01858 434242

Doctor Edward Bach Centre
Tel: 01491 834678

**National Institute of Medical
Herbalists**
Tel: 01392 426022

Society of Homeopaths
Tel: 01604 21400/ 0171 837 9469

British Homeopathy Association
27a Devonshire Street,
London, W1N1RJ
Tel: 0171 935 2163

British Massage Therapy Council
Tel: 01772 881063

**Institute for Complementary
Medicine**
PO Box 194,
London SE16 1QZ
Tel: 0171 237 5165

British Wheel of Yoga
1 Hamilton Place, Boston Road,
Sleaford, Lincolnshire, NG34 7ES
Tel: 01529 306851

**National Health Information
Center**
PO Box 1096,
Washington DC, USA

**International Foundation for
Bowel Dysfunction**
PO Box 17864,
Milwaukee,
Wisconsin 53217, USA
Tel: 414 964 1799

**American Holistic Medical
Association**
4101 Lake Boone Trail,
Suite 201, Raleigh, NC 27607, USA

Patient Support Groups

IBS Network
Northern General Hospital,
Sheffield, S5 7AU
Tel: 0114 261 1531

IBD/IBS Helpline Tel: 01543 492192;
Medical Advisory Service with specialist
nurses available for queries and guidance from 6–8 pm Monday to Fridays

IBS Self Help Group
3332 Yonge Street, PO Box 94074,
Toronto, Ontario, Canada M4N 3RI

IBS Support Group
Los Angeles, Southern California

**Internet web site for irritable bowel
syndrome**
http://www.parkviewpub. com/
irritablebowelsyndrome.html

Chapter 12
Laparoscopic Colorectal Surgery

MARA RITA SALUM MD, Research Resident, Colorectal Surgery, Cleveland Clinic Florida, USA

STEVEN D. WEXNER MD, FACS, FASCRS, Chief of Staff, Chairman, Department of Colorectal Surgery, Cleveland Clinic Florida, Professor of Surgery, Cleveland Clinic Foundation, Florida, USA

NORMA DANIEL RN, MS, CNOR, RNFA, Surgical Nurse Clinican, Colorectal Surgery, Cleveland Clinic Florida, USA

MURALEEN GUSTIN RN, Surgical Nurse, Cleveland Clinic Hospital, Florida, USA.

History of Laparoscopic Colorectal Surgery

As a consequence of the results of laparoscopic cholecystectomy (Reddick and Olsen, 1989; Dubois et al., 1990; Cuschieri et al., 1990), as well as the development of new instruments, surgeons started to apply laparoscopic techniques to treat other gastrointestinal diseases including those of the colon and rectum.

The first laparoscopic appendectomy was performed by DeKok in 1977 (DeKok, 1977). This laparoscopic-assisted procedure included a mini-laparotomy to remove the non-inflamed appendix. Semm achieved the first complete laparoscopic appendectomy in 1983 (Semm, 1983). Laparoscopy subsequently became practical and popular among both general and gynaecologic surgeons for the evaluation and treatment of right lower quadrant pain in women (Schreiber, 1987; Whitworth et al., 1988).

Initially, application of the laparoscopic technique for colorectal surgery was limited by lack of appropriate instrumentation. Therefore the first published laparoscopic colon resection was undertaken as a laparoscopic-assisted one. The introduction of laparoscopic intestinal staplers to the surgeon's armamentarium made it possible for virtually all types of colorectal procedures to be laparoscopically accomplished (Table 12.1).

Table 12.1: Milestones in laparoscopic colorectal surgery

Procedure	Surgeon	Date
Right hemicolectomy	Moises Jacobs	June 1990
Sigmoid resection	Dennis L. Fowler	October 1990
Low anterior resection	Patrick Leahy	November 1990
Abdominal perineal resection	Robert W. Beart	April 1991
Total abdominal colectomy	Steven Wexner/ David G. Jagelman	August 1991
Transverse colectomy	Garth H. Ballantyne	February 1992

Advantages

The acceptable results achieved with laparoscopic cholecystectomy clearly benefited the patient. Specifically as compared with cholecystectomy by laparotomy, laparoscopic cholecystectomy offers less reduction in pulmonary function (Williams and Brenowitz, 1975; Barnett et al., 1992; Poulin et al., 1992), probably less operative pain (Dubois et al., 1990; Bailey et al., 1991; Schirmer et al., 1991; Ure et al., 1994), and a much faster recovery (The Southern Surgeons Club, 1991). Unlike surgery for gallbladder disease, laparoscopic colorectal surgery often requires extensive mobilization and removal of a large section of intestine. Therefore, it is often necessary to reposition personnel as well as to change position of the instruments, monitor and patient. These changes require time and therefore add expense to the procedure. The colon has numerous large vessels encased in an adipose mesentery. Safe, rapid control of the vessels often requires the use of numerous clips or vascular staplers (US Surgical Corp, Norwalk, CT) (Figure 12.1) that can add to the cost of the procedure. An incision, even if small, has to be performed in order to remove the specimen, which may contain a malignancy. An anastomosis must be fashioned in a reliable manner.

Many recent retrospective reports failed to find any differences when laparoscopic technique was compared with standard laparo-

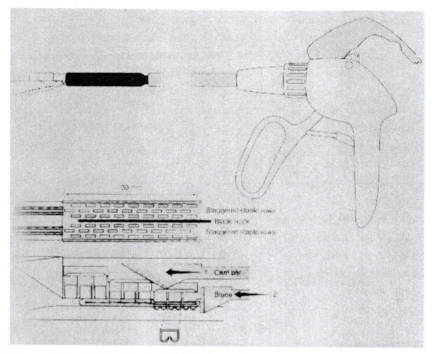

Figure 12.1: Multifire Endo GIA 30 instrument (Longitudinal cut-away view)
Courtesy of US Surgical Corporation, Norwalk, CT) (reprinted with permission).

tomy (Monson et al., 1992; Larach et al., 1993a; Tate et al., 1993; Schmitt et al., 1994), no large prospective randomized clinical trials comparing laparoscopy with conventional surgery have been published. The only well-accepted advantage of laparoscopy on colorectal surgery is improved cosmesis (Guillou et al., 1993; Wexner et al., 1993; Schmitt et al., 1994). Nevertheless, Pfeifer et al. have shown that cosmesis is a very subjective question (Pfeifer et al., 1995). In their study no statistically significant differences existed relative to patient satisfaction with cosmesis between the two groups of patients undergoing laparoscopy or laparotomy.

One of the parameters used to assess the efficacy of a procedure is the length of hospitalization and the patient's ability to return to work. Length of stay has been reported to decrease after laparoscopic colorectal surgery compared with conventional colorectal surgery (Jacobs et al., 1991; Phillips et al., 1992; Franklin et al., 1993; Jenkins et al., 1993).

Shorter postoperative ileus can contribute to shorter hospital stay. It has been hypothesized that laparoscopic colorectal surgery, because of less trauma and manipulation of the bowel, results in earlier recovery of bowel function. One animal study (Böhm et al., 1995) clearly showed an earlier return of bowel myoelectrical activity and normal bowel movement after laparoscopy compared with conventional right colectomy.

However, early return of bowel function in humans is not a unique attribute of laparoscopic surgery. Binderow et al. (1994) and Reissman et al. (1996a) have shown in two separate prospective randomized trials of over 200 patients that the ability to eat soon after surgery is not exclusive to laparoscopy. Approximately 89% of patients can tolerate a diet within one day of laparotomy and colectomy.

In evaluating less pain as a potential benefit to the laparoscopic patient Ramos et al. (1995) showed that patients who underwent standard surgery used patient-controlled analgesia for 6.2 days postoperatively versus 2.9 days if the procedure was laparoscopically performed. However, in a more exacting analysis Pfeifer and colleagues (Pfeifer et al., 1995) demonstrated no statistically different responses regarding pain between patients who had undergone laparotomy or laparoscopic colorectal surgery.

No significant statistical differences in the total cost between the laparoscopic and laparotomy procedure have been found. Both Reiver et al. (1994) and Falk et al. (1993) demonstrated that although the mean hospital stay for patients who underwent laparoscopic sigmoid or right hemicolectomy was significantly shorter, procedure and instrument costs were significantly lower in patients who underwent laparotomy. Thus total costs were similar in both groups. Senagore et al. (1993) reported their overall cost was lower for patients who underwent laparoscopy. They attributed the savings not only to reduction of hospital stay, but also to the use of fewer pharmaceutical agents, intravenous infusions and intramuscular injections as compared with laparotomy.

Even though preliminary results have been encouraging, no prospective randomized trials or other statistically valid data have proven irrefutably the superiority of laparoscopic colectomy as compared with standard laparotomy.

Disadvantages

It is apparent that there is a steep learning curve in laparoscopic colorectal surgery (Cohen et al., 1994). It requires more skill, and presents more challenging issues than does laparoscopic surgery for gall bladder diseases or any other single-quadrant laparoscopy. There exist several differences between laparoscopic colorectal surgery and most other laparoscopic procedures including fundoplication and splenectomy. First, while all other laparoscopic procedures involve one main anatomical region, the laparoscopic technique for colon resection requires dissection and mobilization in more than one region. To obtain the best operating field the surgeon often has to change the position of the camera, instruments, and even the personnel during the procedure. To aid dissection, the mobilized bowel needs to be retracted; however, this manoeuvre is not easily accomplished within the confined space of the abdominal cavity, often resulting in long, tedious surgery. The tactile ability in laparoscopy is compromised and sometimes smaller tumours and large polyps that do not have serosal signs indicative of their location need additional localization techniques. Some surgeons include with initial colonoscopy marking of the lesion with Indian ink, indigo carmine, indocyanine green or methylene blue to allow visualization during laparoscopy. If the site of the lesion is in doubt, an intraoperative colonoscopy to confirm the site of the lesion is performed and the serosal surface is marked with clips. These manoeuvres help to reduce the rate of incorrect segment removal.

Other features unique to colorectal surgery are ligation of vessels and removal of a large specimen. Mesenteric vessels are numerous, large and coarse in a thick layer of opaque fat. Laparoscopically isolating these pedicles and subsequently ligating and dividing them can be much more difficult than in conventional surgery. Most recently, the use of the ultrasonic scalpel (Harmonic Scalpel, Ethicon Endosurgery Inc, Cincinnati, Ohio) (Figure 12.2a, b) has conferred a definite advantage in mesenteric dissection and vascular control by allowing adequate haemostasis without the decreased visibility associated with the smoke created by extensive electrocoagulation. This scalpel can be used as a substitute for the electrosurgery, and employs ultrasonic energy with minimal thermal damage at low temperature under 100°C. To effect removal of a specimen, incisions up to 25 cm in length (Fleshman et al., 1996) have to be made, thereby limiting the cosmetic benefit. Specimen bags have been made available to decrease contamination by bacteria or tumour when the specimen is negotiated through the small wound (Figure 12.3).

An integral part of most colonic resections is fashioning an anastomosis. To achieve a well-vascularized, tension-free, circumferentially intact anastomosis the surgeon needs infinite patience and experience. Nevertheless Phillips, in his report of 51 laparoscopic colectomies, noted that the circular stapled anastomosis was incomplete in 18% of cases (Phillips et al., 1992). This extraordinarily high rate of incom-

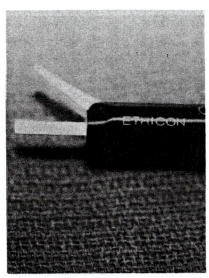
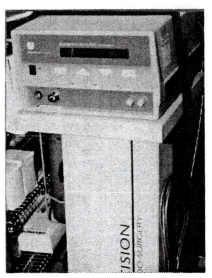

Figure 12.2: (left) The harmonic scalpel and disposable blade which employs ultrasonic energy to achieve precise cutting and controlled coagulation (Ethicon Endosurgery, Inc, Cincinnati, Ohio); (right) the microprocessor-controlled high frequency generator activated by a foot switch (Ethicon Endosurgery Inc, Cincinnati, Ohio).

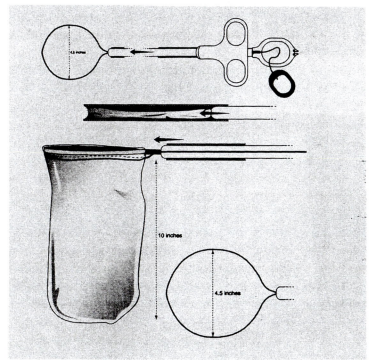

Figure 12.3: Large plastic bag used for retrieval of intestinal segments (US Surgical Corporation, Norwalk, CT) (reprinted with permission).

plete anastomosis compares poorly with the 2–8% rate during laparo-tomy (Lazorthes and Chiotassol, 1986). The development of the endo-scopic linear cutting device, subsequently, would have reduced the need for this step but at a greater cost.

A higher rate of thromboembolic complications has also been reported (Guillou et al., 1993), and is probably related to the increased operative time and pneumoperitoneum.

It is obvious that adequate training is mandatory for laparoscopic colorectal surgery and such guidelines have been published by the Society of American Gastrointestinal Endoscopic Surgeons (SAGES). These principles allow assessment of credentialling and training surgeons in the art of laparoscopy.

Specific Surgical Procedures

Laparoscopic Creation of Stoma

Faecal diversion is a relatively common procedure in a colorectal prac-tice and laparoscopic creation of intestinal stomas is feasible and effec-tive for faecal diversion (Oliveira et al., 1997b). Indications include faecal incontinence, acute sphincter injury, rectovaginal fistulae, colo-vesical or rectourethral fistulae, perineal sepsis due to Crohn's disease or necrotizing fasciitis, and irradiation proctitis (Lange et al., 1991; Romero et al., 1992; Khook et al., 1993; Furhman and Ota, 1994; Teoh et al., 1994; Wexner et al., 1996).

The operative technique is based on standard preoperative prepa-ration of the patient. The stoma site should have been preoperatively selected by the enterostomal therapist or nurse. The initial midline port is placed using either the Veress or Hasson technique (Hasson, 1971). The only caveat for stoma creation is that, to prevent crowding of the instruments, the initial midline camera port should be placed midway between the umbilicus and the xiphoid.

After pneumoperitoneum is established (Figure 12.4) the laparo-scope is inserted under direct vision; a second 10 mm cannula is placed lateral to the rectus sheath through the stoma site. The surgeon then uses a laparoscopic Babcock-type clamp passed through the stoma site to identify the appropriate loop of bowel and lift it to the stoma site.

For sigmoid colostomy formation, the distal sigmoid, usually draped into the pelvis, is usually most easily delivered to the anterior abdominal wall. When creating a loop ileostomy, the terminal ileum may not be immediately apparent; however, by grasping and elevating

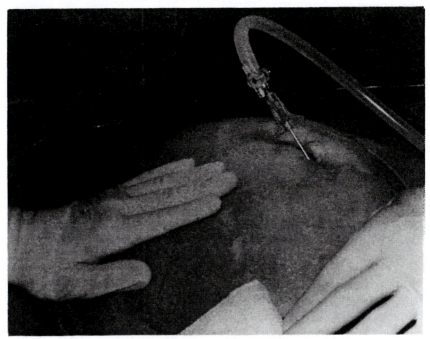

Figure 12.4: Establishing the pneumoperitoneum with the aid of the Veress needle.

the caecum it comes into view and can be proximally traced from the caecum until an appropriate loop is found that easily reaches the anterior wall. This position is usually 15 to 20 cm proximal to the ileocaecal valve. Placing the patient in steep Trendelenburg position with the left side down can also help in locating the terminal ileum by shifting the overlying small bowel loops into the left upper abdomen.

With the bowel firmly grasped with the Babcock clamp, it is brought up to the stoma site cannula. To avoid inadvertent twisting of the bowel one of several manoeuvres can be utilized to ensure appropriate orientation. A small-bore spinal needle can be passed through the abdominal wall medial to the stoma to tattoo the afferent and efferent limbs with methylene blue (one dot proximal and two dots distal) for easy identification. Endoscopy can be performed, an instrument can be passed along both the afferent and efferent limbs of the stoma, or a third port can be introduced through which clips can be applied to the mesentery or appendices epiploicae. Regardless of which mode is selected, the stoma must be delivered for maturation with appropriate anatomic orientation.

After orienting, the bowel is gently grasped with a Babcock clamp through the stoma port. The skin at that site is excised to allow a 2 cm to 3 cm diameter opening. The rectus sheath opening is lengthened by incising along the insulated shaft of the Babcock clamp. The bowel is then withdrawn on to the abdominal wall. With the bowel loop occluding the stoma site, the abdomen is reinsufflated, and the bowel examined once more with the laparoscope to confirm proper orientation. The ostomy is then matured using standard techniques as either an end or a loop stoma.

Appendectomy

Laparoscopic appendectomy is usually performed as an emergency procedure for acute appendicitis or right lower quadrant peritonitis (Pier et al., 1991). One of the major advantages of laparoscopic appendectomy through the traditional McBurney incision is the opportunity to perform an exploratory laparoscopy with thorough inspection of the pelvis and the entire abdomen to exclude concomitant pathology.

The patient is prepared in the standard fashion; after pneumoperitoneum is established, the camera is introduced through the periumbilical port and all subsequent work is undertaken under direct visualization. After a visual exploration of the entire abdominal cavity and pelvis and the diagnosis of acute appendicitis confirmed, additional trocars can be placed. The second 10/12 mm trocar should be placed in a suprapubic position, below the hairline just cephaled to the symphysis pubis. A grasping instrument, scissors or endoscopic stapler can be used through this port and the camera can also be moved to that position prior to extraction of the appendix through the umbilical port. A third trocar (5 mm) should be placed in the right upper quadrant lateral to the rectus muscle. A grasping instrument is used in this port in order to elevate the caecum. If an additional port is necessary for retraction, it should be 5 mm and placed in the right lower quadrant. If the patient has a mobile caecum, an additional port can also be placed in the midline between the first two trocars.

Dissection is initiated by elevating the caecum and identifying the appendix. Complete visualization of the entire appendix from the base to the tip is mandatory to exclude the diagnosis of acute appendicitis. If only a portion of the appendix is visualized it may be necessary to mobilize the peritoneal reflection of the right colon and caecum to properly expose a retrocaecal appendix. If difficulty or excessive bleeding is encountered, the procedure should be converted to an open appendectomy.

Once the mesoappendix is in view, removal of the appendix can be performed. The distal end of the appendix is retracted laterally and a 'window' is made between the vessels in the mesoappendix. Either clips, ligatures, staples or electrocoagulation can be used for securing these vessels. The appendiceal artery should be either proximally secured with two clips or divided with an endoscopic linear cutting stapler.

The stump of the appendix can be managed in a number of ways. Pre-tied vascular sutures can be placed proximally and distally or large haemoclips can be utilized. Usually two clips are placed at the base and the third approximately 2 cm distally to prevent spillage of intraluminal contents; the appendix is then divided with scissors. A more popular expeditious although expensive method is an endoscopic linear cutting stapler instrument.

Removal of the appendix can be performed in several ways. If the appendix is small and non-inflamed, it can be drawn within one of the 10/12 mm trocars and the entire organ and trocar can be removed together. If the appendix is long and thickened from inflammation, a commercially available bag can be placed intraperitoneally and the appendix inserted into this bag prior to removal. This manoeuvre should potentially lessen the chance of wound contamination and appendiceal rupture. Because the bag containing the appendix is too big to be brought into the trocar, the trocar is removed and the bag is grasped with clamps and manually removed. The camera should be moved to the supraumbilical port and the extraction facilitated through the umbilical trocar, as a cosmetically superior result will occur from a slightly enlarged umbilical port as compared with the suprapubic site. Inspection and irrigation of the abdominal cavity can be performed and haemostasis obtained either after the appendix is removed or just prior to extraction. The decision to use an intraperitoneal drain should not be dependent upon the use of the laparoscope. In general, drains are utilized only for the evacuation of an abscess cavity and not to drain the peritoneal cavity.

The trocars should be removed under direct vision to ensure that there is no bleeding or haematoma formation from the port sites. The final umbilical trocar is removed and all incisions are closed. Postoperatively, the nasogastric tube and Foley catheter are removed; the patient should begin to ambulate at the evening of surgery. Antibiotic and pain management is the same as after incisional appendectomy. The diet can be advanced as tolerated, with hospital discharge anticipated generally 2 to 3 days after surgery (Wexner and Cohen, 1996).

Sigmoid Colectomy

For sigmoid colectomy three 10/12 mm ports are used: umbilical, right paraumbilical and right lower quadrant. An optional left paraumbilical port may be needed, especially in obese individuals. Mobilization of the sigmoid colon can be facilitated with the patient placed in the Trendelenburg position with tilt to the right. After mobilization of the colon and identification of the left ureter, the mesenteric vessels are intracorporeally divided. This division can be performed with endoclips or vascular stapling devices. The distal and proximal margins may be marked with hernia staples. For a tension-free anastomosis the splenic flexure may need mobilization.

For introduction of a 60 mm linear stapler device, the right lower quadrant 10/12 mm port is exchanged for an 18 mm port. The segment of colon previously marked as the distal margin is then transected. A trial reach of the intended proximal margin is undertaken and that segment is marked with clips. The left paraumbilical port, if one was used, is replaced with a 33 mm port through which the proximal colon is gently delivered and the diseased segment is extracorporeally resected. If no left-sided (fourth) port was used then the 33 mm port is introduced *de novo*. A purse-string suture is used and a 29 or 33 mm anvil is placed in the proximal end of the colon, which is then returned to the abdominal cavity. The anvil is grasped by a modified Allis clamp (Ethicon Endosurgery Inc, Cincinnati, Ohio). Meanwhile a circular stapler is inserted transanally to reach the rectal stump staple line piercing the rectal wall. To allow the two ends of the colon to be approximated it is helpful at this time to change the position of the laparoscope into the right lower port to confirm the proper orientation, lack of tension and exclusion of extraneous tissue prior to effecting the anastomosis. The procedure is concluded after assessing anastomotic integrity by transanal air insufflation while the pelvis is filled with saline. During the testing, the segment of colon proximal to the anastomosis is occluded with an atraumatic bowel clamp. Finally the tissue rings (donuts) are inspected for completeness. An incomplete anastomosis may be repaired by laparoscopic suturing or hernia clip application (Cohen et al., 1994), redone or by conversion to laparotomy if necessary.

Laparoscopic Abdominoperineal Resection

Laparoscopic proctectomy is a technically feasible alternative for both cancer and colitis (Wu et al., 1997) and may theoretically allow a more precise assessment of excision margins (Darzi et al., 1995a).

After the pneumoperitoneum is established second and third 10/12 mm trocars are placed in the right iliac fossa and right paraumbilical regions. An additional 10/12 mm trocar is positioned in the lower left quadrant at the site pre-marked for the stoma.

The rectosigmoid is mobilized and the left ureter is identified. An endoscopic 30 mm linear cutting stapler device is used to transect the inferior mesenteric vessels. The dissection is completed with mobilization of the rectum and identification and preservation of the presacral sympathetic nerves. The lateral stalks are usually divided by the harmonic scalpel (Ethicon Endosurgery Inc, Cincinnati, Ohio). At this point perineal dissection is performed in the standard fashion and the specimen is retrieved. Creation of an end colostomy and closure of the perineal wound conclude the procedure (Larach et al., 1993b).

Laparoscopic Total Abdominal Colectomy

Laparoscopic total abdominal colectomy with ileoproctostomy and laparoscopic restorative proctocolectomy are both technically feasible (Wexner et al., 1992). Indications include colitis, Crohn's disease, familial adenomatous polyposis and colonic inertia (Bernstein et al., 1996). This procedure is time-consuming and has not yet reduced the length of hospitalization as compared with laparotomy (Rhodes and Stitz, 1994; Schmitt et al., 1994).

Nevertheless laparoscopic total abdominal colectomy may have a role as compared with laparotomy in young patients, in whom improved cosmesis as achieved by the laparoscopically assisted procedure is the major advantage desired.

Five 10/12 mm ports are placed, one in each of the supraumbilical sites, right upper and lower quadrants and left upper and lower quadrants. The incision for the specimen retrieval and the stoma site should both be considered at the time of the port placement. The specimen may be retrieved through a Pfannenstiel incision or through the stoma site, if the stoma is planned. Division of the mesentery and transection of the terminal ileum is preferably extracorporeally performed. The end ileostomy is then delivered through the premarked site and matured.

Laparoscopic Right Hemicolectomy

Indications for this procedure include colonoscopically unresectable polyps, benign lesions such as lipomas or leiomyomas, Crohn's disease and palliation of malignancy.

The selection of port sites depends upon both the patient's body habitus and the type of resection. Two monitors, one on each side of the patient, are used. The surgeon generally stands on the left side, opposite the assistant.

After the initial umbilical port is placed, a second trocar is put in the left iliac fossa, slightly to the left of the epigastric vessels, while a third trocar is introduced at the paraumbilical position. If needed, as in obese patients, an optional fourth port is inserted in the left upper quadrant. Mobilization of the colon is performed and the larger vessels encountered at the flexures are either ligated with surgical clips or divided with the harmonic scalpel (Ethicon Endosurgery Inc, Cincinnati, Ohio). Full mobilization from the ileum to the mid-transverse colon includes visualization of the duodenum and the right ureter. After full mobilization, a 2 to 5 cm transumbilical incision is made, incorporating the incision previously made for the Veress needle. The mesenteric vascular ligation and bowel division are then undertaken as extracorporeal procedures. A side-to-side (functional end-to-end) anastomosis is created with a linear cutting stapler device. The mesenteric defect is repaired, the colon is delivered back to the abdominal cavity and the procedure is concluded with the closure of the incision and the port sites (Cohen and Wexner, 1994).

Laparoscopy for Intestinal Obstruction

Indications for laparoscopic adhesiolysis include patients who have had previous abdominal surgery and present with transient recurrent episodes or an acute progressive onset of intestinal obstruction (Silva and Coghill, 1991). This procedure allows efficient diagnosis and usually effective treatment in cases of an undetermined cause of intestinal obstruction (François et al., 1994; Reissman and Wexner, 1995).

The initial creation of pneumoperitoneum should be carefully planned and executed. When choosing the site for placement of the first trocar, previous incisions, including scars from previous laparoscopy, should be avoided, if possible. After the site is chosen, an open technique is used to insert a blunt-tip Hasson trocar or a 10 mm port with video capability. If the initial site is amid multiple adhesions, an effort should be made to close the fascia to prevent air leakage and an alternative site should be chosen.

After the placement of the first trocar, the laparoscope is inserted, and careful inspection ensues. Most often visibility is limited due to adhesions, and at least one port should be inserted under direct vision before exploration is undertaken. All ports should be 10–12 mm in size to provide flexibility in camera and instrument positioning. As the adhesions are lysed and more of the peritoneal cavity inspected, additional ports are placed. Once the abdominal wall is cleared of adhesions, careful inspection of the bowel is undertaken. As it is often difficult to assess which of the adhesions were responsible for the clinical symptoms, especially in elective cases, sound judgement should be used and all suspected symptomatic adhesions should be lysed. Ideally, collapsed distal bowel and dilated proximal bowel should be confirmed. According to the findings, additional laparoscopic or laparoscopic-assisted procedures such as bowel resection, anastomosis, hernia reduction and repair, or stoma creation is performed (Reissman and Wexner, 1995).

Laparoscopic Surgery for Colorectal Malignancy

Several concerns have arisen regarding adequate laparoscopic excision of a neoplasm, especially for rectal cancer where the surgical technique plays a critical role in the prevention of local recurrence. It has been demonstrated that an incomplete surgical excision of the mesorectum and an inadequate lateral margin clearance (Heald et al., 1982; Cooperman et al., 1991; Irene et al., 1993; Quirke et al., 1986) are both associated with increased locoregional failure and poor prognosis. An improved 5-year survival rate of 78% and local recurrence of 3–5% has been achieved by Heald et al. (Heald and Ryall, 1986), by routine total mesorectal excision, and more recently by many others (Enker et al., 1995; Scott et al., 1995; Arbman et al., 1996; Aitken, 1996).

In our experience and that of others (Guillou et al., 1993), complete mesorectal excision with wide lateral margins is easily done laparoscopically. The rectum, after full mobilization, can be retracted in a cephalad direction, thus facilitating the dissection in the avascular presacral space. Any advantage of radical abdominopelvic lymphadenectomy for rectal cancer, as advocated by several authors (Enker et al., 1979; Koyama et al., 1984), still needs to be determined (Harnsberger et al., 1994). There are only a few experimental reports in the literature of such a lymphatic excision by laparoscopy (Decanini et al., 1994; Karamura et al., 1994).

Some authors (Bacon and Khubchandani, 1964; Sugarbaker et al., 1982) consider high ligation of the inferior mesenteric artery and harvesting of a large number of lymph nodes to be part of a curative resection for colonic neoplasm with improving survival rates. However, some studies have failed to demonstrate any advantages for patients treated by high ligation of the inferior mesenteric artery (Grinnel, 1965; Pezim and Nicholls, 1984).

Many recent studies have demonstrated that there was no significant difference between the number of lymph nodes removed comparing laparoscopy and laparotomy (Kim and Roy, 1994; Franklin et al.,

1995; Lord et al., 1996). However, the number of lymph nodes removed laparoscopically cannot be taken as a criterion for the effectiveness of a surgical excision. The number of lymph nodes collected depends not only on the surgeon, but also on the enthusiasm and technique employed by the pathologist (Cohen et al., 1994).

A critical issue related to laparoscopic surgery for cancer is the problem of port-site tumour recurrence (wound implantation). Since Alexander et al. (1993) first reported a 67-year-old female patient with a wound recurrence after laparoscopic-assisted right hemicolectomy for a Dukes' A carcinoma, many port-site recurrences following laparoscopic procedures for cure of malignancy have been described (Nduka et al., 1994; Wexner and Cohen, 1995). This complication has not occurred only in the port site through which the specimen is delivered, but has involved all port sites. Furthermore, it has not been limited to advanced neoplasia, but has been noted to occur following laparoscopic cholecystectomy for an unsuspected occult gall bladder carcinoma (Clair et al., 1993; Nduka et al., 1994) and after laparoscopic appendectomy in a patient with an occult carcinoma. It has certainly occurred many times in patients with early-stage colon carcinomas. No explanation for this phenomenon has been given. There are experimental data suggesting that surgical wounds are fertile sites for neoplastic growth (Murthy et al., 1989; Murthy et al., 1990), but this complication is virtually absent after laparotomy (Hughes et al., 1983). The actual incidence of port-site recurrence is unknown. Vertruyen and colleagues (Vertruyen et al., 1996) noted an overall 3.5% incidence. Similar numbers were found by other authors (Ngoi et al., 1994; Boulez and Herriot, 1994; Prasad et al., 1994; Fingerhut, 1996; Molenaar et al., 1998). More recently a study showed that 4.6% of members of the American Society of Colon and Rectal Surgeons and Society of American Gastrointestinal Endoscopic Surgeons have seen port-site recurrence (Mavrantonis et al., 1998). At opposite ends of the spectrum Berends (Berends et al., 1994) and Molenaar (Molenaar et al., 1996) reported incidences of 14% and 21%, respectively and Ramos et al. (1994), Fleshman et al. (1996) and Vukasin et al. (1996) demonstrated 1–1.5% port-site recurrence incidences. Putting the problem in perspective, isolated wound implantation without peritoneal carcinomatosis occurs after laparotomy in between 0.1% and 0.3% of cases (Hughes et al., 1983).

Laparoscopic resections for cure of carcinoma are still highly controversial and by no means standard care. In light of this controversy, some institutions and several national societies have started prospective, randomized controlled trials to address questions on the benefits of laparoscopic surgery. Therefore results of laparoscopic cancer resection will not be available for at least 5 years. The consensus is that laparoscopic resection of colorectal carcinoma should be limited to use in prospective randomized externally monitored trials. However, palliation of metastatic disease is a good laparoscopic indication.

Minimal Access Management of Anorectal Conditions such as Rectal Prolapse

Laparoscopic Rectopexy for Rectal Prolapse

Although rectal prolapse is a benign condition it is often debilitating. Surgical therapy is primarily based on transabdominal rectopexy with or without sigmoid resection and transanal proctosigmoidectomy (Altemeier et al., 1971; Keighley et al., 1983). Laparoscopic techniques may have advantages in these procedures (Cuschieri et al., 1994).

For laparoscopic abdominal rectopexy, the rectum is completely mobilized after which a Marlex mesh (C.R. Bard, Massachusetts, USA) or polypropylene mesh (Surgipro mesh, US Surgical Corporation) is stapled to the posterior rectal wall and presacral fascia on both sides of the rectum (Darzi et al., 1995b).

The perineal approach for the surgical treatment of a complete rectal prolapse may be assisted by the laparoscopic technique for transabdominal mobilization of the rectum to facilitate a more extensive perineal resection of the rectosigmoid (Lointier et al., 1993). Furthermore the laparoscope can be introduced transperineally after delivering a sufficiently long segment of prolapsed rectum. The remaining rectum, sigmoid or left colon is now visualized and further mobilization for the resection is undertaken if necessary. The procedure is concluded with resection of the prolapsed segment and subsequent coloanal anastomosis and levatoroplasty (Reissman et al., 1995b). Another laparoscopic update for prolapse treatment is resection rectopexy with coloproctostomy and suture rather than mesh presacral fixation.

Current Controversies in Laparoscopic Colorectal Surgery

Although all the structures such as ureters, mesenteric vessels, rectal vessels and mesorectum can be easily identified during laparoscopic surgery, complications related to iatrogenic injuries of the ureters (Guillou et al., 1993), major vessels (Wexner et al., 1993), and other structures (Phillips et al., 1992; Zucker et al., 1994) have been reported. Probably these complications are related to the loss of tactile sensation through the laparoscope and to the learning curve.

Another concern is the rate of removal of the wrong segment of bowel. Corbitt (1992) converted 3 of 18 procedures because of inability to identify the colonic lesion. Numerous others (Cawthorn et al., 1990; Larach et al., 1993a; Ngoi et al., 1994; Cohen and Wexner, 1995; Fingerhut, 1996) have also reported removal of the wrong segment of bowel.

Nursing Considerations

The practice of perioperative nursing brought new challenges and has grown more complex with the rapid technological advances in laparoscopic surgery. In part, media coverage has been responsible for widespread patient awareness, understanding and acceptance of this minimally invasive surgery. The lay public associate this technique with the benefits of reduced pain, better cosmesis, less trauma, shorter hospital stay and a more rapid return to work (Tucker and Voyles, 1995). As a result patients are more motivated to seek care at facilities that offer this 'new type' of surgery. Laparoscopic colorectal surgery has generated a large assortment of sophisticated equipment and instrumentation in the operating room. Because of this trend, new patterns of nursing care have emerged, motivating nurses to seek additional knowledge and develop new skills to care for patients undergoing laparoscopic bowel surgery.

This delivery of care must be individualized, and must include activities performed during the perioperative period. In order to practise in today's technologically complex environment, the perioperative nurse must be flexible, incorporating knowledge, judgement and skills. In addition, a thorough understanding of the functioning and troubleshooting of the equipment and instruments is vital to the success of any laparoscopic procedure.

Teamwork is important, and the patient must be the focus of attention at all times. From the time the patient is initially seen to the time of discharge and home follow-up, the perioperative nurse plays a significant role in overseeing the care of the patient.

Perioperative Evaluation

Nursing care in the preoperative phase begins at the time the patient makes the decision to have surgery and ends when the patient is transferred to the operating room table (AORN: Standards and Recommendation Practices, 1994). To increase the patient's chance of a positive surgical outcome, emotional and physical preparation is necessary. During this preoperative phase, the nurse establishes rapport with the patient and family, as this interaction builds confidence and trust. At this time, the nurse collects data, and, through patient assessment and interview, organizes and prioritizes this information to implement a plan of care.

Similarly to conventional surgery, patients preparing for laparoscopic surgery experience fears and anxieties, because they are about to undergo a 'new type' of surgery. Nurses should therefore reassure patients, and give an in-depth explanation of the proposed benefits of this approach. The family should be included in the perioperative teaching. The nurse must ascertain their level of knowledge and understanding of the laparoscopic procedure and should then provide the pertinent information to their level of intellect, without causing them to become overwhelmed.

The family should be told that despite the small abdominal incision, laparoscopic colorectal surgery is still major surgery. Despite the expected benefits, the patient should be allowed a safe recuperative period. This protocol includes following the surgeon's instructions regarding rest, diet and physical limitations. The family should be taught how to recognize signs of infection, swelling around the port sites, and if a stoma is made, instructions in stoma care.

A careful history and physical examination are valuable tools with which to assess the patient prior to laparoscopic colorectal surgery. Because of the many different configurations in which the body is positioned during the procedure, any pre-existing medical conditions which may be exacerbated by positioning need to be preoperatively identified.

The patient's age, weight, nutritional status, neurological, respiratory, renal and cardiac function should be documented. It is necessary that the perioperative nurse has a clear understanding of any physiological disturbances and complications that can occur when positioning the patient for laparoscopic bowel surgery.

A detailed explanation of pertinent activities throughout the perioperative phase should be given to the patient and family. This decision helps allay fears and anxieties, as the well-informed patient has a more positive surgical outcome (Brumfield et al., 1996). The nurse should ascertain that the surgeon's explanation of the risks, benefits and alternatives and possible complications of the procedure are understood. Also the patient and family must understand that in the event of any intraoperative complications a traditional laparotomy will be performed. Therefore the nurse should always obtain consent for laparotomy. Should the patient have a diagnosis of rectal neoplasia, the nurse should verify that the patient gives consent for intraoperative colonoscopy as the surgeon may need to identify the tumour location during the procedure.

Preoperative investigations are similar to those of the open procedures. Reports of any investigations such as barium enema, computed tomography (CT) scans, magnetic resonance imaging (MRI) and ultrasounds should be placed in the patient's chart. The perioperative nurse should be familiar with the normal values of blood tests and electrocardiogram (ECG), so that any abnormalities can be brought to the attention of the surgeon. Prior to surgery, the patient's legs are fitted with thigh-high elastic stockings and pneumatic anti-thrombotic intermittent compression stockings (PAS) which help to stimulate venous return.

Bowel Preparation

A clean decompressed bowel is vital to a successful laparoscopic bowel procedure. An unprepared bowel places the patient at risk for injury and spillage of faecal material into the abdominal cavity, potentially increasing the incidence of infectious complications. The day before the surgery, the nurse administers the bowel preparation as ordered. Several preparations are used by surgeons. Several recent large prospective randomized studies have shown that 90 ml of sodium phosphate-based oral solutions (Fleet's phosphosoda – CB Fleet, Lynchburg, VA) is superior to 4 litres of polyethylene glycol. As such, the newer former preparation has replaced the older, less well-tolerated one (Oliveira et al., 1997b). In order to minimize the impact and potential risks of laparoscopic colorectal surgery, the patient should generally be adequately prepared by the use of both mechanical and oral and parenteral antibiotic preparation. Nurses must be vigilant about correctly administering preoperative oral and parenteral antibiotics, as many studies have revealed an association between peri-operative timing and postoperative wound infections (Butts and Woford, 1997).

Operating Room Set-up

Being prepared is the key to a successful laparoscopic procedure. The team must be consistent and familiar with the functioning and troubleshooting of 'high tech' laparoscopic equipment and instrumentation.

Preparation begins with review of the surgeon's preference card. The circulating nurse and scrub nurse must assemble all equipment and instruments, with 'back-up' in case of any malfunctioning. Prior to the patient's arrival in the operating room, all equipment should be verified as being in working order. The basic laparoscopic instruments should be opened and set up. Laparotomy instruments should be also opened on to the same table and counted in case of an immediate conversion. With such a large assortment of high-tech equipment, the operating room should be larger than the traditional procedure room. Equipment should be placed around the sterile field in a manner to maintain the integrity of the sterile field. The major steps in preparing for laparoscopic colorectal surgery are:

1. Assembling the laparoscopic equipment.
2. Instrumentation and handling precautions.
3. Preparing the patient, positioning and safety precautions.

Equipment

The equipment used in laparoscopic bowel surgery includes: video monitors, camera, light source, carbon dioxide insufflation, video recording unit, electrosurgical unit, harmonic scalpel, endoscopy unit, suction and irrigation devices (Ethicon Endosurgery Inc, Cincinnati, OH). Accommodating most of the equipment on one or two units has been very helpful (Figure 12.5). Ceiling-mounted monitors provide for more efficient viewing and decrease the set-up and take-down times.

Laparoscopic surgery permits limited access to the surgical site, therefore the surgeon's direct visual perception is hindered when performing the procedure. Thus the team depends completely on the video equipment to provide intraperitoneal imaging. To facilitate viewing by the assistant, and should technical problems develop, the second monitor is placed opposite the first. Both monitors should be positioned so that they will provide unobstructed views to the surgeon in a direct line of vision. All of the plugs from the video units should be consolidated into an approved transformer, so that one main electrical cord can be used. It is also helpful to have attached to the video unit clear written operating instructions, outlining the steps for assembling the video equipment.

Before use, the camera must first be calibrated by white balancing to provide an accurate colour spectrum (Milsom and Bohm, 1996). The scrub nurse performs this check by attaching the camera to the telescope eyepiece and focusing the camera on a white sponge. The

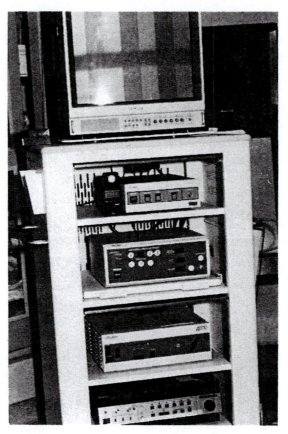

Figure 12.5: Accommodating most of the laparoscopic equipment on one unit has proven to be quite helpful.

circulating nurse presses the white balance button on the camera unit as the scrub nurse watches and adjusts the zoom for the right colour, size and sharpness (Paz-Partlow, 1995). Once white balance is activated, the camera is sensitive to define white, and hence all of the other colours also appropriately appear (Milsom and Bohm, 1996). The scrub nurse must check for condensation of moisture behind the sealed connectors of the camera. Loose connectors can result in lack of sufficient light.

The insufflation uses carbon dioxide or another non-toxic gas to distend the peritoneal cavity to allow visualization of the abdominal organs. In order to maintain pneumoperitoneum, the circulating nurse must ascertain that there are no obvious defects or damage to the equipment. An extra tank of CO_2 should be available on the unit for exchange to avoid the risk of interruption of the procedure for lack of insufflation gas. The intra-abdominal pressure is pre-selected and the rate for gas flow is automatic. A pressure of 10 – 15 mm Hg is optimal. A defective Veress needle or a kinked supply tube should be noticed immediately as an increase registered on the pressure monitor while the gas flow registers '000'.

The circulating nurse is responsible for starting the recording mode once the procedure has begun, so as not to miss documenting important findings. A supply of high-quality blank tapes should be available along with a functional videorecording unit.

Electrosurgery is commonly used in many minimally invasive procedures. It is used to cut and coagulate body tissue with a high radio frequency current. The electrosurgery unit (ESU) is composed of a generator, foot and/or hand control device and electrical cord with plug. Before use, the device should be checked for insulation failure, as any defect in the active electrode can result in unintentional flow of current to the patient's abdominal viscera (Tucker and Voyles, 1995). The circulating nurse should ensure proper connection of the monopolar and/or bipolar electrodes to their corresponding outputs. The power setting should be within range, and it is helpful to turn on the generator volume so that any unintentional activation is immediately recognized. The surgeon should be notified of any defect in the electrode after the procedure, as there could be the potential for unintended injury to the bowel, which can result in a grave postoperative complication.

The harmonic scalpel has no electrical current, and it saves operating time by eliminating multiple ligating and suturing manoeuvres as well as the time needed for smoke evacuation and camera lens cleaning. The blade or the handpiece can be positioned for the use in blunt, flat or sharp modes, therefore the instrument should be passed to the surgeon in the desired position. The unit should be at least 30 cm from the electrosurgical unit to avoid electrical interference. The foot pedal should be identified and placed on the same side as the surgeon using the handpiece.

Instrumentation and Handling

Because laparoscopic surgery allows only limited access to the surgical site, the instruments are designed for easy hand movement. The purpose of the instruments is to establish pneumoperitoneum and entry to the abdomen and manipulation of the tissue. For use on tissue, they are used to manipulate, grasp, dissect, cut, coagulate, retract and isolate the specimen and to provide haemostasis.

The laparoscopic instruments usually used are:

Veress needle;
12 mm trocars;
12 mm blunt trocar – Hasson;
10 mm endoscopic Babcock clamp;
10 mm endoscopic Metzenbaum scissors;
10 mm endoscopic large clips;
LCS harmonic scalpel (Ethicon Endosurgery Inc, Cincinnati, OH);
10 mm endoscopic Kelly clamp;
10 mm endoscopic non-crushing bowel clamps;
10 mm endoscopic modified Allis (anvil grasping) clamps (Ethicon
    Endosurgery Inc, Cincinnati, OH);
18 mm TEC trocar with exchange rod (Ethicon Endosurgery Inc,
    Cincinnati, OH);
EZ45G or ET45B – endoscopic linear cutter 60 mm (Ethicon
    Endosurgery Inc, Cincinnati, OH);
33 mm trocar kit including reducer and exchange rod (Ethicon
    Endosurgery Inc, Cincinnati, OH)
TLC 75;
ECS 29 or 33 endoscopic circular stapler (Ethicon Endosurgery Inc,
    Cincinnati, OH);
ATW35 – endoscopic 35 mm (Ethicon Endosurgery Inc, Cincinnati,
    OH) ;
endoscopic pre-tied loops
18 mm to 10 mm reducer;
10mm diameter high flow suction/irrigation cannula.

The Veress needle is used as the vehicle for instilling carbon dioxide
into the abdomen to establish pneumoperitoneum (see Figure 12.4).
The needle should be checked for blockage before use. Trocars and
cannulas are used to penetrate the abdominal wall and to provide
access for the laparoscopic instruments. The trocar with its spring-
laden shield should be armed before passing the instrument to the
surgeon. The laparoscopic telescope provides an image of the abdominal cavity. Before inserting it into the abdominal cavity, it is helpful to
warm the instrument for at least half an hour before use. It is also
advisable to introduce the CO_2 gas into a port other than that of the
camera, as CO_2 gas is cooler and fogs the lens, obscuring the surgeon's
vision. Periodically opening one of the ports has proven to clear the
smoke. Special anti-fog fluid or hot water should be available to clean
the lens. Grasping instruments can be traumatic or atraumatic, and
the scrub nurse must pass only atraumatic instruments when the
intestines are being handled.

For rapid haemostasis of vessels, intra-abdominal clips are used, and a second application should be ready for quick exchange. Certain clips need to be pre-loaded before first usage. The endoscopic stapler is used to close enterotomies, divide bowel or occlude bleeding vessels. The irrigating/aspirating unit is used to maintain a clear field of vision for the surgeon, as bleeding can result in conversion to a laparotomy if the unit does not accomplish its objective. To avoid unnecessary clutter of instrumentation on the surgical field, the use of a long instrument pouch such as a 1018L Steri-Drape (3M, Medical and Surgical Division, St Paul, MN) has been found to be very helpful (Figure 12.6). A troubleshooting guide (Table 12.2) is provided in the event of any malfunctioning.

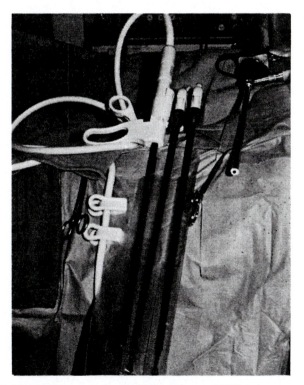

Figure 12.6: The long instrument pouch Steri-Drape 1018L helps to avoid unnecessary clutter of instrumentation on the surgical field (3M, Medical and Surgical Division, St Paul, MN).

Preparing the Patient

As the scope of perioperative nursing continues, the second phase – the intraoperative period – begins with the patient being transferred to the operating room table and ends with admittance to the post-anaesthesia

Table 12.2: Troubleshooting guide

Symptom	Cause	Solution
1. Pneumoperitoneum loss/poor insufflation	CO_2 tank empty	Change tank; have spare in room
	Open accessory port stopcock(s)	Check all trocars; close open stopcocks
	Trocar seal leak or stopcock leak	Exchange for new one
	Too much suctioning	Stop suction; wait for reinsufflation of abdomen
	Insufflator tubing; loose connections at unit or port	Tighten connections
	Loose Hasson stay sutures	Refasten sutures
2. Pressure readings too high	Veress needle not in peritoneal space	Reinsert needle
	Tubing blocked (kinked, cart wheel, too small)	Check all tubing
	Stopcock closed	Open stopcock
	'Light' anaesthesia	More muscle relaxant
3. Dim image/poor lighting	Cable not well connected at port and/or scope	Tighten connections
	Unit on lowest setting	Increase to maximum
	Burned-out bulb	Replace
	Light cable broken	Replace
	Scope light fibres broken	Replace
	Camera auto-iris compensating for overbright reflection	Switch to 'manual' iris or move scope
	Brightness on monitor misadjusted to minimum	Push 'reset' button for factory settings
		Cover fine tuning buttons
4. Overly bright image	'Gain' on camera control unit is set on high	Set to normal
	Light source's 'boost' is on	Turn off 'boost'
	Brightness on monitor misadjusted to maximum	Push 'reset' button for factory settings
5. No monitor image(s)	Monitor, camera control, or other electronic accessory in cart not switched on	Check all power cords. Turn on all units
	Coaxial cable connections to monitor from camera control unit or last electronic item in chain not coupled correctly	Run coaxial cable 'video out' from camera or last item in sequence (i.e. VCR, printer) to 'video in' on monitor
	Coaxial cable between first and second cart monitors not connected	Run cable 'video out' from cart 1 monitor to 'video in' on cart 2 monitor
	Wrong 'input' selection made on monitor	Choose the right 'input' button on monitor's front
6. Inferior monitor image	Scope fogs when introduced into abdominal cavity	Pre-heat scope in warm saline. Keep antifogging solution on sponge in field
	Lens tip smeared with fluids	Clean tip
Intermittent electrical interference, flashes, flickering	Broken coaxial cable	Replace cable
	Inadequate shielding on camera control unit or light source	Isolate electrosurgical unit on separate circuit
	Wet connecting plug on camera cable	Blow dry with compressed air
Fuzzy image	Camera out of focus	Adjust focus ring
	Internal condensation on scope, damaged cover glass	Check lens and camera; exchange

(cont.)

Table 12.2: Cont.

Symptom	Cause	Solution
7. Insufficient irrigation/ suction	Tubing blocked (kinked, tissue, clots)	Check complete length; flush
	Suction/irrigation tip blocked, valves stuck	Flush with syringe; replace
	Suction tubing not connected to wall or canister	Double check and tighten all connections
	Pressure not dialled in; CO_2 or nitrogen valves not open	Check gas source for correct settings
8. Inappropriate/ no cautery current	Insecure grounding pad	Secure pad to patient, ensuring good contact
	Electrosurgical cable partly disconnected to unit or handswitch	Anchor the contacts

Source: With permission from Phillips EH and Rosenthal RJ (Eds) (1995) Operative Strategies in Laparoscopic Surgery. Berlin: Springer-Verlag.

care unit (PACU) (AORN: Standards and Recommended Practice, 1994).

When entering the operating room, the patient may undergo great stress and experience anxiety. Being away from the family and surrounded by masked individuals in a room with multiple high-tech devices, the patient looks to the operating room nurse for reassurance. The nurse needs to reassure the patient, that he or she has entered a safe environment, and will be cared for by a caring team which is knowledgeable in laparoscopic bowel surgery. This nurse should utilize all of his or her knowledge and skills to allow for an efficient performance of the successful laparoscopic procedure.

Positioning

During the intraoperative period, drugs, anaesthetic agents and muscle relaxants depress the pain receptors, resulting in the patient's lack of normal compensatory mechanisms. As a result, the circulating nurse should utilize his or her knowledge of anatomy and physiology, and the patient's history, to position the patient safely. It is in fact the responsibility of the entire laparoscopic team to safely position the patient. During laparoscopic colorectal surgery, the patient is placed in many exaggerated and abnormal positions, in order to offer the optimal exposure. However, these positions can result in undesirable changes that can affect the circulatory and respiratory systems. With improper positioning, the patient can also sustain neurological complications.

The position most often used by surgeons is the modified lithotomy, in which the patient's legs are positioned almost straight to avoid hindrance as the surgeon manipulates the instruments (Figure 12.7).

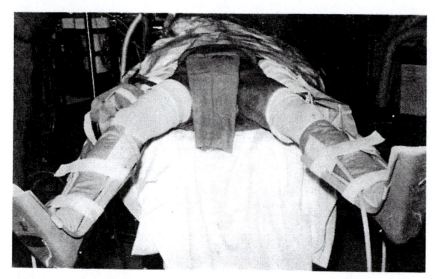

Figure 12.7: The modified lithotomy position with the legs positioned almost straight to avoid hindering the surgeon while manipulating the instruments.

The patient's legs are fitted preoperatively with thigh-high stockings and pneumatic anti-thrombotic stockings (PAS) before placing them on to gel pads in Allen stirrups (Allen Medical Corp, Bedford Heights, OH). These stirrups are preferred to the Lloyd-Davies variety as they do not exert any pressure on the fibular head in the region of the peroneal nerve. The PAS stockings periodically inflate to stimulate venous return and avoid deep vein thrombosis (DVT) (McCammon, 1996) (Figure 12.8).

Bearing in mind that the three forces of pressure, obstruction and stretching account for the majority of injuries because of faulty positioning, the nurse should pad and protect all bony prominences. In the lower extremities, the common peroneal nerve is usually the most frequently damaged (McCammon, 1996). Great care must be taken to avoid compression of the nerve between the head of the fibula and the metal brace of the stirrups. Because of numerous changes of the patient's position during the procedure, the patient's body should be properly secured to the table. Both arms are best secured at the patient's side, with pads or protectors placed at the hands and elbows (Figure 12.9). The hand should not be allowed to touch the metal part of the operating room table, as this could result in neurological damage or electrical current transmission. Continuous monitoring of the patient's position by the circulating nurse should identify any unintended shifts in position that can result in potential intraoperative or postoperative complications. During this intraoperative phase, the circulating nurse also updates the patient's family or significant others of the progress of the surgery.

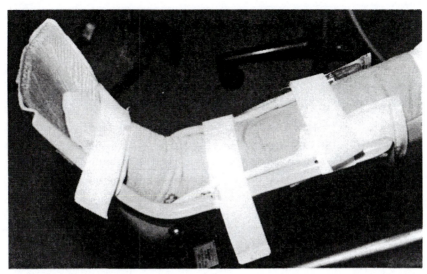

Figure 12.8: The patient's legs are fitted with PAS stockings and placed on gel pads in Allen stirrups.

Postoperative Management

The final stage of perioperative care is the postoperative phase, which begins with the admission to the PACU but does not end until full recovery (AORN: Standards and Recommended Practices, 1994). This period involves caring for the patient in the hospital, in the clinic and at home. Excellence in nursing is continuous until the patient returns to his or her optimum state of health.

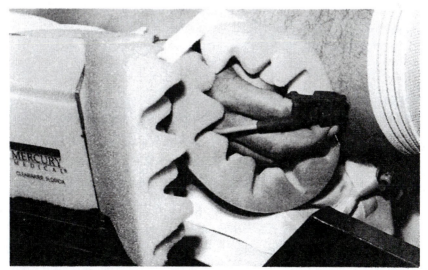

Figure 12.9: The patient's hands are protected with pads and are not allowed to touch the metal part of the operating room table.

The nursing care postoperatively for laparoscopic colorectal surgery is similar to that of conventional open surgery. However, the patient experiences less trauma on the abdominal wall, less bowel dysfunction, improved respiratory function and an earlier return to recovery (McCammon, 1996).

Because of earlier postoperative feeding, the patient should note any signs of gastric distension or eructation. A common complaint of mild shoulder pain is usually experienced for up to 1 week, and is believed to be caused by stretching of the diaphragm during insufflation (McCammon, 1996). Although some authors consider this pain insignificant, others believe that if this pain lasts for more than 24 hours, the patient should be assessed for neurological injury (McCammon, 1996). Analgesics, heat pads or gentle passive exercises have all been found helpful in relieving this pain (Gosling and Mason, 1994).

The patient's respiratory status should be closely monitored as the CO_2 used to distend the abdomen can cause postoperative acidosis from absorbed CO_2, pneumothorax or CO_2 emboli (Pilcher et al., 1996). Therefore monitoring of the respiratory system is vital to avoid these potential complications. The patient should be instructed to cough, deep breathe and use the incentive spirometer. The monitoring of blood gases and pulse monitor readings are important tools with which to assess respiratory status.

Because laparoscopic surgery patients are discharged home earlier, the family and home health nurses should be alerted to the signs and symptoms of any inflammatory reactions, which may present after discharge. The family should be given instructions regarding diet and limitations. Patients experiencing severe abdominal pain after laparoscopic bowel surgery should be aggressively investigated.

Conclusions

With the increased complexity of high-tech procedures in laparoscopic colorectal surgery, perioperative nurses are faced with changing patterns in the delivery of health care. They are assuming new roles and greater responsibilities as they adapt to the rapidly changing, technological and socioeconomic forces. Laparoscopic colorectal surgery demands knowledge and skills to meet the health care needs of the patient effectively, as the outcome of the procedure directly reflects on the quality of perioperative nursing care provided. There must be collaborative efforts to assure the highest quality of care for the patient, therefore perioperative nurses must be encouraged to attend seminars and workshops with surgeons, where they can acquire current knowledge of patient care and become familiar with the use of new laparoscopic equipment and instrumentation.

With the changing scope of nursing practice, nurses must exercise judgement in accepting responsibilities in caring for patients undergoing laparoscopic colorectal surgery. If they lack the education, knowledge, competence and experience to function in this perioperative role, they should not be allowed to fulfil the responsibility of providing nursing care. The patient is always the focus of attention; the patient's welfare should be the greatest concern.

At the moment laparoscopic colorectal surgery is clearly beneficial for the patient with benign disease of the colon. It is also indicated for palliation of metastatic disease. It may confer some advantages in patients with bowel obstruction or with rectal prolapse. It should only be offered for care of carcinoma within the confines of an externally monitored and peer-reviewed prospective randomized trial. When it is offered it must be by a well-trained cohesive team as the outcome of the patient is most directly impacted upon by the experience and integration of the team.

References

Aitken RJ (1996) Mesorectal excision for rectal cancer. British Journal of Surgery 83: 214–16.

Alexander RJ, Jacques BC, Mitchell KG (1993) Laparoscopic assisted colectomy and wound recurrence (letter). Lancet 341: 249–50.

Altemeier WA, Culbertson WR, Schowengerdy C, Hunt J (1971) Nineteen years experience with the one-stage perineal repair of rectal prolapse. Annals of Surgery 173: 993–1006.

AORN (1994) A Model for Perioperative Nursing Practices. AORN Standards and Recommended Practices. Denver: Association of Operating Room Nurses: 57–61.

Arbman G, Nilsson E, Hallbook O, Sjodahl R (1996) Local recurrence following total mesorectal excision for rectal cancer. British Journal of Surgery 83: 375–9.

Bacon HE, Khubchandani IT (1964) The rationale of aortoileopelvic and high ligation of the inferior mesenteric artery for carcinoma of the left half of the colon and rectum. Surgery, Gynecology and Obstetrics 119: 503–8.

Bailey RW, Zucker KA, Flowers JL (1991) Laparoscopic cholecystectomy. Experience with 375 consecutive patients. Annals of Surgery 213: 531–9.

Barnett RB, Clement GS, Drizin GS (1992) Pulmonary changes after laparoscopic cholecystectomy. Surgery, Laparoscopy, Endoscopy 2: 125–7.

Bernstein MA, Dawson JW, Reissman P, Weiss EG, Nogueras JJ, Wexner SD (1996) Is complete laparoscopic colectomy superior to laparoscopic-assisted colectomy. American Surgeon 62: 507–11.

Berends FJ, Kazemier G, Bonjer HJ, Lange JF (1994) Subcutaneous metastases after laparoscopic colectomy (letter). Lancet 344: 344–58.

Binderow SR, Cohen SM, Wexner SD, Nogueras JJ (1994) Must early postoperative oral intake be limited to laparoscopy? Diseases of the Colon and Rectum 37: 584–9.

Böhm B, Milsom JW, Fazio VW (1995) Postoperative intestinal motility following conventional and laparoscopic intestinal surgery. Archives of Surgery 130: 415–19.

Boulez J, Herriot E (1994) Multicentric analysis of laparoscopic colorectal surgery in FDCL group. 274 cases. British Journal of Surgery 81: 527.

Brumfield VC, Kee CC, Johnson JY (1996) Perioperative patient teaching in ambulatory surgery settings. AORN 64 (December): 941–52.

Butts JD, Woford ET (1997) Timing of perioperative antibiotic administration. AORN 65 (January): 109–15.

Cawthorn SJ, Parums DV, Gibbs NM, Ahern RP, Caffarey SM, Broughton CI, Marks CG (1990) Extent of mesorectal spread and involvement of lateral resection margin as a prognostic factor after surgery for rectal cancer. Lancet 335: 1055–9.

Clair DG, Lautz DB, Brooks DC (1993) Rapid development of umbilical metastases after cholecystectomy for unsuspected gallbladder carcinoma. Surgery 113: 355–8.

Cohen SM, Nogueras JJ, Wexner SD (1996) Laparoscopic colorectal surgery: ascending the learning curve. World Journal of Surgery 20: 277–82.

Cohen SM, Wexner SD (1994) Laparoscopic right hemicolectomy. Surgical Rounds: Minimally Invasive Surgery Series (November): 627–35.

Cohen SM, Wexner SD (1995) Laparoscopic colorectal surgery: are we being honest with our patients. Diseases of the Colon and Rectum 38: 723–7.

Cohen SM, Wexner SD, Schmitt SL, Nogueras JJ, Lucas FV (1994) Effect of xylene clearance of mesenteric fat on harvest of lymph nodes after colonic resection. European Journal of Surgery 160: 693–7.

Cooperman A, Katz V, Zimmon D, Bopro G (1991) Laparoscopic colon resection: a case report. Journal of Laparoendoscopic Surgery 1: 79–81.

Corbitt JD (1992) Preliminary experience with laparoscopic-guided colectomy. J Laparo Endosc Surg 2: 79–81.

Cuschieri A, Berci G, McSherry CK (1990) Laparoscopic cholecystectomy. American Journal of Surgery 159: 273–8.

Cuschieri A, Wood RA, Banting S, Shimi SM, Vander Velpen G, Banting S, Wood RA (1994) Laparoscopic prosthesis fixation rectopexy for complete rectal prolapse. British Journal of Surgery 8 (1): 138–9.

Darzi A, Monson JR, Guillou PJ, Menzies-Gow N, Lewis C (1995a) Laparoscopic abdominoperineal excision of the rectum. Surgical Endoscopy 9 (4): 414–17.

Darzi A, Henry MM, Guillou PJ, Shorvon P, Monson JR (1995b) Stapled laparoscopic rectopexy for rectal prolapse. Surgical Endoscopy 3: 301–3.

Decanini C, Milsom JW, Bohm B, Fazio VW (1994) Laparoscopic oncologic abdominoperineal resection. Diseases of the Colon and Rectum 37: 552–8.

DeKok H (1977) A new technique for resecting the noninflamed not-adhesive appendix through a mini-laparotomy with the aid of a laparoscope. Arch Chir Neerl 29: 195.

Dubois F, Icard P, Berthelot G (1990) Coeliscopic cholecystectomy. Preliminary report of 36 cases. Annals of Surgery 211: 60–2.

Enker W, Laffer VT, Block GE (1979) Enhanced survival of patients with colon and rectal cancer is based upon wide anatomic resection. Annals of Surgery 190: 350–60.

Enker WE, Thaler HT, Cranor ML, Polyak T (1995) Total mesorectal excision in the operative treatment of carcinoma of the rectum. Journal of the American College of Surgeons 181: 335–46.

Falk PM, Beart RW, Wexner SD, Thorson AG, Jagelman DG, Lavery IC, Johansen OB, Fitzgibbons RJ Jr (1993) Laparoscopic colectomy: a critical appraisal. Diseases of the Colon and Rectum 36: 28–34.

Fingerhut A (1996) Laparoscopic assisted colonic resection: the French experience. In Jagar R, Wexner SD Laparoscopic Colorectal Surgery. New York: Churchill Livingstone, pp 253–7.

Fleshman JW, Nelson H, Peters WR, Kim HC, Larach S, Boorse RR et al. (1996a). Clinical Outcomes of Surgical Therapy (COST) Study Group. Early results of laparoscopic surgery for colorectal cancer: retrospective analysis of 372 patients treated by COST Study Group. Diseases of the Colon and Rectum 39(Suppl): S53–S58.

Fleshman JW, Fry PD, Birnbaum EH, Kodner IJ (1996b) Laparoscopic assisted and minilaparotomy approaches to colorectal diseases are similar in early outcome. Diseases of the Colon and Rectum 39: 15–22.

François Y, Vignal J, Tomaoglu K, Mouret P (1994) Postoperative adhesive peritoneal disease. The Treatment. Surgical Endoscopy 8 (7): 781–3.

Franklin ME Jr, Ramos R, Rosenthal D, Schuessler W (1993) Laparoscopic colonic procedures. World Journal of Surgery 17: 51–6.

Franklin ME, Rosenthal D, Norem RF (1995) Prospective evaluation of laparoscopic colon resection versus open colon resection for adenocarcinoma. A multicenter study. Surgical Endoscopy 9: 811–16.

Furhman G, Ota DM (1994) Laparoscopic intestinal stomas. Diseases of the Colon and Rectum 37: 444–9.

Gosling M, Mason J (1994) Perioperative care. In Hall FA (Ed.) Minimal Access Surgery for Nurses and Technicians. Oxford: Radcliff Medical Press: 58.

Grinnel RS (1965) Results of ligation of inferior mesenteric artery at the aorta in resections of carcinoma of the descending sigmoid and colon and rectum. Surgery, Gynecology and Obstetrics 120: 1031–6.

Guillou OJ, Darzi A, Monson JR (1993) Experience with laparoscopic colorectal surgery for malignant disease. Journal of Surgical Oncology 2(Suppl 1): 43–9.

Harnsberger JR, Vernava AM, Longo WE (1994) Radical abdominopelvic lymphadenectomy: historic perspective and current role in the surgical management of rectal cancer. Diseases of the Colon and Rectum 37: 73–87.

Hasson HM (1971) Modified instrument and method for laparoscopy. American Journal of Obstetrics and Gynecology 110: 886–7.

Heald RJ, Husband EM, Ryall RD (1982) The mesorectum in rectal cancer surgery: the clue to pelvic recurrence. British Journal of Surgery 69: 613–16.

Heald RJ, Ryall RD (1986) Recurrence and survival after total mesorectal excision for rectal cancer. Lancet 1479–82.

Hughes ESR, McDermott FT, Polglase AL, Johnson WR (1983) Tumor recurrence in the abdominal wall scar after large bowel cancer surgery. Diseases of the Colon and Rectum 26: 571–2.

Jacobs M, Verdeja JC, Goldstein HS (1991) Minimally invasive colon resection (laparoscopic colectomy) Surgery, Laparoscopy, Endoscopy 1: 144–50.

Jenkins DM, Paluzzi M, Scott TE (1993) Postlaparoscopic small bowel obstruction. Surgery, Laparoscopy, Endoscopy 3: 139–41.

Karamura YJ, Savada T, Muto T, Nagai H (1994) Laparoscopic assisted colectomy and lymphadenectomy with abdominal wall lifting method. Diseases of the Colon and Rectum 37: 16.

Keighley MRB, Fielding JWL, Alexander-Williams J (1983) Results of marlex mesh abdominal rectopexy for rectal prolapse in 100 consecutive patients. British Journal of Surgery 70: 229–32.

Khoor E, Montrey J, Cohen MM (1993) Laparoscopic loop ileostomy for temporary fecal diversion. Diseases of the Colon and Rectum 36: 966–8.

Kim HJ, Roy T (1994) Unexpected gallbladder cancer with cutaneous seeding after laparoscopic cholecystectomy. South Medical Journal 87: 817–20.

Koyama Y, Moriya Y, Hojo K (1984) Effects of extended systemic lymphadenectomy for adenocarcinoma of the rectum: significant improvement of survival rate and decrease of local recurrence. Japanese Journal of Clinical Oncology 14: 131–2.

Lange V, Meyer G, Shardey M, Schildberg FW (1991) Laparoscopic creation of a loop ileostomy. Journal of Laparoendoscopic Surgery 1: 307–12.

Larach SW, Salomon MC, Williamson PR, Goldstein E (1993a) Laparoscopic-assisted colectomy: experience during the learning curve. Coloproctology 1: 38–41.

Larach SW, Salomon MC, Williamson PR, Goldstein E (1993b) Laparoscopic-assisted abdominoperineal resection. Surgery, Laparoscopy, Endoscopy 3: 115–18.

Lazorthes F, Chiotassol P (1986) Stapled colorectal anastomosis: perspective integrity of the anastomosis and risk of postoperative leakage. International Journal of Colorectal Diseases 1: 96–8.

Lointier P, Lechner C, Larpent J L, Chipponi J (1993) Laparoscopic assisted perineal rectosigmoidectomy with pull through. Journal of Laparoendoscopic Surgery 3: 547–56.

Lord SA, Larach SW, Ferrara A, Williamson PR, Lago CP, Lube MW (1996) Laparoscopic resections for colorectal carcinoma. A three year experience. Diseases of the Colon and Rectum 39(2): 148–54.

McCammon R (1996) Anesthetic and positional complications. In Jager RM, Wexner SD (Eds) Laparoscopic Colorectal Surgery. New York: Churchill Livingstone, pp 45–53.

Mavrantonis C, Potenti F, Wexner SD (1998) Laparoscopic colorectal surgery – have attitudes changed (abstract). Diseases of the Colon and Rectum 14 (4): A47.

Milson JW, Bohm B (1996) Laparoscopic Colorectal Surgery. New York: Springer, pp 1–5.

Molenaar CBH, Bijnen AB, Lopes-Cardozo AMF, de Ruiter P (1996) Indications for laparoscopic colectomy. Presentation at the XVIth Biennial Congress of the International Society of University Colon and Rectal Surgeons, Lisbon, Portugal, 14–18 April.

Molenaar ChBH, Bijnen AB, Ruiter P(1998) Indications for laparoscopic colorectal surgery. Surgical Endoscopy 12: 42–5.

Monson JRT, Darzi A, Carey PD, Guillou PJ (1992) Prospective evaluation of laparoscopic-assisted colectomy in an unselected group of patients. Lancet 340: 831–3.

Murthy SM, Goldschmidt RA, Rhao LN, Ammirati M, Buchmann T, Scanlon EF (1989) The influence of surgical trauma on experimental metastases. Cancer 64: 2035–44.

Murthy SM, Summaria JL et al. (1990) Experimental metastases at sites of surgical trauma (abstract). Proceedings of the Annual Meeting of the American Association for Cancer Research 31: A393.

Nduka CC, Monson JRT, Menzies-Gow, Darzi A (1994) Abdominal wall metastases following laparoscopy. British Journal of Surgery 81: 648–52.

Ng IO, Luk IS, Yuen ST, Lau PW, Pritchett CJ, Ng M, Poon GP, Ho J (1993) Surgical lateral clearance in resected rectal carcinomas: a multivariate analysis of clinicopathologic features. Cancer 71: 1972–6.

Ngoi SS, Kum CK, Goh PMY et al. (1994) Laparoscopic colon resection; the Singapore experience. Poster presentation at the Tripartite Colorectal Surgery Meeting. Sydney, Australia, 17–20 October.

Oliveira L, Werner SD, Daniel N, DeMarta D, Weiss EG, Nogueras JJ, Bernstein M (1997a) Mechanical bowel preparation for elective colorectal surgery: A prospective, randomized surgeon-blinded trial comparing sodium phosphate and polyethylene glycol-based oral lavage solutions. Diseases of the Colon and Rectum 40: 585–91.

Oliveira L, Reissman P, Nogueras J, Wexner SD (1997b) Laparoscopic creation of stomas. Surgical Endoscopy 11: 19–23.

Paz-Partlow M (1995) Basic instrumentation and troubleshooting. In Phillips H, Rosenthal RJ (Eds) Operative Strategies in Laparoscopic Surgery. Berlin: Springer-Verlag, pp 2–9.

Pezim ME, Nicholls RJ (1984) Survival after high or low ligation of the inferior mesenteric artery during curative surgery of rectal cancer. Annals of Surgery 200: 729–33.

Pfeifer J, Wexner SD, Reissman P, Bernstein M, Nogueras JJ, Singh S, Weiss EG (1995) Laparoscopy versus open colon surgery: costs and outcome. Surgical Endoscopy 9: 1322–6.

Phillips EH, Franklin M, Carroll BJ, Fallas MJ, Ramos R, Rosenthal D (1992) Laparoscopic colectomy. Annals of Surgery 216: 703–7.

Philips EH, Rosenthal RJ (Eds) Operative Strategies in Laparoscopic Surgery. Berlin: Springer-Verlag.

Pier A, Gotz F, Bacher C (1991) Laparoscopic appendectomy in 625 cases: from innovation to routine. Surgery, Laparoscopy, Endoscopy 1: 8–13.

Pilcher CJ, Wesdowski MS, Jawad MA (1996) Laparoscopic applications for abdominal trauma injuries. AORN 64 (September) 365–75.

Poulin EC, Mamazza J, Breton G, Fortin CL, Wabha R, Ergina P (1992) Evaluation of pulmonary function in laparoscopic cholecystectomy. Surgery, Laparoscopy, Endoscopy 2: 292–6.

Prasad A, Avery C, Foley RJG (1994) Abdominal wall metastases following laparoscopy (letter). British Journal of Surgery 81: 1697.

Quirke P, Durdey P, Dixon MF, Williams NS (1986) Local recurrence of rectal adenocarcinoma due to inadequate surgical resection. Lancet 1: 1996–9.

Ramos JM, Beart RW, Goes R, Ortega AE, Schlinkert RT (1995) Role of laparoscopy in colorectal surgery. A prospective evaluation of 200 cases. Diseases of the Colon and Rectum 38: 494–501.

Ramos JM, Gupta S, Anthone GJ, Ortega AE, Simons AJ, Beart RW (1994) Laparoscopic colon cancer: is the port site at risk. A preliminary report. Archives of Surgery 127: 897–900.

Reddick EJ, Olsen DO (1989) Laparoscopic laser cholecystectomy: a comparison with minilaparotomy cholecystectomy. Surgical Endoscopy 3: 131–3.

Reissman P, Teoh TA, Weiss EG, Cohen SM, Nogueras JJ, Wexner SD (1995a) Is early feeding safe after elective colorectal surgery? Annals of Surgery 222: 73–7.

Reissman P, Weiss EG, Teoh TA, Cohen SM, Wexner SD (1995b) Laparoscopic assisted perineal rectosigmoidectomy for rectal prolapse. Surgery, Laparoscopy, Endoscopy 5: 217–18.

Reissman P, Wexner SD (1995) Laparoscopic surgery for intestinal obstruction. Surgical Endoscopy 9: 865–8.

Reiver D, Kmiot WA, Cohen SM, Weiss EG, Nogueras JJ, Wexner SD (1994) A prospective comparison of laparoscopic procedures in colorectal surgery (abstract). Diseases of the Colon and Rectum 37: 22.

Rhodes M, Stitz RW (1994) Laparoscopic subtotal colectomy. Seminars in Colon and Rectal Surgery 5 (4): 267–70.

Romero CA, James KM, Cooperstone LM, Mishrick AS, Ger R (1992) Laparoscopic sigmoid colostomy for perineal Crohn's disease. Surgery, Laparoscopy, Endoscopy, 2: 148–51.

Schirmer BD, Edge SB, Dix J (1991) Laparoscopic cholecystectomy. Annals of Surgery 213: 665–76.

Schmitt SL, Cohen SM, Wexner SD, Nogueras JJ, Jagelman DG (1994) Does laparoscopic-assisted ileal pouch anal anastomosis reduce the length of hospitalization? International Journal of Colorectal Diseases 9: 134–7.

Schreiber J (1987) Early experience with laparoscopic appendectomy in women. Surgical Endoscopy 1: 211–16.

Scott N, Jackson P, Al-Jaberi T, Dixon MF, Quirke P, Finan PJ (1995) Total mesorectal excision and local recurrence. A study of tumor spread in the mesorectum distal to rectal cancer. British Journal of Surgery 82: 1031–3.

Semm K (1983) Endoscopic appendectomy. Endoscopy 15: 59–64.

Senagore AJ, Luchtefeld MA, MacKeigan JM, Mazier WP (1993) Open colectomy versus laparoscopic colectomy: are there differences? American Surgeon 59: 549–54.

Silva PD, Coghill TH (1991) Laparoscopic treatment of recurrent small bowel obstruction. Wisconsin Medical Journal 90: 169–70.

Sugarbaker PH, Corlew S (1982) Influence of surgical technique on survival in patients with colorectal cancer: a review. Diseases of the Colon and Rectum 25: 545–57.

Tate JJT, Kwok S, Dawson JW, Lau WY, Li AK (1993) Prospective comparison of laparoscopic and conventional anterior resection. British Journal of Surgery 80: 1396–8.

Teoh TA, Reissman P, Cohen SM, Weiss EG, Wexner SD (1994) Laparoscopic loop ileostomy (letter). Diseases of the Colon and Rectum 37: 514.

The Southern Surgeons Club (1991) A prospective analysis of 1518 laparoscopic cholecystectomies. New England Journal of Medicine 324: 1073–8.

Tucker RD, Voyles C (1995) . Laparoscopic electrosurgical complications and their prevention. AORN 62(1): 51–3, 55, 58–9..

Ure BM, Tridl H, Spangenberger W, Dietrich A, Lefering R, Neugebauer E (1994) Pain after laparoscopic cholecystectomy. Surgical Endoscopy 8: 90–6.

Vertruyen M, Cadiere GB, Himpens J, Bruyn SJ, Lemper JC, Urbain D (1996) Laparosocpic colectomy for cancer (abstract). Surgical Endoscopy 10: 558.

Vukasin P, Ortega AE, Greene FL, Steele GD, Simons AJ, Anthone GJ, Weston LA, Beart RW (1996) Wound recurrence following laparoscopic colon resection: results of the American Society of Colon and Rectal Surgeons Laparoscopic Registry. Diseases of the Colon and Rectum 39(Suppl): S20–S23.

Wexner SD, Cohen SM (1995) Port site metastases after laparoscopic surgery for cure of malignancy: a plea for caution. British Journal of Surgery 82: 295–8.

Wexner SD, Cohen SM (1996) Laparoscopic appendectomy and colectomy. In Zuidema GD (Ed.) Surgery of the Alimentary Tract. 4th edn. Philadelphia: WB Saunders.

Wexner SD, Cohen SM, Johansen OB, Nogueras JJ, Jagelman DG (1993) Laparoscopic colorectal surgery: a prospective assessment and current perspective. British Journal of Surgery 80: 1602–5.

Wexner SD, Gonzalez–Padron A, Teoh TA, Moon HK (1996) The stimulated gracilis neosphincter for fecal incontinence: a new use for an old concept. Plastic and Reconstructive Surgery 98: 693–9.

Wexner SD, Johansen OB, Nogueras JJ, Jagelman DG (1992) Laparoscopic total abdominal colectomy. A prospective trial. Diseases of the Colon and Rectum 35 (7): 651–5.

Whitworth CM, Whitworth PW, Sanfillipo J et al. (1988) Value of diagnostic laparoscopy in young women with possible appendicitis. Surgery, Gynecology and Obstetrics 107: 187–90.

Williams CD, Brenowitz JB (1975) Ventilatory patterns after vertical and transverse upper abdominal incisions. American Journal of Surgery 130: 725–8.

Wu JS, Birnbaum EH, Fleshman JW (1997) Early experience with laparoscopic abdominoperineal resection. Surgical Endoscopy 11 (5): 449–55.

Zucker KA, Pitcher DE, Martin DT, Ford RS (1994) Laparoscopic-assisted colon resection. Surgical Endoscopy 8: 12–17.

Chapter 13
The Modern Management of Faecal Incontinence

BARBARA STUCHFIELD RGN Clinical Nurse Specialist, Stoma
  Care, The Royal Hospitals NHS Trust, London, UK
A. J. P ECCERSLEY MA, FRCS
  The Royal Hospitals NHS Trust, London, UK

Introduction

Faecal incontinence is a distressing and disabling condition which affects about 2.2% of the population (Nelson et al., 1995). Although not life threatening, it poses a major threat to quality of life and the ability to function in society (Brook, 1991). It may not be linked to a major health problem and the majority of sufferers are fit and well. The degree of incontinence ranges from slight soiling to a total loss of bowel function, and an everyday event such as shopping may be ruled by the availability of a toilet. Relationships may be placed under strain if incontinence during sexual activity causes embarrassment and raises fears of rejection. The shame and stigma of incontinence may lead to low self-esteem and social isolation with the use of pads and plastic pants only serving to magnify the indignity.

Despite greater awareness of continence problems, many people are reluctant to seek medical help. Less than 50% discuss bowel problems with their doctor (Johnson and Lafferty, 1996) and reliable data on incidence and prevalence are unavailable (Enck et al., 1991).

Although most people associate faecal incontinence with the frail and elderly, Nelson et al. (1995) identified that 70% of suffers were under 65 years of age. Faecal soiling in children accounted for 25% of visits to a paediatric gastroenterology clinic in the USA (Taitz et al., 1986). Children may encounter particular difficulties at school (Hassink et al., 1994) and even as adults they may recall episodes of bullying and name-calling.

Common Causes of Faecal Incontinence

The main causes of faecal incontinence are set out in Table 13.1.

Table 13.1: Main causes of faecal incontinence

Cause	Example
Sphincter damage	
Obstetric	
Surgical	Anal stretch procedures
Traumatic	Road traffic accidents
Congenital anomalies	
Anorectal atresia	
Spina bifida	
Intestinal disease	
Inflammatory bowel disease	Ulcerative colitis, Crohn's disease
Irritable bowel syndrome	
Shortened bowel	Colonic resection
Radiation enteritis	Following radiotherapy for carcinoma
Neurological disease	
Denervation of pelvic floor	Spinal injuries
Generalized neuropathy	Multiple sclerosis
Psychological disease	
Chronic soiling	Childhood encopresis
Laxative abuse	
Other causes	
Endocrine	Thyrotoxicosis
Faecal impaction and overflow	Dementia

Obstetric Anal Sphincter Damage

Trauma to the internal and external sphincter experienced during childbirth may result in incontinence soon after pregnancy or later in life. It is estimated that most damage is sustained during the first vaginal delivery, and is more likely following forceps delivery. An episiotomy does not altogether prevent subsequent sphincter damage (Sultan et al., 1993).

Pelvic Floor Neuropathy

Damage to the pudendal nerve may occur during a prolonged or difficult vaginal delivery (Sultan et al., 1994). Although pudendal neuropathy predominantly affects multiparous women, it can occur as a consequence of both chronic constipation and generalized neurological disease, examples of which include multiple sclerosis and diabetic neuropathy (Jameson and Scott, 1997).

Trauma

Road traffic accidents leading to pelvic fractures or perineal lacerations, as well as missile injuries, can cause catastrophic damage to the sphincters and their nerve supply as well as to the rectum. The anal sphincter can also be damaged by some sexual practices (Chun et al., 1997).

Faecal incontinence can also result from any surgical operation on the anal canal. For example, the treatment of fistula *in ano* and anal dilatations for fissures can both lead to permanent continence problems (Lunniss et al., 1994). Temporary or even permanent sphincter damage has been demonstrated following even minor anorectal surgery (Van Tets et al., 1997).

Faecal Impaction

Generally faecal impaction is found in geriatric patients but younger people may have spurious diarrhoea resulting from the effect of impacted faeces in the rectum which can be exacerbated by the use of laxatives and fibre supplements.

Congenital Anomalies

Despite infantile corrective surgery for congenital anorectal atresia (where the anus and the internal sphincter fail to develop in utero) only 25% have complete continence as adults (Rintala et al., 1994).

Psychological Chronic Soiling

Both children and adults may develop soiling as an emotional response to stress. Prolonged laxative abuse, which typically occurs in people with abnormal perception of body image, can also manifest itself as apparent incontinence.

Diarrhoea

Diarrhoea associated with inflammatory bowel disease, irritable bowel syndrome and colonic resections or radiotherapy may lead to symptoms of incontinence and faecal urgency. Both prescribed drugs and medications bought from pharmacists for unrelated illnesses may induce diarrhoea as a side-effect. Hyperthyroidism can also lead to rapid bowel transit and subsequent incontinence.

Many cases of incontinence may be multifactorial, and the natural ageing process in the presence of a previously disrupted sphincter may exacerbate the problem.

Normal Mechanism of Continence Control

The anal canal is surrounded by two sphincters. The innermost is an involuntary smooth muscle sphincter which provides continuous closure of the anus, whilst the voluntary external anal sphincter contracts to further occlude the anal canal in response to rises in abdominal pressure induced by coughing or straining. The pelvic floor muscles such as the levator ani and the puborectalis have an important function in bowel control by encircling the back of the rectum, just above the anus, and creating an anorectal angle.

Nerve endings in the upper anal canal are important in the discrimination of rectal contents and when rectal filling is detected they stimulate the desire to defecate. After infancy this desire can usually be controlled by the central nervous system contracting the voluntary external anal sphincter. In an appropriate environment, the anal sphincters can be relaxed and by a combination of mass contraction of the rectum and the raising of intra-abdominal pressure, rectal contents can be expelled. Any interference either with the sphincters, their complex innervation or the ability of the rectum to store and expel stool appropriately can lead to incontinence.

Team Approach to the Management of Faecal Incontinence

Although the causes of faecal incontinence are well known, its management remains difficult and controversial, with few clinicians and nurses having experience of managing such a complex problem. As well as a thorough medical examination the patient's social and psychological state and family dynamics should be assessed by members of a multidisciplinary team to promote an individualized approach to care. The team (see Table 13.2) must incorporate nursing staff who have experience and interest in continence and stoma care. A clinical psychologist or a trained counsellor can be an invaluable member of this team. The colorectal surgeon should have ready access to facilities for investigation as well as access to expert urological opin-

Table 13.2: Team approach to the management of faecal incontinence

Nurse specialist
     Continence care
     Stoma care
     Biofeedback
     Colorectal nurse practitioner
Colorectal surgeon
General or family practitioner
Physiotherapist
Urologist
Psychologist
Physiologist
Community nurse

ion as around 20% of women who have faecal incontinence also have symptoms of urinary incontinence (Tetzchner et al., 1996)

A good knowledge of anatomy and physiology relating to continence is important, but all members of the team need to develop a sensitive understanding of the patient's experience of living with incontinence. Ongoing assessment in the setting of an open and trusting relationship both within the team and between the patient and the team will allow the development of a holistic plan of care to help the individual patient.

Assessing the Level of Incontinence

In an attempt both to categorize the severity of incontinence and to measure the effect of therapeutic interventions, some form of continence scoring should be used. Perhaps the best method is to ask the patient to record episodes of incontinence and associated phenomena in a diary. This is useful in planning dietary and drug treatments as part of optimizing the medical management of bowel control.

The use of short questionnaires such as the Cleveland Clinic Continence Score (Table 13.3) allows a numerical index of the severity of incontinence to be recorded. This is useful for monitoring individual outcomes and for auditing the overall results of a particular operative intervention.

Investigating the Cause of Faecal Incontinence

Although investigations of sphincter function can be embarrassing, when performed sympathetically by an experienced member of staff

Table 13.3: Cleveland Clinic continence score

Frequency of	Never	Less than once a month	More than once a	More once a week	Daily
Incontinence of solid	0	1	2	3	4
Incontinence of liquid	0	1	2	3	4
Incontinence of flatus	0	1	2	3	4
Use of pads (soiling)	0	1	2	3	4
Lifestyle impact	0	1	2	3	4

Note: Minimum score = 0, maximum score = 20.

they need not be painful and can yield accurate information to plan future treatment and predict prognosis. Common tests are:

1. Sphincter function: This is generally measured by means of a pressure transducer inserted into the anal canal. The pressure is recorded at various positions, both at rest and on active squeeze. The usual resting pressure is between 80 and 120 cm of water with a squeeze pressure of up to 200 cm of water. Much of the resting pressure is provided by the internal sphincter, whilst the majority of the squeeze pressure is provided by the external (voluntary) sphincter.
2. Anorectal sensation: Anal sensation is measured by passing a small electrical current between two miniature electrodes held within the anus which causes the patient to feel a pricking sensation. Reduced anal sensation can cause soiling because the reflex tightening of the external sphincter in response to faecal matter is lost. Rectal sensation is measured with a balloon filled slowly with air or water. The patient is asked to indicate when they feel the balloon filling, at what point they feel the urge to defecate, and at what point they feel they can no longer tolerate further filling. Increased sensitivity can be caused by rectal disease or previous radiotherapy.
3. Imaging: endoanal ultrasonography (Sultan and Stanton, 1997): Thickness of the internal sphincter varies with age, and defects within the internal sphincter are most frequently induced by an obstructed vaginal delivery. Other internal sphincter defects may

arise as a consequence of trauma or surgery. For example, both the lateral anal sphincterotomy and anal stretch procedures used to treat anal fissure can produce permanent defects in the internal anal sphincter.

The external anal sphincter consists of striated or voluntary muscle. Defects in the external anal sphincter are typically related to large obstetric tears as well as trauma. Imaging of the size and position of such a tear is important as part of the planning of any direct sphincter repair.

In defecatory proctography the patient is asked to evacuate barium paste while sitting on a commode in front of an X-ray screening facility. This test is more frequently useful in assessing people who complain of soiling and evacuatory difficulties which may be related to rectal prolapses or rectoceles.

4. The pudendal nerve and electrophysiology: The pudendal nerve controls the external sphincter and nerve damage occurs as a consequence of chronic straining at stool or a difficult vaginal delivery. This causes atrophy of the sphincter muscle. The pudendal nerve conduction is measured by direct electrostimulation of the nerve through the rectal wall. A pudendal neuropathy reduces the chance of surgery leading to a successful restoration of continence (Sangwan et al., 1996).

Management of Faecal Incontinence

There are many therapeutic options in treating faecal incontinence and a combination of managements may help to control the problem and improve quality of life. Dietary manipulation alone may be very effective, and the avoidance of foods that exacerbate diarrhoea such as highly spiced foods, fruit and fibre may reduce the number of episodes of incontinence.

Drug Therapy

The use of constipating agents such as loperamide, codeine phosphate and Lomotil® (diphenoxylate with atropine) may be used to help in solidifying liquid stool. The dosage may be individually titrated according to need, with some advice about the risk of constipation. Care has to be taken when used in the elderly and the immobile because impaction with overflow may be mistaken for diarrhoea. Gelatine as a powder or in a more palatable form may be used as a more natural method of thickening stool. The reduction of dietary fat and the use of cholestyramine may help some people whose recurrent diarrhoea is related to fat intolerance.

For some patients the routine use of suppositories or enemas may be effective in maintaining regular emptying of the rectum to prevent leakage. Although awkward to administer, rectal washouts may be helpful in some patients. Bulk laxatives may also help but the additional faecal volume may worsen the symptoms of soiling related to rectal evacuation disorders.

Biofeedback and Physiotherapy

Some success has been achieved with pelvic floor retraining and sphincter strengthening exercises taught by physiotherapists. Biofeedback training (Enck, 1993), which aims to strengthen the voluntary component of the sphincter muscle, is useful for a select group of patients but compliance may be a problem (Loening Baucke, 1995).

Incontinence Products

In the UK there is little in the way of products for faecal incontinence. Pads used for urinary incontinence are bulky and uncomfortable, and the wrong shape. Many people resort to using sanitary towels, which can become expensive in the long term, and may be embarrassing for men and young children to use.

In some circumstances an anal plug made in a similar shape to a tampon (e.g. by Coloplast, Denmark) may be effective, especially for people with congenital anomalies, where relative insensitivity of the anal canal may make the plug less uncomfortable to use. An anal plug may provide the patient with a degree of confidence for a special occasion (Mortensen and Smilgin Humphries, 1991; Smilgin Humphries, 1993).

Odour and Perianal Care

Faecal soiling frequently leads to odour and can result in breakdown of the perianal skin. The use of regular perineal douches, application of topical cream such as Drapolene to act as a barrier and frequent changes of pads and underwear will minimize these awkward problems. An aerosol deodorant may also be used to mask odour.

Social Support

In the UK some continence products are available on prescription. However, the cost of laundering clothes and bed linen may be considerable; for patients on low incomes financial help is available from the Department of Social Security.

The Surgical Treatment of Incontinence

If the medical management methods described above fail to improve bowel control, the use of appropriate surgical techniques may lead to improvements in continence. The only indication for surgery is a failure of medical management together with a patient's insistence that his/her quality of life is affected by ongoing incontinence.

Preparing the Patient for Surgery

Patients preparing for surgery to improve bowel function deserve to receive a full and frank explanation of the proposed procedure together with information on the possible risks and benefits. Ideally both the surgeon and nurse specialist should fully counsel the patient prior to admission to hospital, with opportunity given to the patient and family to ask questions. The involvement of the family in the decision-making process is important as they will be caring for the patient during the postoperative phase. A supportive spouse, partner or family member is influential in helping patients to adjust to changes in body image (Wade, 1989). The use of literature, videos and the chance to meet other patients may help the individual decide whether to proceed with the surgery. This preoperative counselling is essential if the patient is to be psychologically prepared to cope with a variable functional outcome (Salter, 1990). When in hospital further time should be set aside to give the patient a chance to complete the process of gaining informed consent.

Anorectal surgery is usually performed under general anaesthetic and so every effort must be made to improve other medical symptoms such as cardiac or respiratory disease. Antithrombosis prophylaxis such as heparin and compression stockings must also be used appropriately. Many surgeons will prescribe a bowel preparation regimen using either stimulant or osmotic laxatives for one or two days prior to surgery to reduce faecal contamination of perineal wounds. Whilst copious water (and sometimes electrolyte supplements) is encouraged during bowel preparation, no food is allowed following laxative ingestion. Most surgeons will also give their patients broad-spectrum antibiotics, including cover against anaerobic organisms during and following the operation.

Postoperative management varies between surgeons and many units have standard protocols for the perioperative management of each patient. In our unit the patient is allowed to drink water as soon as he/she has recovered from the anaesthetic, but food is not reintroduced for a several days until the wounds have begun to heal. During this time fluid balance is maintained by the intravenous route. We aim to soften the first bowel motion by introducing regular laxatives around 3 days after surgery, but some units may advocate the use of antidiarrhoeal medication to constipate the patient. The skin is usually closed with interrupted absorbable sutures and if a drain is present this is removed on the third day or when indicated.

Effective pain management is achieved by patient-controlled analgesia administered in response to individual needs, progressing to oral analgesia as required. A urinary catheter remains *in situ* until postoperative monitoring is no longer required. Mobilization under the supervision of a physiotherapist is encouraged to prevent complications such as chest infections or deep vein thrombosis.

Wound infection is a common complication of perianal surgery which can lead to failure of the operation. It may be reduced by effective bowel preparation, good theatre technique and meticulous postoperative wound care by the ward nursing staff. Wound care may need to be continued at home by the district nursing service.

Discharge is planned once bowel function is re-established satisfactorily. It is important that patients are warned that even after a successful procedure they may still have difficulties with bowel control for several weeks. Normal activities can resume when the patient feels able, although avoidance of sexual intercourse for up to 6 weeks may be advised to allow perineal wounds to heal.

Traditional Operations for Incontinence

1. Post-anal repair: This procedure is done under general anaesthetic through a curved incision between the anal canal and the coccyx. The posterior fibres of the pelvic floor are exposed through this incision. A series of non-dissolvable stitches is used to overlap these muscles, so accentuating the anorectal angle. The commonest indication for this operation is the presence of a pudendal neuropathy in a patient who has no specific sphincter defect suitable for a direct sphincter repair. Good initial results may be obtained, but later failures are not unusual and the long-term continence rate is around 50% (Deen et al., 1993).
2. Anterior levatorplasty/pelvic floor repair: In this procedure a perineal incision is made and the levator ani muscles on each side are exposed, overlapped and sutured together to tighten the pelvic

floor. When the levatorplasty is combined with a postanal repair described previously the combined procedure is known as the total pelvic floor repair and is claimed to improve incontinence in over 70% of patients (Korsgen et al., 1997).

3. Direct sphincter repair: This procedure is performed through a perineal incision. The external anal sphincter is dissected free and the defect is identified. The scarred portion of the sphincter is removed and the remaining healthy muscle fibres are overlapped and permanently joined together by a series of interrupted sutures. The wound in a direct sphincter repair is close to the anal canal and so at risk of faecal contamination. For this reason some surgeons routinely perform a defunctioning loop stoma which is closed 3–6 months after the surgery. Alternatively the patient may be kept on a low-residue diet for several days after surgery to reduce the frequency of bowel actions.

   Overlapping sphincter repairs can be used to treat a defect occupying over one-third of the external sphincter and a good improvement in continence can be achieved in around 60% of patients (Ternent et al., 1997). The longer term results may be poorer as the scar tissue around the anal canal stretches somewhat over time. The procedure can, however, be repeated in selected cases.

   Patients may also develop evacuation difficulties after any sphincter repair resulting in the need for laxatives or enemas.

4. Stoma formation: In cases where faecal incontinence has persisted despite optimal medical management, a permanent stoma is a realistic and often overlooked option. It has the benefit of ensuring all faecal matter is retained in a disposable appliance and allows most people to maintain a fully active and independent lifestyle. Stoma formation does necessitate an abdominal operation but this can frequently be done using laparoscopic techniques. Usually an end colostomy is formed with the rectal stump oversewn and left *in situ*. Some patients may choose to learn irrigation techniques to control their stomal output. Occasionally the rectal stump may become inflamed and develop diversion colitis, a condition in which mucus and occasionally blood is passed per anus.

   Clearly some people find the idea of a stoma frightening, but with appropriate support and education from a team incorporating an experienced stoma therapist, many of these fears can be overcome. Up to 30% of people develop moderate to severe psychiatric disturbance after stoma formation (Rubin and Devlin, 1987; Bekkers et al., 1995). This group needs specialist psychological investigation and treatment (White and Hunt, 1997). Other people may find life with a stoma so abhorrent that they seek to undergo one of the complex reconstructive procedures described below.

Recent Advances: Complex Restorative Operations

The Gracilis Neosphincter

For many years (Pickrell et al., 1956) surgeons have attempted to rebuild the sphincter apparatus using the gracilis muscle, a weak adductor of the thigh. In this gracilis neosphincter technique (Figures 13.1, 13.2, 13.3) the inner thigh is opened and the gracilis dissected free with its distal tendon divided at the knee. Through perianal incisions the part of the muscle previously in the leg is tunnelled around the anal orifice and fixed to the bone of the ischial tuberosity. This creates a sling around the anus which at least partially occludes the anal canal at rest. The sling can be contracted by squeezing the knees together. Results indicate moderately successful outcomes, even over prolonged follow up (Corman, 1985; Faucheron et al., 1994)

A problem with the gracilis neosphincter is that a skeletal muscle such as the gracilis is designed for short forcible contractions rather than the sustained contraction that an effective sphincter exerts. It has been shown that low-frequency electrical stimulation of skeletal muscle over several weeks alters muscle physiology from a skeletal fast-twitch

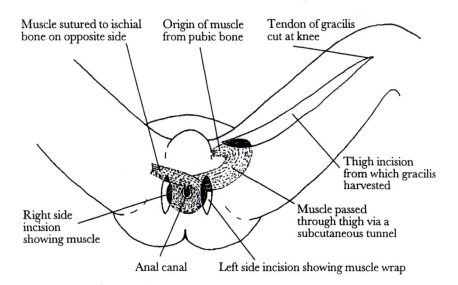

Figure labels:
Muscle sutured to ischial bone on opposite side
Origin of muscle from pubic bone
Tendon of gracilis cut at knee
Thigh incision from which gracilis harvested
Right side incision showing muscle
Muscle passed through thigh via a subcutaneous tunnel
Anal canal
Left side incision showing muscle wrap

Figure 13.1: Formation of gracilis neosphincter showing incisions and muscle wrap.

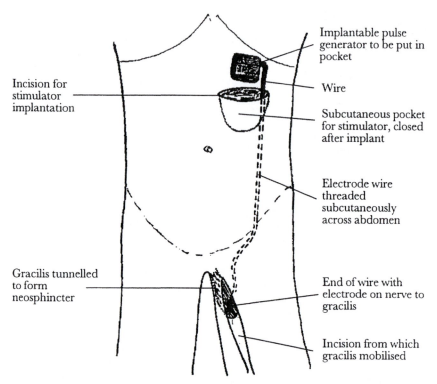

Figure 13.2: Implantation of a stimulator for the electrically stimulated gracilis neosphincter.

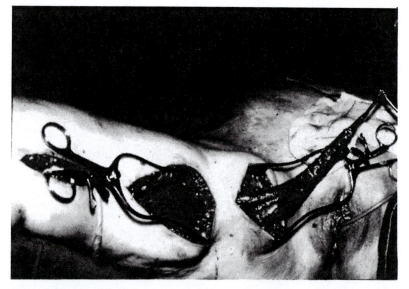

Figure 13.3: Gracilis neosphincter: after division of the distal tendon the muscle is mobilized prior to forming the neosphincter wrap. See colour section.

type to a slow-twitch fatigue-resistant muscle type (George et al., 1993). The induction of this change in muscle type allows continuous occlusion of the anal canal. Continuous low-frequency electrical stimulation can be delivered to the gracilis muscle by an implantable pulse generator (IPG) similar to a cardiac pacemaker, creating an electrically stimulated gracilis neosphincter.

Electrical stimulation may be given either directly into the muscle fibres of the gracilis by implanted electrodes, or alternatively the gracilis can be exposed at operation and a small electrode plate sutured directly over its nerve. These electrodes are connected by a tunnelled wire to the implantable pulse generator (IPG: see Figure 13.4), which is placed subcutaneously in the anterior abdominal wall. A remote-control device is used to programme the IPG by transmitting radio waves through the patient's skin. Using this remote control the voltage and frequency of the electrical stimulation can be modified to adjust the level of contraction within the gracilis and thus the tightness of the anus. The patient is taught how to use a battery-powered hand-held stimulator controller which when placed on the abdominal wall over the IPG can turn the stimulation on or off. This must be used to turn the electrical stimulation off and relax the anus prior to defecation. Alternatively a small magnet can be used with the same effect.

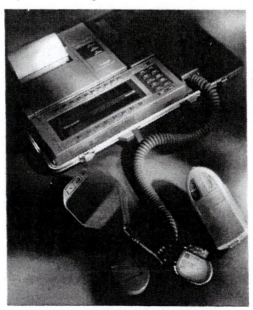

Figure 13.4: Medtronic Interstim 3023 implantable pulse generator, electrode wire and programmer for adjustment of pulse generator. Amplitude, frequency, pulse width and periodicity of stimulation can all be altered by radiotelemetry. See colour section.
Source: Courtesy of Medtronic Interstim, Maastricht, The Netherlands.

Since 1988 over 90 gracilis neosphincter procedures have been performed in our unit in people ranging from teenagers suffering incontinence after atresia or trauma to people in their seventies undergoing sphincter reconstruction after treatment for low rectal cancers. The construction of an electrically stimulated gracilis neosphincter is a complex procedure so careful patient selection and preparation is essential. An information booklet is given out which describes the operation and answers the most commonly asked questions such as how much time off work is required and whether the operation will restrict travel, sexual activity or pregnancy. As stated earlier in this chapter the patients need extensive preoperative counselling in order for them to make well-informed choices. The patient is encouraged to discuss the potential risks and benefits of the procedure with members of the multidisciplinary team including the clinical nurse specialist. It is important that realistic expectations of outcome are offered to the patient; the operation even if successful may still result in some mild incontinence. Counselling about a temporary loop ileostomy is given because a stoma is frequently used to divert faeces until the neosphincter wounds have healed.

At the present time the neosphincter is created over two or three stages, each performed under general anaesthetic. Prior to the first stage, full bowel preparation is performed over 48 hours unless the patient has an existing stoma. The process of gaining informed consent is completed by the surgeon, and appropriate stoma sites are marked with indelible ink by the clinical nurse specialist. Low-dose heparin and thromboembolic deterrent stockings are used.

Anaesthesia is induced without the aid of muscle relaxants (which would temporarily paralyse the gracilis muscle), and the patient placed in the Lloyd-Davies position. A chlorhexidine rectal washout is given and the skin is prepared with a povidone-iodine solution. As described above the gracilis is mobilized from the pre-selected leg and transposed around the anal canal to create the neosphincter. The main nerve to the gracilis is identified and after testing an electrode plate is sutured directly over the nerve as it enters the muscle. This wire from this electrode is tunnelled to the anterior abdominal wall and sheathed in a silastic catheter. The incisions are closed with absorbable sutures and one or two drains may be placed. If a loop ileostomy is deemed necessary it is created at this time. Prophylactic antibiotics including metronidazole, a cephalosporin and gentamicin are given perioperatively and continued for 5 days. A patient-controlled analgesia system using an intravenous opiate is set up, progressing to oral analgesics when appropriate.

Postoperatively the patient is kept on bed rest for 3 days in order to prevent avulsion of the electrode from the nerve before any healing has taken place. After this the patient is encouraged to mobilize but warned not to abduct the thighs excessively. Oral intake is permitted when the stoma, if placed, has begun to function. If there is no stoma, a period of total parenteral nutrition is instituted. Daily wound care is required and any drains are removed on the third day. The urinary catheter is removed when the patient is ambulant.

Two weeks after this first stage the abdominal incision containing the sheathed end of the electrode wire is reopened under a short general anaesthetic. The pulse generator (IPG Model 3023, Medtronic Interstim, Maastricht, The Netherlands) is connected, placed in a previously marked subcutaneous pocket and neosphincter contraction is confirmed by digital examination. When the pulse generator is first implanted the muscle cannot be turned on continuously because its fast-twitch morphology would lead to rapid fatigue and cramp. Therefore the pulse generator is initially programmed to stimulate the muscle intermittently. The percentage of time the stimulation is 'on' is increased at fortnightly intervals until 8 weeks by which time slow-twitch transformation has occurred in the bulk of the muscle and continuous full-strength occlusion of the anal canal can be achieved (see Table 13.4).

Table 13.4: Training regime for electrically stimulated gracilis neosphincter

Time since stimulator implanted	Stimulator 'on'	Stimulator 'off'	Percentage time 'on'
Week 0	1 second	4 seconds	20%
Week 2	1 second	2 seconds	33%
Week 4	2 seconds	2 seconds	50%
Week 6	Continuous	0 seconds	100%
Week 8	Close stoma		

When all perianal wounds have healed any defunctioning stoma can then be closed under general anaesthetic. After stoma closure the patient still needs considerable practical and psychological support over several months in adapting to the neosphincter. To defecate, the stimulation must be turned off. Some people encounter difficulties with rectal evacuation and use laxatives or suppositories. Many patients experience leakage of flatus and use pads for minor soiling, but the majority of the patients in our series had severe incontinence which had failed to respond to other surgical interventions; for many this was the last alternative to a stoma.

There are a number of potential complications which the patient must be warned about (Mander and Williams, 1997). For example, perianal infections are common and may even lead to failure of the procedure. The electrode plate may become dislodged and this can require re-exploration with the risk of neuropraxia (nerve damage). Lymphoedema and sensory loss in the leg which donated the gracilis have also been described. The effects of the stimulator on any future pregnancy are unknown, although the IPG for the gracilis neosphincter may be safely combined with a cardiac pacemaker. The IPG programming can be affected by strong electromagnetic fields and patients should be cautious in passing library and airport security devices. An identity card and telephone support as well as clinic follow-up is provided for all patients.

Continuous electrical stimulation of the muscle is possible and although the stimulator battery may have to be replaced under a short general anaesthetic every 3 to five years, several of our patients have demonstrable gracilis muscle contraction and useful improvement in continence up to 8 years after formation of an electrically stimulation gracilis sphincter.

The procedure is contra-indicated in people with ongoing perineal sepsis and Crohn's disease.

Results of the Royal London Hospital Series

Results of a recent audit of 72 patients who have attended our unit for follow up after gracilis neosphincter reconstruction for a median of 62 (range 3–116) months are given in Table 13.5. Overall, long-term improvements in continence signified by the avoidance of a permanent stoma are achieved in around 60% of patients.

In the patients undergoing total anorectal reconstruction following cancer resections or anorectal atresia the new rectum has deficient sensation (Abercrombie et al., 1996) which leads to poorer evacuatory function. Good function in this group has only been achieved in combination with either regular enemas or antegrade colonic irrigation usually via a conduit to augment evacuation; it is now our policy to combine these procedures in patients with congenital high anorectal atresia.

Two-thirds of those suffering incontinence after obstetric disasters had previously undergone an unsuccessful sphincter or postanal repair prior to neosphincter formation. A high chance of success can also be

Table 13.5: Results of the gracilis neosphincter at the Royal London Hospital 1988–96 (see text for details).

Aetiology	Number	Successful at 1 year follow-up	Number combined with colonic conduit
Anorectal atresia	19	10 (52%)	13
Obstetric trauma	21	15 (71%)	3
Other trauma	10	7 (70%)	1
Neuropathy	10	4 (40%)	0
Post APER	15	7 (44%)	0 (3 had ileal pouch)
Total	75	43 (57%)	17

achieved in this group as well as in those with traumatic incontinence. Sphincter reconstruction for primary neuropathic or idiopathic faecal incontinence has a lower success rate. At least part of this poor outcome is explained by the very high perineal sepsis rates encountered in this group.

Total reconstruction of both the anus and rectum is possible after the abdominoperineal excision of the rectum (APER) for cancer (Mander et al., 1996). Out of twelve patients undergoing the procedure, four did not have their stoma closed because of complications or other medical illnesses, and two patients were forced to return to a permanent stoma because of recurrent sepsis. Six patients achieved long-term continence with the procedure following cancer resections, and one other had success from a neosphincter combined with an ileoperineal pouch after panproctocolectomy for familial adenomatous polyposis.

Formal quality of life evaluation after gracilis neosphincter construction has shown a number of benefits on scales such as the Nottingham Health Profile (Baeten et al., 1995, Eccersley et al., 1997) and a long-term evaluation of the cost–utility of the procedure against permanent stoma formation is currently being undertaken.

Antegrade Colonic Irrigation (ACE) as a Method of Managing Incontinence

The majority of surgical treatments for incontinence aim to prevent soiling by augmenting sphincter function. An alternative management strategy is to ensure regular and complete emptying of the colon and rectum by irrigation techniques so that no soiling can occur between irrigations. This strategy may be particularly appropriate if the cause of incontinence is related to a rectal evacuatory disorder and overflow incontinence (Briel et al., 1997).

Rectal irrigation is awkward and fails to empty the more proximal colon, so the hollow appendix can be used to create a channel or appendicostomy leading from the bowel to the anterior abdominal wall. The patient can then be taught how to pass a catheter via the appendicostomy into the caecum. Water or a variety of medicated enema solutions can then be instilled directly into the colon. These stimulate colonic contractions and act to flush out colonic contents via the rectum and anus. The appendicostomy has yielded good results in children with intractable incontinence as a result of congenital anomalies (Squire at al., 1993). Stenosis of the appendicostomy or reflux of faecal matter can be problems for certain patients, and some surgeons reverse and re-implant the appendix for this reason. If the appendix has previously been removed a segment of tubularized caecum or the ileocaecal valve (Marsh and Kiff, 1996) can be used as a catheterizable access to the colon. Other surgeons have implanted a silastic valve between the caecum and the abdominal wall; a similar technique to a percutaneous gastrostomy (Kalidasun et al., 1997).

The Colonic Conduit

The colonic conduit (Figure 13.5) is an alternative means of colonic access which incorporates an intussuscepted anti-reflux valve within a segment of transverse colon, through which the patient is able to intermittently pass an appropriate catheter for irrigation. Reflux and stomal stenosis are probably less frequent with this technique (Maw et al., 1996), but it requires a laparotomy and construction of a colonic anastomosis.

A patient considering the colonic conduit is counselled by the multidisciplinary team as described earlier. A patient information booklet is available to help answer common questions about the irrigation process and the likely outcome of the procedure.

The patient is admitted 3 days before surgery and further counselling occurs as part of gaining informed consent. The position of the conduit is marked by the clinical nurse specialist and the bowel is prepared as described previously.

Operation is performed under general anaesthetic, with antibiotic and heparin prophylaxis. A midline laparotomy is performed and a section of the transverse colon is mobilized. In this a 5 cm long valve is created by suturing an intussusception or infolding of the colon wall,

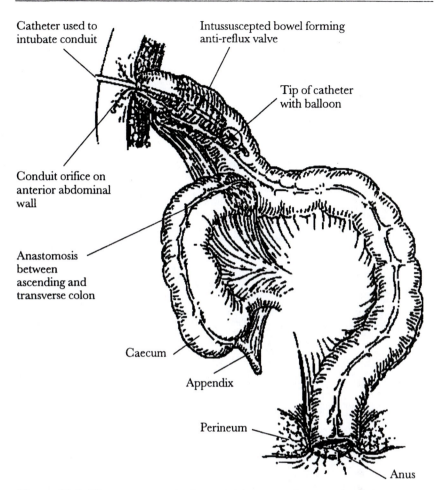

Catheter used to
intubate conduit

Intussuscepted bowel forming
anti-reflux valve

Tip of catheter
with balloon

Conduit orifice on
anterior abdominal
wall

Anastomosis
between
ascending and
transverse colon

Caecum

Appendix

Perineum

Anus

Figure 13.5: The transverse colonic conduit in a case of anorectal atresia.

and the colon forming the conduit is tunnelled through the abdominal
wall and sutured to the skin. The conduit orifice on the abdominal
wall (Figure 13.6) has a diameter of around 1 cm and an irrigation
catheter passing into the colon is left at the end of the procedure. The
abdomen is closed in a routine fashion.

Postoperatively the patient is encouraged to mobilize early and the
urinary catheter is removed when the patient is ambulant. Oral fluids
are permitted when bowel sounds return. A water-soluble contrast
radiological study ('conduitogram') is performed 7 days after the operation, and if all anastomoses are intact the patient is allowed to eat.
After the conduitogram, the patient is taught to irrigate the conduit
daily whilst sitting on the toilet, using between half and one litre of tap
water at 37°C via the catheter placed at surgery (Figures 13.7, 13.8).

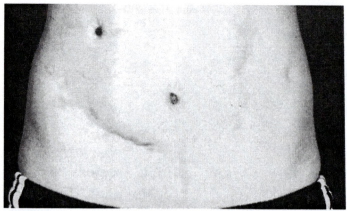

Figure 13.6: Orifice of colonic conduit in a male with a congenital anorectal anomaly. See colour section.

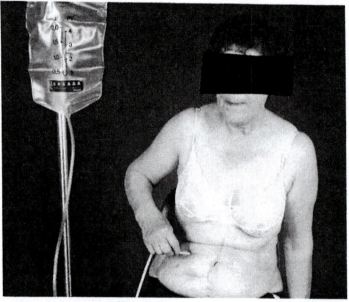

Figure 13.7: Irrigating the colonic conduit. The bag is filled with warmed tap water and hung from a hook. The patient passes the catheter into the conduit and irrigates the colon while sitting on a toilet. See colour section.

This catheter is removed 4 weeks after surgery, when the patient is shown how to intubate the conduit with a catheter each day prior to irrigation. Irrigation takes around 30 minutes to perform and is usually done daily at a time that is convenient to the patient's lifestyle. The catheter is removed from the conduit between washouts for cleaning and re-use.

Usually the conduit does not leak, and can be left uncovered. In a small number of people intermittent leakage of flatus or mucus does

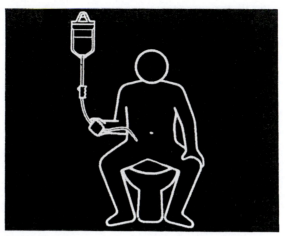

Figure 13.8: Diagrammatic view of conduit irrigation.

occur, and the patient may wish to wear a Band-Aid, gauze square or a stoma cap over the site. Full sexual and physical activity is permitted once wounds have healed, and the conduit orifice is discreet enough to permit swimming. Continued leakage of water per rectum for up to one hour after irrigation is complete can be encountered in those with poor sphincter function, and the use of a pad may be advisable.

The colonic conduit technique has been used in adolescents with incontinence after pull-through procedures for anorectal agenesis, in adults following severe anorectal trauma which has rendered sphincter reconstruction impossible, and in people with rectal evacuatory disorders who frequently suffer overflow incontinence (Williams et al., 1994). It may also have a role in the management of intractable constipation (Stuchfield, 1995) (see Table 13.6 for results of this procedure).

Artificial Bowel Sphincter (ABS)

The ABS (American Medical Systems, Minnesota, USA) (Figure 13.9) is a novel procedure involving the implantation of a hydraulic cuff around the anal canal which when filled occludes the anal orifice. The cuff is filled from a reservoir in the suprapubic region, and the filling is controlled by a valve placed in the scrotum or labia. The cuff must be deflated during defecation. Problems with this technique have included infections, evacuatory difficulties, erosion of the skin overlying the cuff, and fluid leaks. Two recent reports (Lehur et al., 1996; Wong et al., 1996) have described considerable short-term success and the technique offers much future potential.

Table 13.6: Results of the transverse colonic conduit at the Royal London Hospital 1994–7

	Indication for conduit formation		
	Rectal evacuatory disorder with incontinence	Incontinence following high anorectal atresia	Traumatic anorectal injuries
Number of patients having conduit	10	13	8
Number (%) combined with gracilis neosphincter	0 (0%)	11 (84%)	5 (63%)
Success (%)	8 (80%)	11 (84%)	6 (75%)

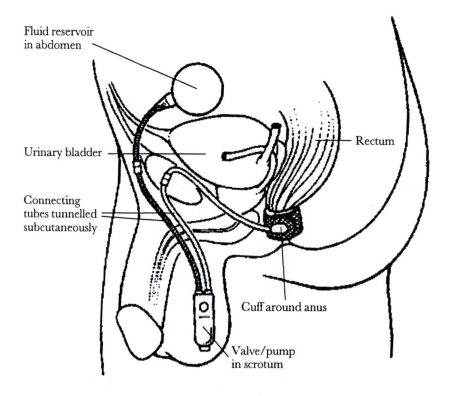

Figure 13.9: The AMS Artificial Bowel Sphincter implanted in a male.
Source: Courtesy of American Medical Systems Inc, Minnetonka, MN; medical illustration by Michael Schenk.

Conclusion

Faecal incontinence is a dire condition which affects at least 2.2% of the population. In the majority of cases simple adjustments to diet and medication may enable the patient to achieve an optimal level of continence that is only interrupted by the occasional accident. Surgical procedures can be performed with varying degrees of success but there will always be patients who will resort to a permanent stoma in order to improve their quality of life.

The assessment, inpatient care and subsequent support of all patients with faecal incontinence should be performed by an experienced multidisciplinary team in order to provide a holistic approach to care. This team should include surgeons and experienced nurse specialists with ready access to diagnostic and support services such as physiologists, psychologists and urologists.

Modern developments in this field have begun to offer a more aesthetic solution to those people in whom conventional treatments have failed. Whilst success is not guaranteed these operations offer a realistic alternative to people with intractable incontinence.

Acknowledgement

The authors would like to thank Joanna Lee for her help in preparing the manuscript.

References

Abercrombie JF, Rogers J, Williams NS (1996) Total anorectal reconstruction results in complete anorectal sensory loss. British Journal of Surgery 83: 57–9.

Baeten CGMI, Geerdes BP, Adang E, Heineman E, Konsten J, Engel GL, Kester ADM, Spaans F, Soeters PB (1995) Anal dynamic graciloplasty in the treatment of intractable faecal incontinence. New England Journal of Medicine 332: 1600–5.

Bekkers M, van Knippenberg F, van den Borne H, Poen H, Bergsma J, van Berge Hengouwen GP (1995) Psychosocial adaptation to stoma surgery: A review. Journal of Behavioral Medicine 18: 1–31.

Briel JW, Schouten WR, Vlot EA, Smits S, van Kessel I (1997) Clinical value of colonic irrigation in patients with continence disturbances. Diseases of the Colon and Rectum 40: 802–5.

Brook A (1991) Bowel distress and emotional conflict. Journal of the Royal Society of Medicine 84: 39–42.

Chun AB, Rose S, Mitrani C, Silvestre AJ, Wald A (1997) Anal sphincter structure and function in homosexual males engaging in anoreceptive intercourse. American Journal of Gastroenterology 92: 465–8.

Corman ML (1985) Gracilis muscle transposition for anal incontinence; late results. British Journal of Surgery 72: S21–2.

Deen KI, Oya M, Ortiz J, Keighley MR (1993) Randomised trial comparing three forms of pelvic floor repair for neuropathic faecal incontinence. British Journal of Surgery 80: 794–8.

Eccersley AJP, Maw A, Williams NS (1997) Quality of life can be improved by anorectal reconstruction. International Journal of Colorectal Disease 12: 130.

Enck P (1993) Biofeedback training in disordered defecation – a critical review. Digestive Diseases and Sciences 38: 1953–60.

Enck P, Bielefeldt R, Rathmann W, Purmann J, Tschope D, Erckenbrecht JF (1991) Epidemiology of faecal incontinence in selected patient groups. International Journal of Colorectal Disease 6: 143–6.

Faucheron JL, Hannoun L, Thorne C, Parc R (1994) Is faecal continence improved by non stimulated gracilis muscle transposition? Diseases of the Colon and Rectum 37: 979–83.

George BD, Williams NS, Patel J, Swash M, Watkins ES (1993) Physiological and histochemical adaptation of the electrically stimulated gracilis muscle to neoanal sphincter function. British Journal of Surgery 80: 342–6.

Hassink EAM, Rieu PNMA, Brugman ATM, Festen C (1994) Quality of life after operatively corrected high anorectal malformation: A long-term follow-up study of patients aged 18 years and older. Journal of Pediatric Surgery 29: 773–6.

Jameson JS, Scott AND (1997) Medical causes of faecal incontinence. European Journal of Gastroenterology and Hepatology 9: 428–30.

Johnson JF, Lafferty J (1996) Epidemiology of faecal incontinence: the silent affliction. American Journal of Gastroenterology 91(1): 33–6.

Kalidasun V, Elgabroun MA, Guiney EJ (1997) Button caecostomy in the management of faecal incontinence. British Journal of Surgery 84: 694.

Korsgen S, Deen KI, Keighley MR (1997) Long-term results of total pelvic floor repair for post obstetric faecal incontinence. Diseases of the Colon and Rectum 40: 835–9.

Lehur PA, Michot F Denis P, Grise P, Leborgne J, Teniere P, Buzelin JM (1996) Results of artificial sphincter in severe anal incontinence. Diseases of the Colon and Rectum 39: 1352–5.

Loening Baucke V (1995) Biofeedback treatment for chronic constipation and encopresis in childhood. Pediatrics 96: 105–10.

Lunniss PJ, Kamm MA, Phillips RKS (1994) Factors affecting continence after surgery for anal fistula. British Journal of Surgery 81: 1382–5.

Mander BJ, Abercrombie JF, George BD, Williams NS (1996) The electrically stimulated gracilis neosphincter as part of total anorectal reconstruction after abdominoperineal excision of the rectum. Annals of Surgery 224: 702–11.

Mander BJ, Williams NS (1997) The electrically stimulated gracilis neosphincter. European Journal of Gastrology and Hepatology 9: 435–41.

Marsh BJ, Kiff ES (1996) Ileocaecostomy: an alternative surgical procedure for antegrade colonic enema. British Journal of Surgery 83: 507–8.

Maw A, Eccersley AJP, Williams NS (1996) Ileocaecostomy. British Journal of Surgery 83: 1304–5.

Mortensen N, Smilgin Humphries M (1991) The anal continence plug: a disposable device for patients with ano-rectal incontinence. Lancet 338: 295–7.

Nelson R, Norton N, Cautley E, Furner S (1995) Community based prevalence of anal incontinence. Journal of the American Medical Association 274(7): 556–9.

Pickrell K, Georgiade N, Maguire C, Crawford H, Durham NC (1956) Gracilis muscle transplant for faecal incontinence. Surgery 40: 349–63.

Rintala R, Mildh L, Lindahl H (1994) Faecal continence and quality of life for adult patients with an operative high or intermediate anorectal malformation. Journal of Pediatric Surgery 29: 777–80.

Rubin GP, Devlin HB (1987) Quality of life with a stoma. British Journal of Hospital Medicine 38(4): 300–6.

Salter M (1990) Altered Body Image – The Nurse's Role. Chichester: Wiley.

Sangwan YP, Coller JA, Barrett RC, Roberts PL, Murray JJ, Rusin L, Schoetz DJ (1996) Unilateral pudendal neuropathy: impact on outcome of anal sphincter repair. Diseases of the Colon and Rectum 39: 686–9.

Smilgin Humphries M (1993) WC Enterostomal Therapists Journal 13: 15–16.

Squire R, Kiely EM, Carr B, Ransley PG, Duffy PG (1993) Clinical application of the malone antegrade colonic enema. Journal of Pediatric Surgery 28: 1012–5.

Stuchfield B (1995) The continent colonic conduit in the management of severe constipation. British Journal of Nursing 4(17): 1012–16.

Sultan AH, Kamm MA, Hudson CN (1994) Pudendal nerve damage during labour: prospective study before and after childbirth. British Journal of Obstetrics & Gynaecology 101: 22–8.

Sultan AH, Kamm MA, Hudson CN, Thomas JM, Bartram CI (1993) Anal sphincter disruption during vaginal delivery. New England Journal of Medicine 329: 1905–11.

Sultan AH, Stanton SL (1997) Occult obstetric trauma and anal incontinence. European Journal of Gastrology and Hepatology 9: 423–7.

Taitz LS, Water JKH, Urwin OM, Molner D (1986) Factors associated with outcome in management of defecation disorders. Archives of Disease in Childhood 61: 472–7.

Ternent CA, Shashidaran M, Blatchford GJ, Christensen MA, Thorson AG, Sentovich SM (1997) Transanal ultrasound and anorectal physiology findings affecting continence after sphincteroplasty. Diseases of the Colon and Rectum 40: 462–7.

Tetzchner T, Sorensen M, Lose G, Christiansen J (1996) Anal and urinary incontinence in women with anal sphincter rupture. British Journal of Obstetrics & Gynaecology 103: 1034–40.

Van Tets WF, Kuijpers JHC, Tran K, Mollen R, Van Goor H (1997) Influence of Parks anal retractor on anal sphincter pressures. Diseases of the Colon and Rectum 40: 1042–5.

Wade B (1989) Patient adaptation. In A Stoma is For Life. London: Scutari Press, pp 151–70.

White C, Hunt JC (1997) Psychological factors in postoperative adjustment to stoma surgery. Annals of the Royal College of Surgeons of England 79: 3–7.

Williams NS, Hughes SF, Stuchfield B (1994) Continent colonic conduit for rectal evacuation in severe constipation. Lancet 343: 1321–4.

Wong WD, Jensen LJ, Bartolo BCC, Rothenberger DA (1996) Artificial anal sphincter. Diseases of the Colon and Rectum 39: 1345–51.

Chapter 14
Sexually Transmitted Diseases and the Acquired Immune Deficiency Syndrome

STEPHANIE L. SCHMITT MD, Assistant Professor of Surgery, University of South Florida, Tampa General Hospital, Tampa, Florida, USA

Sexually transmitted diseases (STDs) and acquired immune deficiency syndrome (AIDS) continue to constitute a major public health concern. Despite efforts to educate the public, the incidence of these illnesses continues to rise faster than that originally predicted. It is important for those involved in health care to be aware of presenting signs and symptoms to facilitate diagnosis and treatment. This chapter will cover some of the more common STDs and colorectal manifestations of AIDS.

Gonorrhoea

Gonorrhoea, caused by *Neisseria gonorrhoeae*, produces a non-ulcerating inflammatory proctitis. It can infect the mucosal surface of all body orifices. Transmission occurs by anal receptive intercourse with symptoms developing after an incubation period of approximately 7 days. Most women, however, develop gonococcal proctitis via autoinoculation of vaginal gonorrhoea into the rectum.

Most patients are asymptomatic. Others may present with bloody or mucopurulent discharge or pruritis ani. Tenesmus may be severe, making the examination difficult for the patient. It is important to remember to avoid the use of lubricants, using only water to moisten the instruments, as some lubricants contain antibacterial agents and interfere with culture results (Adams and Huber, 1984).

Culture is performed on Thayer-Martin agar or Stuart's medium.

Gram-stain preparation will reveal gram-negative intracellular diplo-
cocci in pairs or clusters. It is important to obtain culture to determine
whether the strain is drug resistant. A high index of suspicion
mandates empiric treatment prior to obtaining final culture results.

Treatment options include aqueous procaine penicillin G, ceftriaxone, cefixime, ceftizoxime, ciprofloxacin (Miles, West Haven, CT) and
spectinomycin (*The Medical Letter*, 1996) Repeat screening in 3 months
is necessary as initial treatment failure occurs in 35% of cases (Klein et
al., 1977). As with other STDs, in order to prevent recurrence all
sexual contacts must be treated.

Syphilis

Syphilis is caused by a motile spirochete, *Treponema pallidum*. The initial
lesion, or chancre, usually develops within 2 to 6 weeks of exposure
(Catterall, 1975). These lesions are raised, circular and 1 to 2 cm in
diameter and are often associated with inguinal lymphadenopathy. The
ulcers may also be multiple or have irregular borders. Two ulcers may be
located opposite each other in a kissing configuration. If left untreated,
the ulcer may heal in 3 to 4 weeks (Hughes et al., 1983). Primary syphilis
can be diagnosed with dark-field examination of scrapings of the chancre base, which demonstrates motile cork-screw shaped organisms.
Additional tools for diagnosis include the Venereal Disease Research
Laboratory (VDRL) which is positive in 75% of patients at the time of
presentation. The fluorescent treponemal antibody (FTA) assay is positive approximately 4 to 6 weeks after infection (Knapp et al., 1990).

Secondary syphilis will appear 6 to 8 weeks after the chancre has
healed in untreated patients. The lesion at this stage is a condyloma
latum, a raised, thickened verrucous lesion. Again, spirochetes may be
found in this lesion. Another presentation may be a maculopapular
rash, most obvious on the palms of the hands. It is possible for the
primary and secondary lesions to coexist. Both the VDRL and the
FTA will be highly positive at this stage.

Treatment options include penicillin G, tetracycline, and ceftriaxone
(*The Medical Letter*, 1996) It is mandatory that all sexual contacts for the
preceding year receive treatment. Those infected should abstain from
sexual contact until proven non-infective on follow-up laboratory studies.

Chlamydia

Chlamydia is the most common infectious disease reported to state
health departments and the Centers for Disease Control (CDC).

Chlamydia trachomatis is a small intracellular organism with multiple immunotypes; serotypes D to K cause proctitis and serotypes L1, L2 and L3 cause lymphogranuloma venereum (LGV). Inguinal lymphadeno-pathy occurs with serotypes D to K and L1 through L3. Prolonged inflammation may lead to lymphoedema of the lower extremities or formation of chronic sinus tracts from the involved lymph nodes to the skin. Symptoms include malaise, anorexia, headache, fever, joint pain and rectal pain. If untreated, a rectal stricture or mass may be present on exam. As *Chlamydia* is an obligate intracellular organism, culture is usually unsuccessful. Complement fixation testing relies on an intact immune system and thus may be inactive in human immunodeficiency virus (HIV) positive. Microimmunofluorescent antibody titre testing is most sensitive but is not widely available (Centers for Disease Control, 1996; Wang et al., 1975).

Treatment is undertaken with azithromycin or a tetracycline. Both rectal strictures and skin fistulae may heal with antibiotic therapy. If strictures fail to improve and remain symptomatic, sphincter-sparing surgical excision may be necessary.

Herpes Simplex Virus

Most cases of anorectal herpes are caused by herpes simplex virus type 2 (HSV-2). After inoculation, the viral particles travel along neurons to the nucleus. The virus may then lie dormant in the nucleus, only to be reactivated at a later date. After the initial infection, the risk of recurrent episodes is greater than 80% with HSV-2 (Reeves et al., 1981). Recurrences range from infrequent and subclinical in individuals with normal immune systems to severe and progressive in those with compromised immune systems (Corey et al., 1988). Normally, symptoms last for 7 to 10 days with the infection persisting and progressing in immunocompromised individuals unless therapy is begun.

During the initial outbreak, the patient usually complains of severe pain in the perianal region. Constipation and tenesmus may be reported. In fact, the pain may be so excruciating that the patient may fear defecation and develop faecal impaction. Systemic symptoms include malaise, fever, chills and headache (Goldmeier, 1980).

In the early days of the episode, inspection of the area will reveal painful vesicles or ulcerations of the perianal skin, anal canal or distal rectum. Tender inguinal adenopathy may be present. A direct swab of the involved area should be performed and will document infection in 90% of HSV-2 cases (Fife and Corey, 1990). Thus it is important that viral culture swabs and medium should be available in the office to facilitate diagnosis. If no culture medium is available, scrapings of the ulcer base may be obtained, placed on a glass microscope slide and the Tzanck preparation method utilized to document the multinucleated giant cells typical of this infection.

Treatment includes symptomatic relief with warm sitz baths, stool softeners and pain medication. Medication utilized includes acyclovir, valcyclovir and famciclovir. Long-term administration of oral acyclovir decreases the frequency of symptomatic recurrences and asymptomatic HSV shedding (Wald et al., 1997). Topical acyclovir ointment may be used in conjunction with oral therapy. Oral acyclovir has been shown to decrease pain by 4 days, viral shedding by 8 days, and time to healing by 1 week (Corey et al., 1983). Immuno-compromised patients will require higher doses of acyclovir with continued suppression thereafter. It has been suggested that once suppressive therapy has begun in these patients, it should continue indefinitely (Mertz, 1990).

Human Papilloma Virus

More than 50 types of human papilloma virus (HPV) have been recognized through DNA hybridization techniques (Eron, 1992). Benign condylomata and low-grade dysplasia of the anogenital region are most commonly associated with HPV types 6 and 11. Anogenital condylomata, more severe dysplasia and invasive squamous cell carcinoma are associated with HPV types 16 and 18.

The incidence of anogenital warts is only an indirect indicator of the true incidence of this STD. Subclinical and latent infections as well as minimally symptomatic lesions are known to occur. The vast majority of patients, 80% to 90%, with anal condylomata are homosexual (Oriel, 1971; Brown and Fife, 1990).

The primary mode of transmission is via sexual intercourse. Relative ease of transmission is apparent in that more than 70% of the male partners of women with clinical HPV infections will show evidence of infection (Rosenberg et al., 1987).

Subclinical HPV infections are present in a large number of sexually active individuals (Koutsy et al., 1988). Incubation periods of 1 to 3 months to years have been reported for development of symptoms after sexual contact (Oriel, 1971). The lesion may appear flat or as a papillary excrescence. The surface character ranges from smooth to rough with finger-like projections. Condylomata of the perianal skin may be pigmented whilst those of the anal canal appear pink to white. Several scattered individual condylomata to numerous coalescing lesions with the appearance of large growths may be seen. Symptoms include pruritus ani, increased moisture of the perianal area, and passage of small amounts of bright red blood per rectum with defecation.

Buschke–Lowenstein tumours or giant condyloma accuminata are variants of anogenital condylomata, presenting as a rapidly growing, fungating squamous cell carcinoma. Another variant seen with HPV infection is Bowenoid papulosis. Multiple small reddish-brown to purple papules are present on inspection. Several studies have now shown an association between anal condyloma and dysplasia or carcinoma (Croxson et al., 1984; Nash et al., 1986).

Various options exist for the treatment of condylomata. Topical applications include podophyllin and bichloroacetic acid (BCAA). Both solutions are applied directly to the warts as they are toxic to normal skin. Six to eight hours after the application of podophyllin, the patient should be instructed to wash the entire area thoroughly to prevent damage to the surrounding skin. Unlike podophyllin, BCAA may be used to treat anal canal condylomata. Other treatment options include excision, electrocoagulation, laser ablation and cryotherapy.

Epithelium adjacent to involved areas may contain HPV while having a normal histologic and colposcopic appearance. This undoubtedly is responsible for the high rate of recurrence seen. This has brought about interest in immunotherapy for treatment of all infected epithelium, not just the areas of clinical involvement. Autologous vaccine from the patient's own wart tissue and interferon have been shown to be effective (Abcarian and Sharon, 1977; Gall et al., 1986; Friedman-Kien et al., 1988).

Cytomegalovirus

In the homosexual AIDS population, cytomegalovirus (CMV) is ubiquitous. Seropositivity for CMV has been found in over 90% of healthy homosexual men (Drew et al., 1981; Lange et al., 1984). Active infection is estimated to be present in 14% of homosexuals between the ages of 18 and 29 years (Drew et al., 1981).

Symptomatic CMV ileocolitis is the most common intestinal infection in AIDS patients, occurring in at least 10% of patients (Drew et al., 1988). Symptoms include weight loss, fever, diarrhoea, and sometimes melaena or haematochezia. Colonoscopic evaluation with biopsies can confirm the diagnosis. Findings range from patchy erythema with or without shallow ulcers to multiple wide, deep ulcers. Due to the multifocal nature of the disease, biopsies should be obtained from multiple sites to facilitate diagnosis (Frank and Raicht, 1984). Histopathologic examination reveals the pathognomonic findings of large basophilic intranuclear inclusions. These microscopic features are particularly visible in vascular endothelial cells. The diagnosis may be confirmed by either viral culture of biopsy specimens or antigen assay of washings taken from ulcers.

Although CMV can be diagnosed by the above methods, it is not known whether CMV is the true cause of the ulcer or merely inhabits an existing ulcer. Coexisting gastrointestinal (GI) pathogens have been reported in more than 70% of homosexual AIDS patients (Quinn, 1985; Morris, 1990). These other organisms include *Candida, Cryptosporidium, Mycobacterium, Salmonella* and *Shigella*. It is unclear whether CMV infection increases susceptibility to these other pathogens or whether mucosal damage secondary to these synchronous infections promotes replication of CMV (Wexner, 1990).

Because of the resultant vasculitis, ischaemic ulcerations may occur (Balthazar et al., 1985). Perforation may develop secondary to transmural infarction.

Bleeding and perforation of multifocal CMV ulcerations are the most common indications for surgical intervention (Kram et al., 1984; Wexner, 1988; Dieterich and Rahmin, 1991).

Complications of CMV infection account for the majority of emergency laparotomies in AIDS patients. As the disease is multifocal in nature, ulcerations may be found in the ileum, abdominal colon and rectum (Wexner et al., 1988; Kram and Shoemaker, 1990). In one study, a postoperative morbidity rate of 90% was noted with postoperative mortality rates of 28%, 71% and 86% at 1 day, 1 month and 6 months, respectively (Wexner, 1988). These statistics emphasize the 'malignant' nature of this infection. Because of the high mortality rate associated with emergency abdominal procedures in AIDS patients, it is important that the patient, their family, and other physicians involved in their care understand the guarded prognosis.

There have been several reports of AIDS patients who underwent laparotomy for presumed appendicitis (Binderow and Shaked, 1991; Dieterich et al., 1991; Valderiz-Casasola and Pardo-Mindan, 1991; Thuluvath et al., 1991). On histopathologic examination, CMV appendicitis was found to be the cause.

Medical therapy of CMV infections includes ganciclovir, foscarnet and cidofovir. One recent study has noted that ganciclovir may be of benefit in the resolution of the 'wasting syndrome' associated with CMV colitis (Kotler, 1991).

Mycobacterium Avium-Intracellulare

Infection with atypical mycobacterium has become a significant health problem as the AIDS epidemic progresses. *Mycobacterium avium-intracellulare* (MAI) is an opportunistic infection seen in AIDS patients. Presentations of the infection range from an asymptomatic carrier state to profuse watery diarrhoea, dehydration and severe abdominal pain. Colonoscopy with ileal biopsies is the best way to confirm the diagnosis. The characteristic finding on histopathologic examination is macrophages laden with acid-fast mycobacteria. In addition, stool samples may be positive for acid-fast bacilli.

Markedly enlarged mesenteric lymph nodes, ulcerations and obstruction of the terminal ileum may occur (Schneebaum et al., 1987; Waisman et al., 1987; Wexner, 1989).

Medical treatment of intestinal MAI is a significant challenge. This may be secondary to the organism load present at the time the patient becomes symptomatic (Rathbun et al., 1991). Unfortunately, resistance to standard antituberculosis drugs is a common finding. Medications utilized include azithromycin or clarithromycin plus one or more of the following: ciprofloxacin, clofazimine, ethambutol, rifabutin and rifampin.

Other Infectious Proctocolitides

In healthy individuals, proctocolitis secondary to *Cryptosporidium* and *Isospora belli* produces a self-limited infection. However, in AIDS patients these organisms may produce a life-threatening proctocolitis (Judson et al., 1980). The mucosal surface of the small and large bowel will reveal adherence of the cryptosporidial protozoans rather than invasion of the involved tissues. Cryptosporidiosis was previously recognized as a causative agent of gastroenteritis in birds and animals (Tzipori, 1983). After an incubation period of 5 to 10 days, immuno-competent individuals develop a self-limited watery diarrhoea associated with fever, nausea, vomiting and abdominal pain lasting up to 2 weeks. AIDS patients exhibit a profuse watery diarrhoea with resultant electrolyte imbalance, dehydration and prostration (Current et al., 1983; Daul and DeShazo, 1983). Up to 15 or 17 litres/day of watery stools may be produced without blood or mucus and without chills or fever (Rodgers and Kagnoff, 1987; Soave et al., 1984) Significant weight loss may occur prior to diagnosis (Soave et al., 1984).

Histopathologic evaluation of rectal biopsies revealing characteris-tic oocytes can confirm the diagnosis. These organisms appear as minute blue, round structures adherent to microvilli.

Supportive intervention is instituted with hydration and nutrition as the cornerstones of therapy. Antiparasitic medications such as metronidazole, furazolidone, spiramycin and thiabendazole have been utilized. Unfortunately, these agents have been largely unsuccessful (Soave et al., 1984).

Isospora belli produces symptoms similar to those seen with cryptosporidiosis. The diagnosis is confirmed by the identification of oocysts on faecal smears. The oocysts are acid-fast, elliptical and are approximately tenfold larger than those of cryptosporidia.

As opposed to cryptosporidiosis, isosporiasis responds readily to treatment with trimethoprim-sulfamethoxazole (TMP-SMX) (DeHovitz et al., 1986; Restrepo et al., 1987). Owing to a high rate of recurrence, prophylaxis is recommended (Soave et al., 1984). Other options for treatment are quinacrine and metronidazole (Faust et al., 1961).

Parasitic colitis is transmitted primarily through oroanal intercourse with an infected partner. *Entamoeba histolytica* infection is relatively common among homosexual or bisexual men in the United States (Pomerantz et al., 1980). *E. histolytica* is a protozoan that inhabits the colon in either trophozoite or cyst form. When ingested, cysts pass into the small intestine where trophozoites are released. Although some patients may be asymptomatic, some will present with malaise, fever, abdominal pain and bloody diarrhoea with tenesmus. On endoscopy, findings range from normal to friable mucosa, oedema and 'hour-glass' ulcers laden with trophozoites (Pittman et al., 1973). Stool specimens should be obtained as 90% of symptomatic patients' stools contain trophozoites (William, 1980). The diagnosis may also be established with indirect haemagglutination testing. Treatment is with metronidazole with diodohydroxyquin (Peppercorn, 1989).

Another protozoan, *Giardia lamblia*, is also transmitted through oroanal intercourse. Its prevalence in the homosexual population is lower than that of *E. histolytica* (Quinn et al., 1983). A variety of symptoms may be present including anorexia, bloating, weight loss and severe cramps with frequent foul-smelling, greasy, loose stools. Endoscopy usually reveals normal mucosa, but diffuse ulcerations may be seen (Knapp et al., 1990). Microscopic examination of stool specimens or scrapings of an ulcer base may be diagnostic. For both *E. histolytica* and *G. lamblia*, the specimens must be examined within an hour of collection. Therapeutic agents include metronidazole, quinacrine, furazolidone, tinidazole and paramomycin (Peppercorn, 1989) .

Shigella flexneri is another common infection in the homosexual population (Bader et al., 1977; William et al., 1977; Allason-Jones and

Mindel, 1987). Transmission is by direct or indirect faecal–oral route. As few as 10 organisms may produce infection (Knapp et al., 1990). Patients may present with the abrupt onset of nausea, fever, abdominal cramping and bloody diarrhoea. Stool cultures will reveal *Shigella*. Hydration and the avoidance of anticholinergic antidiarrhoeal agents are important supportive measures. The above-noted medications may prolong symptoms and shedding of the organism or precipitate toxic megacolon (Dupont and Hornick, 1973). The antibiotic of choice is double-strength trimethoprim-sulfamethoxazole, with tetracycline and ampicillin as additional options. Treatment continues until repeat stool cultures are negative (Knapp et al., 1990).

Anal Ulcerations in the HIV-positive Patient

Special consideration needs to be given to ulcerative lesions in the HIV-positive patient. Trauma secondary to anoreceptive intercourse as well as bacterial, viral and fungal infections and even some malignancies may lead to the development of these lesions. The ulcers are unique in that they may extend well up into the anal canal and invade deeply into the anal sphincters.

Bacterial infections which may present as ulcers include *Mycobacterium tuberculosis*, syphilis, chancroid and LGV (Centers for Disease Control, 1986; Nunn and McAdam, 1988). Viral causes of anal ulcerations include CMV and HSV. HIV is now more frequently identified in gastrointestinal tract ulcers (Nelson et al., 1988; Levy et al., 1989). The appearance of HIV ulcers is no different from that of other ulcers of various causes. It remains unclear as to whether there is a direct cause and effect relationship between HIV and anal ulcers. However, it does have important ramifications for diagnosis and treatment. The parasite *E. histolytica* may cause anal ulcerations.

The most frustrating of all ulcers for the clinician is the idiopathic ulcer, which may be deep and extremely painful. Unfortunately, treatment is usually ineffective in obtaining a cure. Instead, relief of symptoms is the therapeutic goal. Intralesional steroid injection may be of some benefit. Debilitating pain, haemorrhage, and anal incontinence made intolerable by intractable diarrhoea may necessitate a diverting colostomy for symptomatic relief.

To facilitate diagnosis and treatment, biopsies of these ulcerations should be obtained with specimens sent for bacterial, viral and acid-fast culture, and routine and acid-fast staining. Treatment can then be tailored to the defined cause.

General Considerations

It is important to have available appropriate equipment and culture medium to facilitate the diagnosis and treatment of these various infectious processes. As some infections may be exquisitely tender rendering the patient unable to cooperate with the examination in the outpatient setting, examination under anaesthesia may be required. Regardless of where the patient is seen and examined, several considerations are of vital importance. All individuals should be considered to be HIV positive and therefore universal precautions instituted. It is advisable that only one individual's hands be present on the patients anogenital region during the use of any sharp instruments. Again, no sharp instruments should ever be passed directly from one individual to another. Testing to determine seropositivity in order to reduce the risk of transmission of HIV within the health care setting has not been shown to be effective and is no substitute for universal precautions (Tokars et al., 1992).

Counselling of the individuals presenting for evaluation remains of utmost importance. A significant number of patients continue to delay seeking treatment in the hope that the symptoms will simply 'go away' (Hook et al., 1997). Recently, it has been shown that treatment of concomitant STDs reduces the HIV viral load in semen and thus the risk of transmission during unprotected sexual intercourse (*AIDS Weekly*, 1997a, 1997b). In addition, HIV seropositive individuals require immunologic monitoring, screening for concurrent STDs, antiretroviral therapy, prophylaxis against opportunistic diseases and other services (Centers for Disease Control, 1993; Jewett and Hecht, 1993).

Conclusion

As the prevalence of heterosexually transmitted STDs and AIDS continues to increase, vigilance will be required to detect changes in colorectal manifestations which may develop among this population. It is imperative that those involved in coloproctology remain up to date in order to optimize diagnosis and treatment of these challenging patients.

References

Abcarian H, Sharon N (1977) The effectiveness of immunotherapy in the treatment of anal condyloma acuminatum. Journal of Surgical Research 22: 231–6.

Adams R, Huber P (1984) Anal syphilis. South Medical Journal 77: 1368–70.

AIDS Weekly Plus (1997a) New study proves treating STDs reduces infectiousness of HIV. Aids Weekly Plus 14 July: 28.

AIDS Weekly Plus (1997b) Treatment for other STDs should be part of HIV prevention. AIDS Weekly Plus 7 July: 30.

Allason-Jones E, Mindel A (1987) Sex and the bowel. International Journal of Colorectal Disease 2: 32–7.

Bader M, Pederson AHB, Williams R, et al. (1977) Venereal transmission of shigellosis in Seattle – King County. Sexually Transmitted Diseases 4: 89–91.

Balthazar EJ, Meigbow AJ, Hulnick DH (1985) Cytomegalovirus esophagitis and gastritis in AIDS. American Journal of Radiology 144: 1201–4.

Binderow SR, Shaked AA (1991) Acute appendicitis in patients with AIDS/HIV infection. American Journal of Surgery 162: 9–12.

Brown DR, Fife KH (1990) Human papillomavirus infections of the genital tract. Medical Clinics of North America 74: 1455–85.

Catterall RD (1975) Sexually transmitted diseases of the anus and rectum. Clinical Gastroenterology 4: 659–69.

Centers for Disease Control (1986) Tuberculosis and the acquired immunodeficiency syndrome –Florida. Morbidity and Mortality Weekly Report 35: 587–90.

Centers for Disease Control (1996) Ten leading nationally notifiable infectious diseases – United States, 1995. Morbidity and Mortality Weekly Report 45: 883–4.

Centers for Disease Control and Prevention (1993) Recommendations for HIV testing services for inpatients and outpatients in acute care settings. Morbidity and Mortality Weekly Report 42: 1–17.

Corey L, Ashley R, Benedetti J et al. (1988) The effect of prior HSV-1 infection on the subsequent natural history of genital HSV-2. Paper presented at the Programs and Abstracts of the 28th Interscience Conference on Antimicrobial Agents, Chemotherapy; American Society for Microbiology, Washington DC.

Corey L, Benedetti J, Critchlow C et al. (1983) Treatment of primary first-episode genital herpes simplex virus infections with acyclovir: results of topical, intravenous and oral therapy. Journal of Antimicrobial Chemotherapy 12(Suppl. B): S79–88.

Croxson T, Chabon, AB, Rorat E et al. (1984) Intraepithelial carcinoma of the anus in homosexual men. Diseases of the Colon and Rectum 27: 325–30.

Current WL, Reese NC, Ernst JV et al. (1983) Human cryptosporidiosis in immunocompetent and immunodeficient persons. Studies of an outbreak and experimental transmission. New England Journal of Medicine 308: 1252–7.

Daul CB, DeShazo RD (1983) Acquired immunodeficiency syndrome: an update and interpretation. Annals of Allergy 51: 351–61.

DeHovitz JA, Pape JW, Boncy M et al. (1986) Clinical manifestations and therapy of Isospora belli infection in patients with acquired immunodeficiency syndrome. New England Journal of Medicine 315: 87–90.

Dieterich DT, Kim MH, McMeeding A, Rotterdam H (1991) Cytomegalovirus infection of the appendix in a patient with the acquired immunodeficiency syndrome. American Journal of Gastroenterology 86: 904–6.

Drew WL, Buhles W, Erlich KS (1988) Herpes virus infections (cytomegalovirus, herpes simplex virus, varicella-zoster virus) Infectious Disease Clinics of North America 2: 495–509.

Drew WL, Mintz L,Miner RC et al. (1981) Prevalence of cytomegalovirus infection in homosexual males. Journal of Infectious Diseases 143: 188–92.

DuPont HL, Hornick RB (1973) Adverse effect of lomotil therapy in shigellosis. Journal of the American Medical Association 2: 475–84.

Eron LJ (1992) Human papillomavirus and anogenital disease. In Gorbach SL, Bartlett JG, Blecknow NR (Eds) Infectious Disease. Philadelphia: WB Saunders, pp 852–6.

Faust EC, Giraldo LE, Caicedo G et al. (1961) Human isosporiasis in the Western hemisphere. American Journal of Tropical Medicine and Hygiene 10: 343–5.

Fife KH, Corey L (1990) Herpes simplex virus. In Sexually Transmitted Diseases. 2nd edn. New York: McGraw-Hill, p 941.

Frank D, Raicht RF (1984) Intestinal perforation associated with cytomegalovirus infection in patients with acquired immune deficiency syndrome. American Journal of Gastroenterology 79: 201–5.

Friedman-Kien AE, Eron LJ, Conant M et al. (1988) Natural interferon alpha for treatment of condylomata acuminata. Journal of the American Medical Association 259: 533.

Gall SA, Hughes CE, Mounts P et al. (1986) Efficacy of human lymphoblastoid interferon in the therapy of resistant condylomata acuminata. Obstetrics and Gynecology 67: 643–7.

Goldmeier D (1980) Proctitis and herpes simplex virus in homosexual men. British Journal of Venereal Disease 56: 111–14.

Hook EW, Richey CM, Leone P et al. (1997) Delayed presentation to clinics for sexually transmitted diseases by symptomatic patients: a potential contributor to continuing STD morbidity. Sexually Transmitted Diseases 24: 443.

Hughes E, Cuthbertson AM, Killingback MK (1983) Venereal diseases of the anal canal and rectum. In Hughes E, Cuthbertson AM, Killingback MK (Eds) Colorectal Surgery. New York: Churchill Livingstone, pp 203–8.

Jewett JF, Hecht FM (1993) Preventive health care for adults with HIV infection. Journal of the American Medical Association 269: 1144–53.

Judson FN, Penley KA, Robinson ME et al. (1980) Comparative prevalence rates of sexually transmitted diseases in homosexual men. American Journal of Epidemiology 112: 836–43.

Klein EF, Fisher LS, Chow AD, Guz LB (1977) Anorectal gonococcal infection: a clinical review. Annals of Internal Medicine 86: 340–6.

Knapp JS, Zenilman JM, Thompson SE (1990) Gonorrhea. In Morse SA, Moreland AA, Thompson SE (Eds) Sexually Transmitted Diseases. Philadelphia, PA: JB Lippincott, pp 512–22.

Kotler DP (1991) Cytomegalovirus colitis and wasting. Journal of Acquired Immune Deficiency Syndromes 4(Suppl 1): S36–S41.

Koutsy LA, Galloway DA, Holmes KK (1988) Epidemiology of genital human papillomavirus infection. Epidemiology Reviews 10: 122–63.

Kram HB, Hino ST, Cohen RE, DeSantis SA et al. (1984) Spontaneous colonic perforation secondary to cytomegalovirus in a patient with acquired immune deficiency syndrome. Critical Care Medicine 12: 469–71.

Kram HB, Shoemaker WC (1990) Intestinal perforation due to cytomegalovirus infection in patients with AIDS. Diseases of the Colon and Rectum 33: 1037–40.

Lange M, Klein EB, Kornfield H et al. (1984) Cytomegalovirus isolation from healthy homosexual men. Journal of the American Medical Association 252: 1908–10.

Levy JA, Margaretten W, Nelson J (1989) Detection of HIV in enterochromaffin cells in the rectal mucosa of an AIDS patient. American Journal of Gastroenterology 84: 787–9.

Mertz GJ (1990) Genital herpes simplex virus infections. Medical Clinics of North America 74: 1433–54.

Morris DJ (1990) Is human immunodeficiency virus (HIV) rather than cytomegalovirus the cause of retinitis and colitis in HIV-infected patients? Reviews of Infectious Diseases 2: 557–9.

Nash G, Allen W, Nash S (1986) Atypical lesions of the anal mucosa in homosexual men. Journal of the American Medical Association 256: 873–6.

Nelson JA, Wiley CA, Reynolds-Kohler C, Reese CE, Margaretten W, Levy JA (1988) Human immunodeficiency virus detected in bowel epithelium from patients with gastrointestinal symptoms. Lancet 1 (8580): 259–62.

Nunn PP, McAdam PK (1988) Mycobacterial infections and AIDS. British Medical Bulletin 44: 801–13.

Oriel JD (1971) Anal warts and anal coitus. British Journal of Venereal Disease 47: 373–6.

Peppercorn MA (1989) Enteric infections in homosexual men with and without AIDS. Contemporary Gastroenterology 2: 23–32.

Pittman FE, El-Hashimi WK, Pittman JC (1973) Studies of human amebiasis, I: Clinical and laboratory findings of eight cases of acute amebic colitis. Gastroenterology 56: 581–7.

Pomerantz BM, Marr JS, Goldman WD (1980) Amebiasis in New York City 1958–1978: Identification of the male homosexual high risk population. Bulletin of the New York Academy of Medicine 56: 232–44.

Quinn TC (1985) Gastrointestinal manifestations of AIDS. Practical Gastroenterology 9: 23–34.

Quinn TC, Stamm WE, Goddell SE et al. (1983) The polymicrobial origin of intestinal infections in homosexual men. New England Journal of Medicine 309: 576–82.

Rathbun RC, Martin ES 3rd, Eaton VE, Matthew EB (1991) Current and investigational therapies for AIDS-associated mycobacterium-avium complex disease. Clinical Pharmacology 10: 280–91.

Reeves WC, Corey L, Adams HG et al. (1981) Risk of recurrence after first episodes of genital herpes: relation to HSV type and antibody response. New England Journal of Medicine 305: 315–19.

Restrepo C, Macher AM, Radany EH (1987) Disseminated extraintestinal isosporiasis in a patient with acquired immune deficiency syndrome. American Journal of Clinical Pathology 87: 536–9.

Rodgers VD, Kagnoff MF (1987) Gastrointestinal manifestations of the acquired immunodeficiency syndrome. Western Journal of Medicine 146: 57–67.

Rosenberg KS, Greenberg MD, Reid R (1987) Sexually transmitted papilloma viral infection in men. Obstetrics and Gynecology Clinics of North America 14: 495–512.

Schneebaum CW, Novick DM, Chabon AB et al. (1987) Terminal ileitis associated with mycobacterium avium-intracellulare infection in homosexual men with the acquired immune deficiency syndrome. Gastroenterology 92: 1127–30.

Soave R, Danner RL, Honig CL et al. (1984) Cryptosporidiosis in homosexual men. Annals of Internal Medicine 100: 504–11.

The Medical Letter (1996) The choice of antibacterial drugs The Medical Letter 38(971 – 29 March).

Thuluvath PJ, Connolly GM, Forbes A, Gazzard BG (1991) Abdominal pain in HIV infection. Queensland Journal of Medicine 78: 275–85.

Tokars JI, Bell DM, Culver DH et al. (1992) Percutaneous injuries during surgical procedures. Journal of the American Medical Association 267: 2899–904.

Tzipori S (1983) Cryptosporidiosis in animals and humans. Microbiology Reviews 47: 84–96.

Valderiz-Casasola S, Pardo-Mindan FJ (1991) Cytomegalovirus infection of the appendix in a patient with the acquired immunodeficiency syndrome. Gastroenterology 101: 247–9.

Waisman J, Rotterdam H, Niedt GN et al. (1987) AIDS: an overview of the pathology. Pathology, Research and Practice 182: 729–54.

Wald A, Corey L, Cone R, Hobson A et al. (1997) Frequent genital herpes simplex virus shedding in immunocompetent women. Effect of acyclovir treatment. Journal of Clinical Investigations 99: 1092–7.

Wang SP, Grayston JT, Alexander ER, Holmes KK (1975) A simplified microimmunofluorescent test with trachoma-lymphogranuloma venereum (Chlamydia trachomatis) antigen for use as a screening test for antibody. Journal of Clinical Microbiology 1: 250–5.

Wexner SD (1988) Major emergent and urgent abdominal surgery in AIDS patients. South Medical Journal 18: S89.

Wexner SD (1989) AIDS: What the colorectal surgeon needs to know. Perspectives on Colon and Rectal Surgery 2: 19–54.

Wexner SD (1990) Cytomegalovirus ileocolitis and Kaposi's sarcoma in AIDS. In Fazio VW (Ed.) Current Therapy in Colon and Rectal Surgery. Toronto: BC Decker, pp 217–21.

Wexner SD, Smithy WB, Trillo C, Hopkins BS, Dailey TH (1988) Emergency colectomy for cytomegalovirus ileocolitis in patients with acquired immune deficiency syndrome. Diseases of the Colon and Rectum 31: 755–61.

William DC (1980) The sexual transmission of parasitic infections in gay men. Journal of Homosexuality 5: 291–4.

William DC, Felman YM, Marr JS et al. (1977) Sexually transmitted enteric pathogens in male homosexual populations. New York State Journal of Medicine 77: 2050–2.

Chapter 15
Colorectal Problems in Paediatric Patients

ALBERTO PEÑA MD, FACS, Chief, Pediatric Surgery, Schneider
    Children's Hospital, Long Island Jewish Medical Center, New
    Hyde Park, NY, USA
KATHLEEN O'CONNOR GUARDINO RN, MSN, Pediatric
    Surgery Nurse Clinican, Schnider Children's Hospital, Long Island
    Jewish Medical Center, New Hyde Park, NY, USA

Introduction

Anorectal malformations represent a spectrum of defects, ranging
from benign, non-complex with a good functional prognosis, to more
severe involving malformations in the genitourinary and sexual structures and with poor prognosis for bowel and urinary function.
Generally, children with complex malformations present with poor
sphincter tone, flat perineum, and no clear midline intergluteal groove
and need a three-stage surgical repair, that is, colostomy, main repair
(pull-through) and colostomy closure. The most frequent surgical
approach for the main repair is termed posterior sagittal anorectoplasty – PSARP. Those children with relatively benign malformations,
hence 'low' defects, do not need such extensive surgical repair, they
simply receive an anoplasty, without a colostomy.

The nurse plays a very important role in the care of these patients
from the time of the initial diagnosis, pre-colostomy and post-
colostomy care, as well as before and after the main repair of the
malformation and the colostomy closure. These patients also need
strong nursing support during the process of anal dilations.

Many patients achieve very satisfactory bowel and urinary control,
whereas others either remain faecally incontinent or suffer from important functional disorders. These last two groups require a great deal of

help, and the participation of the nurse is essential during their management. The nurse plays an important role in the emotional support of the parents of children with anorectal malformations.

The nursing care of the child born with an anorectal malformation is essential in order to achieve optimal results in all stages of surgical repair. The natural history of these defects, diagnostic methods, and medical and surgical therapy are reviewed here with special emphasis on those aspects relevant to nurses taking care of these children.

The purpose of this chapter is to take the nurse through the various stages of assessment and management of these children.

Introduction and Incidence

Anorectal malformations occur in 1 in every 4000 newborn (Brenner, 1915; Santulli, 1952; Truffler and Wilkinson, 1962). The term *anorectal malformation* encompasses multiple congenital defects of the rectum or of urinary and/or sexual structures with varying degrees of complexity that require different types of treatment with different prognosis for bowel and urinary control as well as sexual function. Most children with anorectal malformations have an abnormal communication between the rectum and the genitourinary tact or the perineum; this communication is called a fistula.

Classification

The following classification is proposed because it is therapeutic and prognosis oriented (Peña, 1990a).

Males

No colostomy required	Colostomy required
Low defects (perineal fistula)	Rectourethral bulbar fistula
	Rectourethral prostatic fistula
	Rectobladder neck fistula
	Imperforate anus without fistula
	Rectal atresia and stenosis

Females

No colostomy required	Colostomy required
Perineal fistula	Vestibular fistula
	Vaginal fistula

Colostomy required (cont.)

Imperforate anus without fistula
Rectal atresia and stenosis
Persistent cloaca

Initial Approach

An anorectal malformation represents a diagnosis that is rarely missed, even by a non-medical person. The physical examination of the newborn must always include the perineum, the genitalia and the patency of the anus.

Once the diagnosis of imperforate anus (anorectal malformation) has been established, the efforts of the medical team, including nurses, neonatologists and paediatric surgeons, are centred on the following goals:

1. to provide general medical support;
2. to determine whether or not the baby suffers from other associated defects that require immediate attention;
3. to determine whether the baby needs a temporary colostomy (high defects) or whether the defect can be treated by a minor operation called an anoplasty;
4. to give moral and psychological support to the parents, providing relevant information concerning the diagnosis, tests, treatment and prognosis.

During this initial stage the role of the nurse is invaluable. Besides the routine nursing examination, the following information must be assessed in the baby with an imperforate anus:

- abdominal distension;
- vomiting;
- presence of meconium in the perineum of a male baby or in the genitalia of a female baby;
- voiding pattern;
- presence of meconium in the urine of a male baby as detected by filtering the urine through a gauze placed at the tip of the penis or by urinalysis.

This information, plus a meticulous examination of the perineum and genitalia, as well as some special tests, will help the surgeon decide about the next therapeutic action.

General Support

General support includes: administration of antibiotics, keeping the baby nothing by mouth (NPO), insertion of an nasogastric (NG) tube to prevent vomiting, administration of vitamin K, administration of intravenous fluids and strict monitoring.

Associated Defects

The most frequently associated defects that may require immediate attention are those of the urinary tract. Therefore, every baby with an anorectal malformation requires an ultrasound examination of the abdomen to detect a urinary obstruction. This test is the most valuable initial screening test of the urinary tract; if this test is abnormal, a more specialized urological evaluation will be indicated. Other associated defects may include those of the gastrointestinal tract, including oesophageal atresia, duodenal atresia or atresia in other locations; cardiovascular anomalies are also frequently associated. Cardiac evaluation with ECG and echocardiogram will be performed only if the baby shows any cardiovascular symptoms.

Colostomy Opening Versus Anoplasty

The opening of an intestinal diversion called colostomy is considered necessary to decompress the bowel, also often to save the baby's life and, eventually, to avoid infection during the postoperative period of the main repair of the defect. This operation is indicated in some malformations as mentioned in the classification. This decision is taken after 24 hours of observation. In general, indications for a colostomy include:

- flat perineum (no intergluteal groove);
- meconium in urine (male patients);
- vestibular or vaginal fistula (females);
- single perineal orifice as evidence of a persistent cloaca (females);
- an X-ray film showing a rectum located more than 1 cm away from the perineal skin.

Indications for an anoplasty (no colostomy) include:

- meconium in the perineum (male);
- perineal fistula (male or female);
- an X-ray film showing a rectum located closer than 1 cm from the perineal skin.

Radiological Evaluation to Determine the Height of the Defect

As previously mentioned, in 80–90% of cases the decision concerning the opening of a colostomy versus anoplasty can be taken on purely clinical grounds. However, there are babies in whom the above-mentioned signs are not present or are not prominent enough, and then a specific X-ray study is indicated. Traditionally, this study is an 'invertogram' or upside-down film (Wangensteen and Rice, 1930), and must be taken after 24 hours of life in order for the baby to have enough intraluminal pressure in the bowel to distend with gas the most distal blind portion of the rectum. At the present time, it is no longer necessary to turn the baby upside down to take this film; the same good quality image is obtained with a cross-table lateral film taken with the baby placed in prone position with the pelvis elevated (Narasimharao et al., 1983). The gas inside the distended blind rectum gives a radiolucent image; the distance between the radio-opaque marker (skin) and the blind rectum is measured, and that provides valuable information concerning the height of the defect. During the study, the nurse must remain close to the baby to prevent hypothermia and to assist the baby in cases of vomiting or cyanosis.

Moral and Psychological Support

The nurse plays a key role in providing moral and psychological support. Very frequently, the nurse can perceive and transmit emotions from and to the parents. She detects more subtle manifestations of anxiety from them and acts as a liaison to alert the physicians about this. The constant presence of the nurse next to the baby allows the possibility of establishing a good rapport with the parents, and her attitude must be directed to provide confidence, affection, understanding and support.

Specific Defects

Male Defects

Perineal Fistula

When the rectum opens into the perineum, it is said to be a low malformation called perineal fistula; this is a benign condition, does not require a protective colostomy and has an excellent prognosis for future bowel function. It is best treated with a small operation called anoplasty which is usually performed during the newborn period.

During the first 24 hours of life these babies usually pass meconium through a small fistula orifice located somewhere in the midline, anterior to the anal dimple, in the perineum, at the base of the scrotum, or sometimes at the base of the penis. Sometimes they show a midline 'black-ribbon-like' subepithelial meconium fistula (Figure 15.1), and at other times they have a prominent midline skin tag located in the anal dimple, below which one can pass an instrument. This last defect is called 'bucket handle' malformation (Figure 15.2).

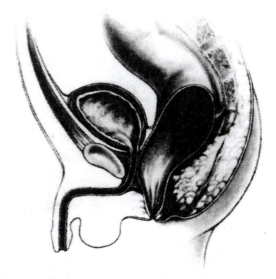

Figure 15.1: Low malformation in a male patient (perineal subepithelial fistula).

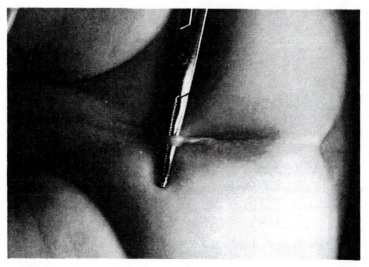

Figure 15.2: Low malformation in a male patient ('bucket handle' malformation).

About 80% of the male patients with anorectal malformations have an abnormal communication between the rectum and the urinary tract called a rectourinary fistula. The specific location of the fistula has important therapeutic and prognostic implications.

Rectourethral Bulbar Fistula

In rectourethral bulbar fistula, the rectum communicates with the lower posterior portion of the urethra called bulbar. Most frequently meconium can be detected in the urine as filtered through a gauze placed at the tip of the penis or confirmed at urinalysis. The passing of meconium through urine usually occurs after 16–24 hours of life, once enough intraluminal bowel pressure has been developed to force the meconium through the fistula. A colostomy is indicated followed by a final repair usually called a posterior sagittal anorectoplasty (PSARP) done on an elective basis later in life (Wangensteen and Rice, 1930).

Rectourethral Prostatic Fistula

In rectourethral prostatic fistula, the rectum communicates with the upper portion of the posterior portion of the urethra, passing through prostatic tissue. The passing of meconium through the urethra follows the same pattern described for rectourethral bulbar fistulae cases. The therapeutic approach is the same as described for the bulbar-urethral fistula but the prognosis for future bowel control is not good (Wangensteen and Rice, 1930).

Rectobladder Neck Fistula

Rectobladder neck fistula is the highest defect in male patients. The rectum communicates with the bladder neck, and the sacrum is usually abnormal, indicating the existence of a very serious nerve deficiency, which will translate into a poor prognosis for future bowel control; sometimes, such patients also suffer urinary incontinence. The main repair in these cases is performed later in life on an elective basis and includes a PSARP plus a laparotomy to mobilize a rectum that cannot be reached from below. Furtunately, this defect represents only approximately 10% of all the male cases (Peña, 1988).

Imperforate Anus without a Fistula

Imperforate anus without fistula is an unusual malformation that occurs in less than 10% of all patients (Narasimharao et al., 1983). The rectum is completely blind and ends approximately 2 cm from the perineum. There is no meconium in the urine, and therefore these patients are usually the ones who are subjected to a radiological study to determine the height of the malformation. This defect is frequently associated with Down's syndrome. The treatment, prognosis, perineal appearance, characteristics of the sacrum and frequency of associated urological defects are the same as in cases of rectourethral bulbar fistulas.

Rectal Atresia and Stenosis

Rectal atresia and stenosis is an unusual defect that occurs in approximately 1% of all cases of anorectal malformations (Peña, 1988); there is no communication with the urinary tract. The perineum looks normal including a normal-looking anus. There is complete obstruction (atresia) or a decrease in the calibre (stenosis) of the rectum approximately 2 cm above the anal opening. These are the cases in which the diagnosis is frequently delayed and established by a nurse while trying to take a rectal temperature. The sacrum is normal, the sphincters are normal and therefore the prognosis for bowel function is excellent. A temporary colostomy is indicated followed by a main repair (PSARP) performed later in life on an elective basis.

Female Defects

The clinical diagnosis of the specific type of defect as well as the decision concerning the opening of a colostomy in cases of female patients is usually easier than in male patients as approximately 95% of these patients have a fistula to the genitalia or to the perineum.

Perineal Fistula

Perineal fistula is the most benign of all the defects seen in female patients (Figure 15.3). The rectum opens through an abnormal orifice (fistula) located in the perineum, that is, between the genitalia and the anal dimple (Truffler and Wilkinson, 1962). These patients have an excellent functional prognosis.

Vestibular Fistula

Vestibular fistula is by far the most frequent defect seen in females. The rectum opens through an abnormally narrow orifice, located in the vestibule of the genitalia, that is, immediately outside the hymen (Figure 15.4). More than 90% of these patients will achieve bowel

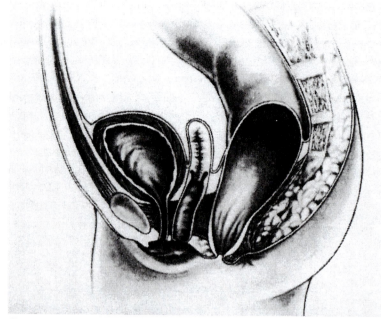

Figure 15.3: Low malformation in a female patient (perineal fistula).

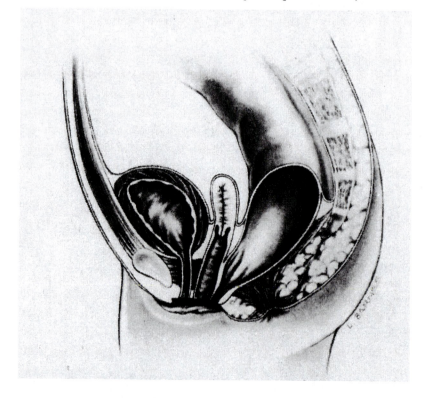

Figure 15.4: Vestibular fistula.

control when adequately managed. A colostomy is indicated during the first few days of life. Even when these patients have a fistula, one must not expect to see meconium coming out through the genitalia before 20 hours of life.

Vaginal Fistula

Vaginal fistula is an exceptionally rare malformation. Most of the cases reported in the literature as 'vaginal fistulae' are cases of vestibular fistulae that have been erroneously diagnosed. In order to establish this diagnosis, one must see the meconium coming out through the vagina, that is, from inside the hymen orifice. These patients must also receive a colostomy and subsequently a PSARP as in cases of vestibular fistula.

Imperforate Anus without a Fistula and Rectal Atresia and Stenosis

The characteristics of these two defects, as well as treatment and prognosis, are identical to those previously discussed in male patients.

Persistent Cloaca

Persistent cloaca, a complex malformation, is defined as a defect in which rectum, vagina and urinary tract are fused together into a single common channel that communicates exteriorly through a single perineal orifice located at the normal urethral site (Figure 15.5).

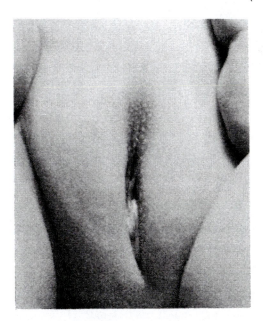

Figure 15.5: Perineum of a patient with a persistent cloaca.

Perhaps the most important fact to remember is that a patient suffering from a cloaca has about a 90% chance of having an associated urological defect that may require immediate attention (Rich et al., 1988), therefore, as in the cases of bladder neck fistulae in males, these patients represent a potential urological emergency, so an abdominal ultrasound examination must always be performed prior to the opening of a colostomy, followed by a urological work-up when necessary. These babies need a diverting colostomy, and frequently, during the same procedure, some sort of urinary diversion (vesicostomy, ureterostomy) or vaginal diversion (vaginostomy), in cases of obstructed, distended vaginas. When the baby is older than 6 months, the entire malformation is repaired with an operation called posterior sagittal anorectovaginourethroplasty (PSARVUP). This is a long, complex, meticulous operation done in a few specialized centres. About 40% of the time, it is necessary to open the abdomen simultaneously with the posterior approach to search for and mobilize a very highly located rectum and/or vagina.

Treatment

Anoplasty

Anoplasty is performed in babies with low defects or perineal fistulae and who do not require a protective colostomy (Peña, 1988). The technique in newborns does not involve a complex preoperative and postoperative course. Prior to the operation, the child remains NPO for 3–4 hours. During the operation the fistula opening is moved back and placed at the centre of the sphincter and, at the same time, the opening is made bigger. The postoperative care consists of application of an antibiotic ointment to the perineum three times per day for 2 weeks. Intravenous antibiotics are administered for 2–3 days. The baby can be fed immediately after surgery. At the 2-week check-up, a programme of anal dilation is initiated. The dilation schedule is described in detail later. A diet to prevent constipation is stressed. For example, if the baby is breast fed, the baby is less likely to be constipated; on the other hand, the baby who is having a synthetic formula may need a stool softener and occasionally a laxative.

Colostomy Creation

The best type of colostomy is a descending type with stomas separated enough to be able to use a stoma bag in the functional site (Wilkins and Peña, 1988) (Figure 15.6). These children generally have a benign

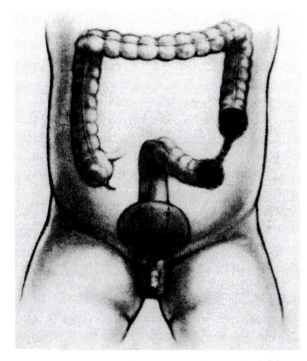

Figure 15.6: Descending colostomy with separated stomas in left lower quadrant of the abdomen.

hospital stay postoperatively with nursing care focused specially on hydration status and measuring input and output (with emphasis on the output on the colostomy). The minimal acceptable urinary output is 1–2 ml per kg/hr. These children are hydrated with an amount of fluid equivalent to one to one and a half times the maintenance requirement. The child has an NG tube for approximately 48 hours and receives IV antibiotics such as ampicillin, gentamycin and clindamycin. Colostomy and skin care, as well as vital signs, are important during the postoperative care. Postoperative pain is generally managed with morphine. At this time, the nurse clinician, who often functions as an enterostomal therapist, assesses and implements the learning needs for the family. The postoperative course generally lasts 4–5 days.

Females born with a cloaca defect are much more complex to manage. What remains essential is that the care of a newborn female baby with a cloaca defect focuses on two goals: first, that any urinary problem, mainly obstructive, be addressed and corrected. These children are fequently born with defects such as absent kidney, vesico-ureteral reflux, hydronephrosis, ureteropelvic obstruction, or megacysto and/or neurogenic bladder, to name a few. During the newborn period, it is sometimes necessary to decompress the urinary tract or a very distended vagina (hydrocolpos) on a temporary basis, for example by forming a ureterostomy, suprapubic cystostomy or vaginostomy. Later in life, the entire urological defect will be corrected. Second, the opening of a colostomy is performed.

After patients recover from the colostomy opening (and the urinary diversion when necessary), they are discharged and followed up by the paediatrician. The mother must learn stoma care prior to the baby's discharge. It is very important for the surgeon who performs the colostomy to work in a coordinated way with the nurse clinician or enterostomal therapist in charge of colostomy care. In that way the nurse will provide feedback to the surgeon regarding the stoma. The surgeon can then improve the characteristics of the stoma to facilitate the use of stoma appliances. Some institutions do not use stoma bags in infants; they claim that these babies will be using nappies (diapers) anyway. In fact, some mothers do prefer to do this. It is our conviction that the use of a stoma bag in a regular, neat, well-built colostomy is really beneficial for patients since they will not suffer from skin irritation.

The initial reaction from a mother who sees her baby's colostomy for the first time and is informed that she will be responsible for the care of it, is one of anxiety. Such mothers frequently state that there is no way that they can do this. Again, the nurse plays a key role in reassuring and teaching the mother. With patience, affection, support, understanding and clarity from the nurse, the mothers learn the stoma management, and it is surprising how, in a few months, they reach an acceptable degree of expertise.

Pre-PSARP Care

Nursing care and assessment are essential during the preoperative stage. A distal colostogram is the most important radiological study to determine the location of the most distal part of the bowel and document the presence and location of a fistula between the bowel and the urogenital tract. This test is generally done as an outpatient (Gross et al., 1991). The child is then admitted 1 day prior to the PSARP procedure. The child may have a normal diet before the operation, and must stop eating solids 8 hours before surgery but may have clear liquids or breast milk up to 3 hours before. Antibiotics are administered on call to the operating room. During the preoperative day in hospital, it is imperative that the nurse irrigate the distal stoma with warm normal saline solution with the aid of a Foley catheter. The purpose of this irrigation is to remove all the faecal matter left in the colon distal to the colostomy and to avoid contamination at the time of the pull-through. There is no written rule about how much saline solution to use or how frequently to irrigate, but it is important to keep in mind that the distal colon must be cleaned. One may use the formula of 20 kg of saline per irrigation; however, sometimes it is necessary to use more or less. Some children may need irrigation of the distal stoma every 3 hours while others need it only every 6 hours. In any event, the goal is to clean the distal bowel, as evidenced by a clean water return during the irrigation. Irrigation is easiest with a double-barrel descending colostomy with well-separated stomas, because the distal bowel most probably is very clean since the chances of stool passing from the proximal to the distal stoma are very slim. Therefore, a child with a loop colostomy or with stomas placed very close to one another has a greater chance of stool passing from the proximal to distal stoma. Thus, these children will generally require more frequent irrigation with larger volumes of fluid to achieve total cleansing of the bowel to prevent postoperative infection. The distal colostogram performed prior to the PSARP shows how much stool was left in the bowel distal to the colostomy, and on that basis the nurse will determine how aggressive the irrigation must be.

Posterior Sagittal Anorectoplasty (PSARP)

The posterior sagittal anorectoplasty is more commonly referred to as PSARP, or the 'Peña procedure'. Generally, this second stage of the surgical repair is performed in patients more than 1 month of age, provided the baby is growing and developing normally. In some institutions, however, they prefer to wait until the baby is 6–12 months old. It entails a midline posterior sagittal incision running from the middle portion of the sacrum to the anterior edge of the external sphincter. The sphincter mechanism is divided in a midline incision, therefore preserving the nerve fibres and decreasing the amount of postoperative pain. The back of the child's buttocks is opened like a book and all internal structures are exposed. The rectum is meticulously separated from the genitourinary tract, dissected, and freed enough to reach its normal site without tension. The fistula site is then closed. With the use of an electrical muscle stimulator, the limits of the sphincteric mechanism are determined and the rectum is placed in its optimal location to achieve the best functional results. The operation is performed in the prone position (face down) and with a Foley catheter inserted in the bladder. If the child is known to have a very high defect, or the child's rectum is not able to be reached with this procedure, then the abdomen must also be opened.

The postoperative course for this surgical procedure is relatively benign. If a laparotomy was not needed, the child may drink fluids after the surgery and have a regular diet the next day. The IV line must be preserved for the administration of antibiotics (ampicillin, gentamicin, clindamycin) for 2–3 days. After that, oral ampicillin is given for 5 more days. In males and in cases of cloacas, the patients are left with a Foley catheter that must remain in place for 5–10 days. If the catheter comes out accidentally, no attempt should be made to replace it, and the surgeon must be notified; if the baby is unable to void, a suprapubic tube is put in place. The children do not need to be positioned in any particular way; we simply let them find the best position for themselves. The nurse needs to teach the parents to use bacitracin ointment on the perineum with every nappy change. This process goes on for two weeks until the child's first post-operative visit. The child's post-operative stay in hospital generally lasts 2–3 days.

Postoperative Care in Cases of PSARP plus Laparotomy

The post-operative course is a bit more painful and lengthened if a laparotomy is needed. A laparotomy is generally performed if the rectum is too high to be visualized and mobilized from a posterior approach. These children return from theatre with an IV, antibiotics, NG tube for 3–4 days and some degree of pain, managed with morphine. They do not eat or drink for 48 hours. The skin care of the perineum remains the same, with bacitracin ointment as previously mentioned.

Two-week Postoperative Visit

At this visit, the stitches are removed and the bacitracin ointment is discontinued. At this time, the process of anal dilations is initiated. Each family must buy their own set of Hegar dilators. This is a very significant stage in the continual healing phase, postoperatively. The dilations prevent anal stricture from scar tissue formation around the anus. It is imperative for the family to adhere to the guidelines given to them. Basically, the surgeon passes the first lubricated anal dilator approximately 3–4 cm and simultaneously shows the mother the importance of holding the child with the knees flexed close to the chest. This process is to be repeated twice a day, lasting about 30 seconds. Every week the mother advances to the next size dilator. Eventually, after about 6–8 weeks, the mother will reach the 'desired size' which is predetermined by the surgeon. Any time after the desired size has been reached, the colostomy may be closed. However, the dilations will continue, decreasing the frequency as stated below. The total process of dilations lasts approximately 6 months after the PSARP. The desired size of dilators is:

1–4 months old	No. 12 Hegar
4–8 months old	No. 13 Hegar
8–12 months old	No. 14 Hegar
1–4 years old	No. 15 Hegar
Older than 4 years	No. 16 Hegar

Dilation Schedule (After the Desired Size has been Reached)

The mother must continue passing the last dilator twice a day, until she finds that the dilator passes easily and without pain, at which point she can start decreasing the frequency of dilations as follows:

once a day for 1 month;
every other day for 1 month;
twice a week for 1 month;
once a week for 1 month;
once a month for 3 months.

Colostomy Closure

The child is admitted 1 day before the operation and maintained only on clear liquids by mouth, until 3 hours prior to the operation. Irrigation of the proximal stoma is begun with the same frequency and consistency as with the preoperative procedure for the PSARP. One must remember that the bowel distal to the colostomy was irrigated prior to the PSARP and therefore it is assumed to be clean and does not have to be irrigated unless otherwise indicated by the surgeon, or in cases of loop colostomy, in which it is conceivable that stool from the proximal stoma spilled over to the distal stoma. Therefore, it may be necessary to irrigate both stomas. Antibiotics are indicated on call to the operating room. The operation entails taking down both stomas and performing a bowel anastomosis to re-establish the colon continuity. Postoperatively, the child experiences more pain than after the initial operation. The child returns to the ward with intravenous fluids and nasogastric tube. Intravenous antibiotics are routinely given for 2–3 days followed by oral ampicillin to complete 1 week. Pain medication is given as needed. The child remains NPO and with an NG tube for 1–3 days; IV fluids are administered during the time that the patient remains NPO. The average length of stay for the colostomy closure is 5–6 days, provided the child's postoperative course is uneventful. The parents may also expect to see the child have his or her first bowel movement through their 'new anus', 1–3 days postoperatively. This seemingly wonderful event may eventually turn frustrating as the child's skin perineum begins to break down. Nappy rash seems to be correlate with multiple postoperative bowel movements. As time goes by, the number of bowel movements per day decreases and the skin then heals nicely. This may take days and sometimes weeks. Skin care is discussed with the family several weeks before the colostomy closure. The child is expected to have a rather severe nappy rash, so we prescribe a variety of 'butt pastes' to prevent and heal the perineum. For example, the most popular paste in the authors' unit consists of: Vitamin A & D ointment, aloe, desitin and mylanta (to help the ointment stick to the skin and help form a paste). Nystatin (only by prescription) may need to be added if the rash is yeast in origin. One relatively natural way to toughen the skin is to coat the perineum with a little stool from the colostomy for 15 minutes three times a day for approximately 2 weeks prior to the colostomy closure. A variety of remedies are given to the families which have been used by other parents because what works for one child may not for another. Eventually, the number of bowel movements decreases and the parents are very happy not to have to deal with the problem of nappy rash. However, at that point, one starts to be concerned about the problem of constipation, which is the most frequent sequela seen in those patients born with anorectal malformations and subjected to a type of surgical repair in which the rectum and sigmoid have been preserved, such as is done in cases subjected to PSARP (Peña and Ell Behery, 1993). Constipation and faecal impaction must be avoided, so a laxative type of diet must be prescribed. This includes a variety of fibre-rich foods and a detailed list is given to the families. If the diet is not enough, one should not hesitate to prescribe laxative medication to be sure that the child empties his or her rectum every day.

Postoperative Bowel Function

Patients operated on for anorectal malformations may achieve bowel control or may suffer from different degrees of faecal incontinence. The surgeon may know in advance which patients have a good functional prognosis and which patients have a poor prognosis.

Indicators of good prognosis for bowel control are:

- normal sacrum;
- prominent midline groove (good muscles);
- rectal atresia;
- vestibular fistula;
- most patients with imperforate anus without a fistula;
- low cloacas;
- most patients with urethral bulbar fistula;
- low defects (perineal fistulas).

Indicators of poor prognosis for bowel control are:

- abnormal sacrum (more than two vertebrae missing);
- flat perineum (poor muscles);
- rectobladder neck fistula;
- some rectoprostatic fistulae;
- some rectovaginal fistulae.

Children born with anorectal malformations are not expected to become toilet trained for stool before 2 ½ to 3 years of age. Before that age, however, there are some signs that have a prognostic value concerning the possibility for the patient becoming toilet trained.

Good prognostic signs are:

- good bowel movement pattern: 1–3 bowel movements per day, and remains clean in between (no soiling);
- urinary control;
- evidence of sensation when passing stool (pushing, making faces).

Bad prognostic signs are:

- urinary incontinence, dribbling of urine;
- constant soiling and passing stool;
- no sensation (no pushing).

Patients born with good prognostic types of malformations and showing good prognostic signs are expected to become toilet trained. On the other hand, patients born with poor prognostic malformations or showing bad prognostic signs are offered a Bowel Management

Program (Peña, 1990a, b, 1992; Peña et al., 1998), which is a way to keep them clean, and make them socially accepted as it is unlikely they will become toilet trained.

Toilet Training

Between 2 and 3 years of age, mothers are instructed to sit the child on their potty after every meal. They are encouraged to do this as a game and not as a punishment. The child must sit in front of a little table on which the parents must put the child's favourite toys. The parents must remain with the child since he or she does not like to be left alone. If he or she decides not to stay on the potty, parents must not fight with them; instead they must pick up the toys and put them away until the child decides to sit again. If it happens that the child has a bowel movement or a voiding episode in the potty, the parents must celebrate and reward the child. If the mother is unsuccessful in training her child and the time is coming for him/her to attend school, we usually give the parents two alternatives: (a) do not send the child to school for 1 more year and keep trying to toilet train him/her; or (b) try the Bowel Management Program (Peña et al., 1998) for 1 year, assuming that it will be implemented on a temporary basis. This will allow the child to be clean and to attend school like a normal child. During the next summer vacation, while at home, the parents can again attempt to toilet train the child.

In any event, we consider it unacceptable to send a child to school in nappies, suffering from faecal incontinence while his/her classmates are already toilet trained. This exposes the child to embarrassing accidents with important psychological sequelae.

Bowel Management Program

It is important to know the three specific factors that need to be present in order to be faecally continent. First, the child needs to have sensation (within the rectum); children born with anorectal malformations lack the intrinsic sensation to feel stool or gas passing through their rectum. Therefore, frequently the child may unknowingly soil.

Second, the child needs to have good motility of the colon. Normally, the rectosigmoid remains quiet for periods of 24–48 hours, then a massive peristaltic wave allows the complete emptying of it and it becomes quiet again. In patients operated on for anorectal malformations, most commonly the rectosigmoid is slow and the stool stays stagnant, hence constipation occurs and the patient may suffer from encopresis (overflow incontinence). On the other hand, a very active colon may provoke a constant passing of stool which may significantly interfere with bowel continence.

Third, the child needs to possess good voluntary muscles, or sphincteric mechanism. These muscles allow for good control and retention of stool. Often the child with an anorectal malformation lacks one or all three of these essential elements of faecal continence.

Patients suffering from faecal incontinence consecutive to the treatment of imperforate anus can be divided into two well-defined groups:

(a) *with constipation:* these are mainly cases subjected to operations in which the rectum was preserved (anoplasties, PSARP and sacroperineal pull-throughs);

(b) *with diarrhoea:* these are mainly cases subjected to operations in which the rectum and sometimes the sigmoid colon was resected (abdominoperineal procedures, endorectal resections), or else the patient lost a portion of the colon for some other reason or suffers from some sort of condition that causes diarrhoea.

Each of these groups of patients must be treated in a different way. The basis of the Bowel Management Program consists of teaching the parents or patient (when more than 12 years old), to clean the colon every day by the use of enemas or colonic irrigations, followed by finding a mechanism to keep the colon quiet for the following 24 hours, so as to avoid soiling episodes and involuntary bowel movements; this last goal is achieved by the use of specific diets and/or medications such as Lomotil or Imodium, usually within a week, by a process of trial and error (Peña et al., 1998).

Patients with Constipation

The parents are asked at what point during the day they would be able to relax and concentrate on the child's enema programme. Often the families say the most convenient time is after dinner and it has been found that children have the most effective emptying of their colon at this time. The enema should be given 1 hour after dinner and the child should remain on the toilet for 30–45 minutes. Fleet's (Fleets Corp., Lynchburg, VA) enemas are used mostly by the authors because of their convenience. However, pure saline enemas are often just as effective and, of course, more economical. Most US insurance companies will reimburse families for Fleet's enemas if a prescription is written. Children over 8 years of age may receive one adult Fleet enema daily. Children between 3 and 8 years may receive only one paediatric Fleet enema a day. Patients should never receive more than one Fleet enema a day; more than that exposes the child to phosphate intoxication and hypocalcaemia. The Fleet enema administered in a routine way is expected to provoke a bowel movement followed by a period of 24 hours of complete cleanliness, in which case there is no further treatment required. However, if one enema is not enough to clean the colon, then the patient requires a more aggressive treatment. High colonic washings are indicated with a Foley catheter attached to the tip of the bottle of the Fleet enema. A No. 20–24 Fr. Foley catheter is lubricated and gently introduced through the anus as high as possible (Figure 15.7a). The authors have found that the Foley catheter manoeuvre is especially useful in severely impacted children. Sometimes it is not possible to pass the tube all the way up into the bowel, at which time the

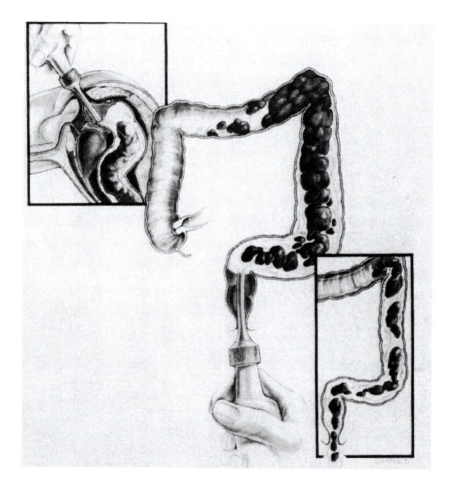

Figure 15.7 (a): Colonic irrigation technique: without a tube.

tube is inserted only a few centimetres and the balloon (which is attached to the end of the catheter) inflated with 20 ml of water. By putting on the catheter, one occludes the colonic lumen with the balloon acting as a plug and enables the enema solution to go up into the bowel with minimal leakage (Figure 15.8). If the child soils at any point during the following 24 hours, it means that the bowel was not washed out enough and, therefore, a more aggressive technique must be conducted which may include increasing the volume of the enema, or administering a second saline enema 30 minutes later. The programme is very individualized and the parents learn (as does the child if old enough), to look at the consistency and amount of stool obtained after the enema. After a period of time, the parents will know when the enema was not effective and when they need to repeat it with saline solution.

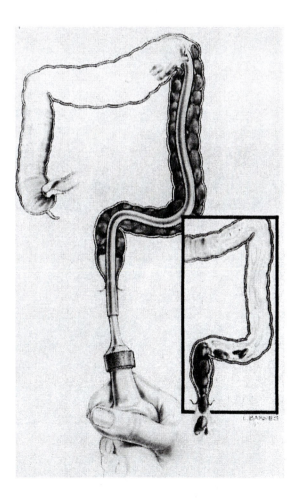

Figure 15.7 (b): Colonic irrigation technique: with a tube.

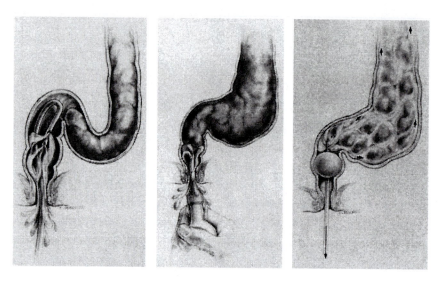

Figure 15.8: Enema and colonic irrigation technique with a Foley balloon inflated.

The position of the child receiving the enema is also important. The purpose of this is to take advantage of the effect of gravity and to try to wash the colon as high as possible. Young children can be held over the parents' lap. In older children, the enemas are best done with the child on their parents' knees, with the buttocks up and the head close to the floor. It is suggested that the patient remain seated on the toilet for 30–45 minutes after the administration of the enema until he/she feels that the colon is empty. For example, some families take a portable TV into the bathroom, some children read a book or do their homework, others play with games; these activities make the time pass quickly. Constipated patients have, by definition, a colon and a rectosigmoid suffering from hypomotility and, therefore, all they may need to remain clean for 24 hours is a good enema or colonic irrigation (Peña et al., 1998).

There is one specific type of patient who, having been subjected to a surgical repair of an anorectal malformation, is assigned a good prognosis based on the quality of the sacrum and type of sphincters. In such cases, the operation is performed in a technically correct manner and the rectosigmoid is preserved. This patient is expected to be toilet trained for stool and to suffer from some degree of constipation. Yet some patients have very severe constipation association with a megasigmoid (Peña and Ell Behery, 1993). They may sometimes go a week without bowel movements. They are referred to the doctor with the diagnosis of 'faecal incontinence'. A contrast enema demonstrates the presence of a giant megasigmoid. They require a very aggressive programme of enemas to be clean. Another alternative is to offer them an operation consisting in resecting the most dilated portion of their megasigmoid. This may not only make them more manageable, but may also make them faecally continent, which demonstrates that they were not really faecally incontinent but rather they suffered from severe constipation, encopresis or overflow pseudo-incontinence (Peña and Ell Behery, 1993). In those cases in whom the constipation is not very severe, sometimes a programme of administration of laxatives has the same effect as the operation.

Patients with Diarrhoea

This group of patients, by definition, have an overactive colon. Most of the time, they have undergone rectosigmoid resection during the repair of their defect. In other words, they do not have a reservoir. As a consequence, even when an enema may clean their colon, they pass stool fairly soon after the application of the enema due to the fact that the stool travels rather fast from the caecum to the descending colon and the anus. To prevent this, the authors recommend a constipating diet and/or medication to slow down the colon, such as loperamide (Imodium). A list of constipating meals is given to the parents to be promoted as part of the regular diet of the patient, as well as a list of laxative meals to be avoided, which must be part of their 'black list'. Most sensitive parents know which meals provoke diarrhoea and which constipate their child. This group of children with diarrhoea is the most difficult to manage. Sometimes, in spite of all efforts, the patient may have a very active or a very short colon and it has to be accepted that the patient is non-manageable. In this last circumstance, the patient is offered a permanent colostomy. Fortunately, this situation is an exception (Peña et al., 1998).

Most patients can be controlled, some of them with only enemas and a constipating diet; others with enemas, diet and a low dose of a medication; and others with enemas, a very strict diet and a high dose of medication. To determine this, in a practical way, what the authors do is to start the treatment with enemas, a very strict diet, and a high dose of Imodium. Most patients respond to this aggressive management within 24 hours. The meals which the patient misses the most are then introduced, in a gradual manner, observing the effect on colonic activity; eventually, the most liberal possible diet is found for the patient. If the patient continues being clean with a regular diet, an attempt is made to reduce, gradually, the dose of medication so as to find the lowest effective dose to keep the patient clean for 24 hours. Again, this is found by a process of trial and error. This strict diet does not need to last forever. Families are told that after about 2 months when the child has remained clean for 24 hours, he/she may have one of the 'black list' foods that they have been craving. If the child soils after eating that food, he/she knows they must stay away from it. They must only introduce one new food a week and observe the bowel movement pattern.

In those cases of patients subjected to a successful Bowel Management Program (Peña, 1990a, b, 1992; Peña et al., 1998) with enemas, the parents frequently ask if this programme will be needed for life. The answer is 'yes' for those patients born with a poor prognosis type of defect (very high defect, poor sacrum and poor sphincters). However, since one is dealing with a spectrum of defects, there are cases with some degree of bowel control; they are subjected to the Bowel Management Program to avoid exposing them to occasional embarrassing accidents of uncontrolled bowel movements at school. However, as time goes by, the patient becomes more cooperative and more interested and concerned about his/her problem. It is then conceivable that, later in life, a patient may stop using enemas and remain clean, following a specific regimen of a disciplined diet with regular meals to provoke bowel movements at a predictable time. Thus, every summer, the patients with some potential for bowel control can try, on an experimental basis, to find out how well they can control their bowel movements without the help of enemas. This is done during the summer vacations to avoid accidents at school. The parents and patients are expected to stay at home, to socialize very little, and to have a regular diet with a regular schedule. The patient must sit on the toilet after every meal and try to pass stool. In addition, he/she must remain alert all day while trying to learn to discriminate the feeling of an imminent bowel movement. If the patient belongs to the 'constipated' group, it is usually suggested they take a laxative every day in a single dose, so as to try to provoke an effect that is as controlled as possible; ideally, that is, a single bowel movement per day. The dose of the laxative is adjusted by trial and error. Too much laxative may have a counterproductive effect which is uncontrolled diarrhoea. Too small a laxative effect will fail to avoid constipation. It is best to try the less aggressive and natural types of laxative first, and then, depending on the patient's response, move on to medication with more active ingredients. The first choice, of course, must be a laxative type of diet; the next is either a bulk-forming product or else a stool softener. If these do not work, a laxative with an active ingredient is indicated. After a few days or weeks, the family and the patient are in a position to decide whether they want to continue with that regimen or if they would prefer to go back to the Bowel Managment Program. This decision is theirs and is based on the quality of life that they experience with each type of method.

This description does not, by any means, give an example of the entire Bowel Management Program; there are many variations depending upon patient needs. What has been found is that it takes dedication, determination, consistency and love on the part of everyone involved. Children who have completed the Bowel Management Program and remain clean for 24 hours experience a new sense of confidence based on an improved quality of life.

References

Brenner EC (1915) Congenital defects of the anus and rectum. Surgery, Gynecology and Obstetrics 20: 579–88.

Gross GW, Wolfson PJ, Peña A (1991) Augmented-pressure colostogram in imperforate anus with fistula. Pediatric Radiology 21: 560–2.

Narasimharao KA, Prassad GR, Katariya S (1983) Prone cross-table lateral view: an alternative to the invertogram in imperforate anus. AJR 140: 227–9.

Peña A (1988) Posterior sagittal anorectoplasty: results in the management of 332 cases of anorectal malformations. Pediatric Surgery International 3: 94–104.

Peña A (1990a) Quote. In Atlas, Surgical Management of Anorectal Malformations. New York: Springer-Verlag, p 1.

Peña A (1990b) Advances in the management of fecal incontinence secondary to anorectal malformations. In Nyhus LM (Ed.) Surgery Annual. Connecticut: Appleton & Lange, pp 143–67.

Peña A (1992) Current management of anorectal anomalies. Surgical Clinics of North America 72(6): 1393–416.

Peña A, Ell Behery M (1993) Megasigmoid: a source of pseudo incontinence in children with repaired anorectal malformations. Journal of Pediatric Surgery 28: 1–5.

Peña A, Guardino JM, Tovilla MA, Levitt G, Rodriguez G, Torres R (1998) Bowel management for fecal incontinence in patients with anorectal malformations. Journal of Pediatric Surgery 33(1): 133–7.

Rich MA, Brock WA, Peña A (1988) Spectrum of genitourinary malformations in patients with imperforate anus. Pediatric Surgery International 3: 110–13.

Santulli TV (1952) Treatment of imperforate anus and associated fistulas. Surgery, Gynaecology and Obstetrics 95: 601–14.

Truffler GA, Wilkinson RH (1962) Imperforate anus; a review of 147 cases. Canadian Journal of Surgery 5: 169–77.

Wangensteen OH, Rice CO (1930) Imperforate anus: a method of determining the surgical approach. Annals of Surgery 92: 77–81.

Wilkins S, Peña A (1988) The role of colostomy in the management of anorectal malformations: Pediatric Surgery International 3: 105–9.

Chapter 16
Infectious Colitis

MARGARET J. GORENSEK MD, FACP, FAAP, Chairman,
Department of Infectious Diseases, Cleveland Clinic Florida,
Florida, USA

Introduction

Colitis is defined as inflammation of the colon. When this inflammation is caused by micro-organisms, it is called infectious colitis. Diarrhoeal diseases are a significant cause of morbidity and mortality worldwide, especially in underdeveloped countries, where they remain a leading cause of childhood death. This chapter will attempt to give an overview of the infectious causes of colitis, which can be classified into three groups (see Table 16.1):

1. bacterial;
2. viral;
3. parasitic.

Each pathogen will be briefly discussed according to aetiology and epidemiology, pathophysiology, signs and symptoms, diagnosis, and treatment. In addition, there are non-infectious causes, such as ulcerative colitis and Crohn's disease. Only the infectious aetiologies are described in this chapter. Farmer (1990) provides details for the differential diagnosis of infectious and non-infectious colitis.

Bacterial Infections

Aeromonas

Aetiology and Epidemiology

Aeromonas bacteria live in fresh water or water that is a mixture of fresh water and seawater. Humans become infected by drinking, swimming

Table 16.1: Major micro-organisms responsible for infectious colitis

Bacterial
  Aeromonas
  Campylobacter
  Clostridium difficile
  Escherichia coli
  Escherichia coli O157: H7
  Salmonella
  Shigella
  Vibrio species
  Yersinia

Viral
  Astroviruses
  Caliciviruses
  Enteroviruses (non-polio)
  (HIV)
  Rotavirus

Parasitic
  Cryptosporidiosis
  Cyclosporiasis
  Entamoeba histolytica
  Giardia lamblia
  Isosporiasis
  Strongyloides

or bathing in contaminated water. The resulting disease, *Aeromonas* gastroenteritis, is seen mostly in young children. *Aeromonas* bacteria generally live in the presence of oxygen (aerobic) but under certain conditions can live without oxygen (anaerobic), and are classified as gram-negative.

Pathophysiology

Aeromonas infections cause diarrhoea by producing toxins that cause damage to the colon.

Symptoms and Signs

Patients generally have watery diarrhoea, fever and vomiting.

Diagnosis

Diagnosis is made by isolating *Aeromonas* from a stool culture but this organism can be difficult to identify and may require several samples.

Treatment

Aggressive rehydration is the primary treatment. Fluoroquinolones, tetracycline, trimethoprim-sulfamethoxazole, chloramphenicol and third-generation cephalosporins are generally effective.

Campylobacter Infections

Aetiology and Epidemiology

Campylobacter infection (campylobacteriosis) is an infection of the gastrointestinal tract or blood caused by the bacterium *Campylobacter*. The name *Campylobacter* refers to the shape of the organism, which is derived from the Greek words for 'curved rod'. *Campylobacter jejuni*, the more common strain of this bacteria, causes sudden gastroenteritis. (*Campylobacter fetus* is less common and is found in infants.) Transmission occurs by ingestion of contaminated food or contact with faecal material from an infected animal or person. Contaminated foods include unpasteurized milk, untreated water and improperly cooked poultry or meat. *Campylobacter* bacteria can also cause diarrohea among travellers in developing countries. It has become one of the most common causes of infectious diarrhoea.

Preventive measures include hand washing and washing of cutting boards that come in contact with poultry. Proper cooking of poultry is also essential. Unpasteurized milk and non-chlorinated municipal water from endemic areas should be avoided.

Pathophysiology

The time from ingestion to first symptoms (incubation period) is generally 1 to 7 days. Mild infections last 2 days and most patients recover within 1 week. *Campylobacter jejuni* invades the lining of the intestines and secretes toxins that cause the diarrhoea.

Symptoms and Signs

Symptoms are cramping abdominal pain, diarrhoea, malaise and fever. Stools often contain blood, and there may be tenesmus, or urgency to evacuate the bowel, due to rectal inflammation.

Diagnosis

Diagnosis is made by stool culture but the laboratory should be notified that *Campylobacter* is suspected, as special media are required to grow the organism.

Treatment

Both erythromycin and tetracycline are effective. For patients over 18 years of age, ciprofloxacin may also be used. Again, aggressive rehydration is very important (Peter, 1997).

Clostridium difficile

Aetiology and Epidemiology

Infectious colitis can be caused inadvertently by the use, or 'over-use', of many antibiotics, such as the third-generation cephalosporins (Settle and Wilcox, 1996). In efforts to treat serious infections in other parts of the body, the normal bacteria that colonize the colon are destroyed. This allows overgrowth of *Clostridium difficile*, a Gram-positive anaerobic bacterium that lives in the colon. Overgrowth of this organism can lead to a very severe form of colitis called 'pseudomembranous colitis'. Older people and children are most susceptible to *Clostridium difficile*. This is becoming a growing problem in hospitals and nursing homes. If this form of colitis is left untreated it can result in severe complications and death (Fekety and Shah, 1993). Preventive measures include hand washing and proper handling of faecal material, such as nappies (diapers), as well as careful and judicious use of antibiotics.

Pathophysiology

When antibiotics kill the normal bacteria in the intestines, *Clostridium difficile* can grow unchecked causing severe inflammation of the intestines. This bacterium then produces two toxins (A and B), which can damage the lining of the large intestines. A toxin is a poisonous substance, usually a protein, that is produced by living cells or organisms. Toxin A is an enterotoxin and Toxin B is a cytotoxin. The cause of this inflammation is related to the effect of the lamina propria neuroimmune cells on the intestinal epithelial cells (Pothoulakis, 1996).

Symptoms and Signs

Diarrhoea, abdominal pain, cramps, tenderness and fever are common. Stools may contain blood, mucus and pus. If not treated, toxic megacolon and death may occur.

Diagnosis

The diagnosis is made by detecting *Clostridium difficile* toxins in stool samples. It can also be grown in stool culture.

Treatment

If the patient has severe diarrhoea or colitis, the current antibiotic treatment should be discontinued. In most cases the diarrhoea stops within 12 days. Metronidazole should be used as the antibiotic of choice for *Clostridium difficile* colitis. Vancomycin is also effective but should be reserved as a last resort to minimize the risk of developing subsequent vancomycin-resistant infections. For guidelines for the diagnosis and management of *Clostridium difficile*-associated diarrhoea and colitis, see Fekety (1997).

Escherichia coli

Aetiology and Epidemiology

The bacteria *E. coli* are commonly found in the intestines of humans and generally cause no problems. There are five main strains of *E. coli* that cause diarrhoea in humans:

1. EHEC	enterohaemorrhagic *E. coli*	O157:H7;
2. EPEC	enteropathogenic *E. coli*	diarrhoea in infants;
3. ETEC	enterotoxigenic *E. coli*	traveller's diarrhoea;
4. EIEC	enteroinvasive *E. coli*	dysentery from food;
5. EAggEC	enteroaggregative *E. coli*	diarrhoea in infants.

Certain strains of *E. coli* infect the large intestines by producing high levels of toxins, which are similar to those produced by the bacteria *Shigella*. These toxins damage the lining of the large intestines resulting in bloody diarrhoea and sometimes death. This type of gastroenteritis is called haemorrhagic colitis. In the United States, haemorrhagic colitis is most often caused by the strain *E. coli* O157:H7. Strains of *E. coli* are identified by special proteins termed somatic (O) and flagellar (H) antigens. Healthy cattle often have this strain in their intestines. Humans most often become infected by eating improperly cooked beef. Ingestion of unpasteurized milk, and food or water contaminated by faecal material of cattle are also sources of infection. Swallowing lake water while swimming has recently been implicated as a cause of infection by both *E. coli* O157:H7 and *Shigella sonnei* (Keene et al., 1994). Prevention includes proper hand washing and hygiene. Beef must be thoroughly cooked until juices run clear. Unpasteurized milk and unpasteurized apple juice should be avoided. Proper sanitary procedures in the commercial preparation and packaging of beef, lettuce, other raw vegetables and salami is essential. Children should be warned not to swallow water while swimming.

Pathophysiology

E. coli is a Gram-negative chiefly aerobic bacterium. A subdivision of this species (or serovar) is capable of producing disease in the intestinal tract (enteropathogenic). These strains of *E. coli* cause diarrhoea due to entero-toxins, substances that damage cells of the intestinal mucosa. *E. coli* enterotoxins are produced by certain strains (serotypes) of *E. coli*, seem-ingly associated with a transferable genetic particle. For a comparison of pathologic differences in the various strains of *E. coli*, see Moon (1997).

Symptoms and Signs

With *E. coli* O157:H7, patients develop non-bloody diarrhoea that often leads to bloody diarrhoea in 24 hours. There is associated severe abdominal pain of acute onset as well as fever. Generally the duration of diarrhoea is 1 to 8 days. Haemolytic-uraemic syndrome occurs in about one in twenty patients infected with *E. coli* O157:H7. This is more common in young children and in the elderly. These patients experience microangiopathic haemolytic anaemia (a narrowing of the small blood vessels resulting in red blood cell destruction), thrombocy-topenia, and kidney failure.

Diagnosis

Stool samples, especially from children with bloody diarrhoea, should be tested within 7 days of illness for *E. coli* O157:H7 and the presence of Shiga-like toxins, which are toxins very similar to those produced by *Shigella* (Su and Brandt, 1995).

Treatment

Correction of electrolyte problems and rehydration are the primary treatment measures. Antibiotics are not generally required unless systemic infection is suspected. Trimethoprim-sulfamethoxazole is usually used in this case.

Salmonella

Aetiology and Epidemiology

Typhoid fever is the well-known infection caused by the Gram-negative bacterium, *Salmonella typhi*. However, many other strains of *Salmonella*, such as *Salmonella enteridis*, cause widespread, costly infections and public health problems. It is spread by ingestion of contaminated meat, eggs and milk products. Prevention includes thoroughly cooking eggs and meat. Raw eggs and food with raw eggs should not be eaten. Proper hand washing and sanitary facilities for food preparation are important, especially in endemic areas. Travellers in these areas should avoid raw leafy vegetables and tap water. Turtles should not be kept as pets.

Salmonella can be acquired when a person touches a reptile, such as a turtle or iguana, and then puts his/her fingers in his/her mouth. Contaminated marijuana has also been a source of *Salmonella* infections. Oral vaccines are available to people at high risk. There are approximately 2000 carriers in the USA. These are mostly elderly women with chronic gall bladder disease.

Pathophysiology

Salmonella secretes cytotoxins but also penetrates the epithelial cells of the intestines (Rampal et al., 1989). It can invade the bloodstream, and once in the blood it can spread to other body sites, such as the meninges, bones or other organs, causing severe disease. The incubation period for gastroenteritis is from 6 to 72 hours. These infections are sometimes referred to as enteric fever.

Symptoms and Signs

Within 1 to 2 days after ingesting most *Salmonella* bacteria, gastrointestinal symptoms may begin. *Salmonella typhi* symptoms usually begin within 8 to 14 days after infection. These include headache, joint pain, sore throat, constipation, loss of appetite, diarrhoea, abdominal cramps, tenderness and fever.

Diagnosis

The diagnosis is made by culturing the organism from stool, blood, urine or other body sites.

Treatment

Ampicillin, amoxicillin, trimethoprim-sulfamethoxazole, cefotaxime or ceftriaxone are recommended for patients who require treatment. These are patients who have invasive disease or are at increased risk for serious disease, such as young infants or immunosuppressed patients. Antimicrobial therapy is not indicated for patients with uncomplicated, non-invasive gastroenteritis.

Shigella

Aetiology and Epidemiology

Shigella is a Gram-negative aerobic bacterium, which is very similar to *E. coli*. The normal habitat is human intestines. When the *Shigella* bacteria invade the human intestines, severe diarrhoea results called shigellosis or 'bacillary dysentery'. The source of infection is faeces from infected humans. Except for monkeys, animals are not thought to carry *Shigella*. Prevention includes hand washing, especially in child care centres, keeping flies away from food, and ensuring proper sanitary conditions for food processing, water supply and sewage.

Pathophysiology

Incubation is generally 1 to 4 days. Biopsy studies of the colon mucosa have shown that shigellosis results in more pronounced inflammation compared with other causes of colitis (Shcherbakov et al., 1995). *Shigella* is not only an invasive diarrhoeal disease that penetrates the epithelial cells of the intestines and invades the bloodstream but it also secretes cytotoxins that can cause seizures, encephalopathy, arthritis and haemolytic-uraemic syndrome (destruction of red blood cells and renal failure).

Symptoms and Signs

In children symptoms are fever, irritability, drowsiness, loss of appetite, nausea, vomiting, diarrhoea, abdominal pain and bloating. In adults, fever may be absent. They may experience abdominal pain and an increasing urge to defecate. Many only experience mild watery diarrhoea.

Diagnosis

The diagnosis is made by culture of faeces or rectal swab specimens.

Treatment

Antibiotics, such as trimethoprim-sulfamethoxazole, norfloxacin, ciprofloxacin and furazolidone, can be used in young patients or patients with severe disease. Possible drug resistance for the population and strain being seen must be considered in the treatment, and appropriate changes made in the antibiotic therapy. Aggressive replacement of fluid and electrolytes is critical.

Vibrio species

Aetiology and Epidemiology

Vibrio cholerae bacteria can infect the small intestines, resulting in cholera, a very devastating diarrhoeal disease. Other vibrios can cause less severe infectious colitis. *Vibrio fluvialis*, for example, is a species similar to *Aeromonas*, which commonly causes diarrhoea. *Vibrio* bacteria are transmitted by ingestion of water or food contaminated by excrement of infected people. The disease is more common in children, during warm weather, in Asia, the Middle East, Africa and Latin America. People who have a deficiency of stomach acid are also more susceptible. Prevention includes proper sanitation for water supply and sewage. In endemic areas water should be boiled and care should be taken to avoid uncooked vegetables and undercooked seafood.

Pathophysiology

Vibrio cholerae bacteria produce a toxin, which causes the small intestines to produce large amounts of fluids. This is called toxinogenic diarrhoea, as opposed to invasive diarrhoea, where the bacteria invade the bloodstream. Some species of *Vibrio*, such as *Vibrio vulnificus*, can cause fatal septicaemia in patients with underlying liver disease.

Symptoms and Signs

The incubation period is 1 to 3 days. Symptoms begin as sudden, painless, watery diarrhoea and vomiting. Severe cases result in extreme dehydration with severe thirst, muscle cramps, and weakness. By 3 to 6 days symptoms usually resolve.

Diagnosis

Diagnosis is made by identifying the *Vibrio cholerae* bacteria in stool culture or from rectal swab cultures. The laboratory should be notified that *Vibrio* is suspected so special culture media are prepared.

Treatment

Patients with cholera must have their body fluids and electrolytes replaced as rapidly as possible. Oral rehydration therapy must be aggressive and special formulae are available in areas of the world where this is endemic. People living with the infected person can take tetracycline to minimize their risk of contracting the disease.

Yersinia

Aetiology and Epidemiology

The bacterium *Yersinia pestis* causes the plague (Black Death). This bacterium is a Gram-negative rod and was named after the Swiss bacteriologist, A.J.E. Yersin (1862–1943). Other forms of *Yersinia*, such as *Yersinia enterocolitica* cause enterocolitis. *Yersinia pseudotuberculosis* causes fever, rash and abdominal symptoms.

Transmission of *Yersinia pestis* normally involves flea bites. *Yersinia enterocolitica* and *Yersinia pseudotuberculosis* are transmitted by eating contaminated food such as uncooked pork or unpasteurized milk. Prevention includes avoiding unpasteurized milk, undercooked meat, and contaminated water. Proper hygiene when handling pork intestines is also critical.

Pathophysiology

The incubation period is generally 4 to 6 days. *Yersinia* invades the lining of the intestines and secretes toxins that cause the diarrhoea.

Symptoms and Signs

Patients may have fever, diarrhoea, a rash and abdominal symptoms.

Diagnosis

Diagnosis can be made from stool samples but the laboratory should be notified that *Yersinia* bacteria are suspected, as special 'cold enrichment' culture techniques are required. Diagnosis can also be made by cultures of blood, peritoneal fluid and throat swabs.

Treatment

Aminoglycosides, cefotaxime, tetracycline, chloramphenicol, and thrimethoprim-sulfamethoxazole are all effective for treatment of *Yersinia*.

Viral Infections

Astroviruses

Aetiology and Epidemiology

Astroviruses get their name from their star shape. Outbreaks of astrovirus-associated gastroenteritis commonly occur among children in hospitals and day-care centres. Improvements in detection of astroviruses have proved them to be more prevalent than previously thought. Among patients hospitalized for diarrhoea, astroviruses have been detected in 2.5% to 9% (Glass et al., 1996). Prevention includes proper hand washing. Little is known about the mechanism of infection.

Pathophysiology

Incubation is 3 to 4 days. The virus is a non-enveloped, single-stranded RNA virus. The infection generally occurs in children less than 2 years of age and, once infected, patients appear to develop an immunity to repeat infections.

Symptoms and Signs

For approximately 6 days patients have abdominal pain, diarrhoea, vomiting, nausea, fever, and malaise.

Diagnosis

Diagnosis generally requires that a stool sample be sent to a research laboratory for electron microscopic confirmation.

Treatment

Fluid replacement is the primary treatment.

Caliciviruses

Aetiology and Epidemiology

Caliciviruses can also cause viral gastroenteritis. Transmission is generally from person to person, usually faecal–oral but may be respiratory. Common sources are contaminated water and food, especially salads and shellfish. Oysters, in particular, have been implicated as a source of this infection (MMWR, 1997). Child care centres can also be a source of outbreaks.

Caliciviruses are non-enveloped RNA viruses. Calici-like viruses include:

1. Norwalk-like;
2. Snow Mountain-like;
3. Sapporo-like;
4. Hepatitis E.

Prevention includes hand washing and proper sanitation.

Pathophysiology

The incubation period is 12 hours to 4 days. These viruses cause damage to the lining of the intestines causing subsequent diarrhoea.

Symptoms and Signs

The following symptoms may last from 1 to 14 days: diarrhoea, vomiting, fever, headache, malaise, myalgia (general muscular pain or tenderness) and abdominal cramps.

Diagnosis

Diagnosis generally requires sending a stool sample to a research facility for electron microscopy studies.

Treatment

The most common treatment includes replacement of fluid and symptomatic therapy with antidiarrhoeal agents.

Enteroviruses (Non-polio)

Aetiology and Epidemiology

There are many forms of non-polio enteroviruses that cause infectious colitis, especially in children. Transmission is either faecal–oral or respiratory. Generally, these viruses are found only in humans. Prevention includes hand washing and proper handling of nappies. Enteroviruses can live at room temperature for days and are resistant to alcohol and detergents. Therefore proper infection-control measures are very important to prevent further spread, especially in day-care centres.

Pathophysiology

The incubation period is 3 to 6 days. Non-polio enteroviruses are single-stranded RNA viruses that have the ability to multiply in the gastrointestinal tract.

Symptoms and Signs

Patients present with vomiting, diarrhoea, abdominal pain and sometimes hepatitis.

Diagnosis

Diagnosis is made by identifying or growing the virus from stool samples.

Treatment

There is no specific treatment, except fluid replacement and symptomatic therapy with antidiarrhoeal agents.

Human Immunodeficiency Virus (HIV)

Aetiology and Epidemiology

Human immunodeficiency virus (HIV) is a cytopathic retrovirus that causes acquired immunodeficiency syndrome (AIDS). Because HIV destroys white blood cells and impairs the immune system, as well as directly damaging the lining cells of the gastrointestinal tract, it can lead to infectious colitis. Prolonged diarrhoea is a common presenting symptom in these patients.

People with AIDS often have severe forms of common gastrointestinal infections. For example, the parasites, *Crypotosporidium*, *Microsporidium*, *Isospora* and *Cyclospora* often infect people with AIDS and can cause profound, severe and chronic disease. These are covered in the chapter on sexually transmitted diseases and AIDS.

Rotavirus

Aetiology and Epidemiology

Rotaviruses are named for their wheel shape ('rota' is Latin for wheel). Infection usually occurs from person to person and is primarily found in young children. Rotaviruses are thought to be the most common virus causing gastroenteritis in children worldwide, and a major cause of dehydration and death in children in underdeveloped countries (Glass et al., 1996). One study showed that nearly 40% of children hospitalized for gastroenteritis had rotavirus (Barnes et al., 1998). Animal to human transmission has not been demonstrated. Transmission can be feacal–oral or respiratory. Rotaviruses are RNA viruses. This group includes human gastrointestinal viruses, duovirus, infantile gastroenteritis virus, gastroenteritis virus type B and a rotavirus-like agent.

Pathophysiology

The incubation period is one to three days. Rotavirus infections result in less pronounced inflammation of the mucosa of the colon compared with other types of infection (Shcherbakov et al., 1995). They are responsible, however, for destruction of villous epithelial cells (Moon, 1997), and subsequent ongoing diarrhoea.

Symptoms and Signs

The symptoms are diarrhoea and fever, as well as vomiting and abdominal pain. Dehydration can be profound and can quickly lead to shock in small infants.

Diagnosis

Diagnosis is made by detecting rotavirus antigen using enzyme immunoassay or latex agglutination.

Treatment

Fluid and electrolyte replacement must be rapid and aggressive. There is no antoviral drug but an effective vaccine will hopefully soon be available.

Parasitic Infections

Cryptosporidiosis

Aetiology and Epidemiology

Cryptosporidium parvum is an intestinal parasite that has re-emerged as an important infectious disease. This coccidian protozoan is an important pathogen of calves, birds, reptiles and other domestic animals. When the human immune system is weakened, these viruses can thrive and the infection can be severe or even fatal.

Drinking contaminated water is the most common source of this infection. It can be transmitted from farm animals or pets to humans. Swimming pools and child care centres can also be sources of outbreaks. Prevention requires filtration of drinking water because the organism may not be killed by the level of chlorine used to treat drinking water. In problematic areas drinking water should be boiled.

Pathophysiology

The incubation period is two to 14 days. *Cryptosporidia* are found in intestinal epithelial cells but the mechanism that results in diarrhoea is not well understood. It causes a severe secretory diarrhoea that can be very refractory to therapy especially in AIDS patients. This organism can sometimes be found in the lungs of infected patients.

Symptoms and Signs

Patients have watery diarrhoea, abdominal cramps, nausea, vomiting and sometimes fever.

Diagnosis

Diagnosis is made by identifying the oocysts (encysted form) from a stool sample, by a special stain.

Treatment

Infected patients must have their fluids and electrolytes aggressively replaced. Antimotility agents are helpful. Paromomycin and azithromycin have been inconsistently effective in patients with HIV. Oral gammaglobulin, octreotide (Somatostatin) and bovine colostrum have all been used.

Cyclosporiasis

Aetiology and Epidemiology

Cyclospora cayetanensis is a protozoan, coccidian parasite that causes infectious colitis. This parasite has been transmitted through imported food, particularly raspberries from Guatemala (Herwaldt and Ackers, 1997) and has caused recent outbreaks in the United States.

Pathophysiology

Incubation is generally one to two days but can be several weeks. Patients may be ill for as long as six weeks. *Cyclospora* can shorten and widen the intestinal villi and cause diffuse oedema, (Ortega et al., 1997), leading to severe watery diarrhoea.

Symptoms and Signs

Patients may be asymptomatic or may periodically suffer from watery diarrhoea, flu-like symptoms, flatulence and burping. Weight loss, abdominal discomfort, bloating and nausea have also been reported among these patients.

Diagnosis

Diagnosis can be made by detecting the oocysts in the stool with ultra-violet light microscopy but it may require an electron microscope. A modified Ziehl-Neelsen acid-fast stain can also detect this organism (Brennan et al., 1996).

Treatment

Trimethoprim-sulfamethoxazole is the current treatment of choice.

Entamoeba histolytica

Aetiology and Epidemiology

Amoebiasis is an infection of the large intestine caused by *Entamoeba histolytica*, a protozoan, amoeba single-celled parasite (Petri, 1996). This organism is transmitted via the stool of infected patients in the form of cysts (dormant phase) or trophozoites (active phase). Contaminated food, water and enema equipment are common sources of infection.

The prevalence is 4% in the USA, 10% worldwide and as high as 50% in tropical areas. Risk factors include: low socioeconomic status, crowded living conditions, tropical climate, inadequate plumbing, male homosexual activity, immunosuppression, malnutrition, and young age.

Preventive measures include hand washing, careful disposal of faecal material, treatment of drinking water, and use of condoms.

Pathophysiology

The incubation period is generally 1 to 4 weeks. Although this parasite can exist in the intestines without causing harm, if it penetrates the epithelial lining of the colon it can cause ulcers and lead to tropical (amoebic) dysentery (*Amoeba dysenteriae*).

Occasionally, this organism can travel to the liver causing abscesses (hepatic amoebiasis). From the liver the parasite can also travel to the lungs, brain, kidney or skin and cause disseminated infection, which is often fatal.

Symptoms and Signs

Entamoeba histolytica infection can have many symptoms. Some patients have no symptoms, others have mild symptoms, such as abdominal distention, flatulence, constipation or loose stools. Abdominal cramps and diarrhoea are present in more severe infections. In cases where the organism travels to the liver the symptoms may include fever, abdominal pain and tenderness around the liver.

Diagnosis

Diagnosis is made by identifying the *E. histolytica* cysts or trophozoites in a stool sample. Computed tomography (CT) scan or ultrasound is used to diagnose liver abscess.

Treatment

Asymptomatic patients can be treated with oral amoebicide drugs, such as iodoquinol, paromomycin or diloxanide furoate. Mild to severe cases can be treated with metronidazole or hehydroemetine, followed by a luminal amoebicide to completely eradicate the infection.

Giardia lamblia

Aetiology and Epidemiology

Giardiasis is a common parasitic infection of the small intestines caused by *Giardia lamblia*, a single-celled parasite that attaches to the lining of the intestines with a pair of sucking organs. The organism is flat and heart-shaped with eight flagellae which provide whip-like propulsion.

Transmission occurs via cysts in contaminated food or water. It may also be transmitted between children or sex partners. Prevention measures include careful selection of food and water when travelling in developing countries. Children should be cautioned not to drink water from streams, ponds or lakes when swimming or hiking. Water must be boiled to kill the cysts. Proper filtration of drinking water is also essential because chlorination does not kill the cysts. Prevention in child care centres requires proper hygiene and handling of nappies.

Pathophysiology

The incubation period is 1 to 4 weeks. The pathophysiology of giardiasis is not well understood but it does invade intestinal cells and causes enterocyte damage and malabsorption. Giadiasis is also called lambliasis.

Symptoms and Signs

Patients may be asymptomatic in the early stages. The late stage of infection causes problems absorbing fats which results in flatulance, steatorrhoea and abdominal pain.

Diagnosis

Diagnosis is made by identification of cysts *Giardia lamblia* in stool samples. There is also an antigen detection stool test now available that is more sensitive.

Treatment

Metronidazole and furazolidone are both effective. Quinacrine hydrochloride can cause gastrointestinal upset and is no longer available in the USA.

Isosporiasis

Aetiology and Epidemiology

Isospora belli is a coccidian protozoan, which can infect human intestines. In patients with AIDS or other immunosuppressed conditions this infection may cause severe diarrhoea and be life-threatening. Isosporiasis is often found in tropical and subtropical regions with poor sanitary conditions. This organism is frequently responsible for 'travellers' diarrhoea'.

Pathophysiology

The incubation period is 8 to 14 days.

Symptoms and Signs

Common symptoms, which can last for weeks or months, are fever, watery diarrhoea, abdominal pain, anorexia and weight loss.

Diagnosis

Diagnosis is made by identifying the oocysts in a stool sample, with a special stain.

Treatment

Patients can be treated with trimethoprim-sulfamethoxazole or pyrimethamine-sulfadoxine.

Strongyloides and other helminth infections

Aetiology and Epidemiology

Helminth is a general term for an intestinal worm-like parasite. A common species that causes infectious colitis is called *Strongyloides* or threadworms. These small roundworms (nematodes) are parasites found in intestines of many mammals. They are commonly found in tropical regions.

Prevention requires proper disposal of human waste and avoiding contact with human skin. Walking barefoot in tropical regions with poor sanitary disposal of waste products should be avoided.

Pathophysiology

Strongyloidiasis, infection with *Strongyloides*, can occur from drinking contaminated water or by the organism entering intact skin directly, usually through the feet when people walk barefoot on contaminated areas. The organism passes through the intestinal mucosa into the bloodstream. It can then pass into the lungs and return back into the bloodstream; this is called 'autoinfection'. In immunosuppressed patients this autoinfection, called 'hyperinfection', can cause severe disseminated disease involving all organs as well as the central nervous system and is usually fatal (Nishimura and Hung, 1997).

Symptoms and Signs

Symptoms include diarrhoea, abdominal pain, skin rashes and sometimes fever.

Diagnosis

The diagnosis is made by identifying the worm larvae in stool specimens or duodenal aspirates. In disseminated disease the organism can even be seen in sputum specimens.

Treatment

Thiabendazole is effective therapy in most patients, though disseminated disease often leads to secondary bacterial sepsis and is usually fatal.

Summary

Infectious colitis remains a major cause of morbidity and mortality worldwide. New pathogens surface and old pathogens re-emerge (Bryan et al., 1994). In addition, HIV infections and AIDS have weakened the immune systems of millions of people around the world, putting them at increased risk of severe infections, including infectious colitis. Although new more powerful antimicrobials and vaccines are being developed, basic public health measures involving proper sanitation and disposal of human waste, as well as access to prompt medical care, are still lacking in many parts of the world, contributing to the spread of disease. Furthermore, pathogens continue to develop increasing resistance to many of our available treatments, making the battle against these diseases a constant challenge.

References

Barnes GL, Uren E, Stevens KB, Bishop RF (1998) Etiology of acute gastroenteritis in hospitalized children in Melbourne, Australia, from April 1980 to March 1993. Journal of Clinical Microbiology 36(1): 133–8.

Brennan MK, MacPherson DW, Palmer J, Keystone JS (1996) Cyclosporiasis: a new cause of diarrhea. Canadian Medical Association Journal 155(9): 1293–6.

Bryan RT, Pinner RW, Berkelman RL (1994) Emerging infectious diseases in the United States, improved surveillance, a requisite for prevention. Annals of the New York Academy of Sciences 15(740): 346–61.

Farmer RG (1990) Infectious causes of diarrhea in the differential diagnosis of inflammatory bowel disease. Medical Clinics of North America 74(1): 29–38.

Fekety R (1997) Guidelines for the diagnosis and management of Clostridium difficile-associated diarrhea and colitis. American College of Gastroenterology, Practice Parameters Committee. American Journal of Gastroenterology 92(5): 739–50.

Fekety R, Shah AB (1993) Diagnosis and treatment of Clostridium difficile colitis. Journal of the American Medical Association 269(1): 71–5.

Glass RI, Noel J, Mitchell D, Herrmann JE, Blacklow NR, Pickering LK, Dennehy P, Ruiz-Palacios G, de Guerrero ML, Monroe SS (1996) The changing epidemiology of astrovirus-associated gastroenteritis: a review. Archives of Virology, Supplement 12: 287–300.

Herwaldt BL, Ackers ML (1997) An outbreak in 1996 of cyclosporiasis associated with imported raspberries. The Cyclospora Working Group. New England Journal of Medicine 336(22): 1548–56.

Keene WE, McAnulty JM, Hoesly FC, Williams LP Jr, Hedberg K, Oxman GL, Barrett TJ, Pfaller MA, Fleming DW (1994) New England Journal of Medicine 331(9): 579–84.

Moon HW (1997) Comparative histopathology of intestinal infections. Advances in Experimental Medicine and Biology 412: 1–19.

Morbidity and Mortality Weekly Report (1997) Addressing emerging infectious disease threats: a prevention strategy for the United States. Executive summary. Morbidity and Mortality Weekly Report 46(47): 1109–12.

Nishimura K, Hung T (1997) Current views on geographic distribution and modes of infection of neurohelminthic diseases. Journal of the Neurological Sciences 145(1): 5–14.

Ortega YR, Nagle R, Gilman RH, Watanabe J, Miyagui J, Quispe H, Kanagusuku P, Roxas C, Sterling CR (1997) Pathologic and clinical findings in patients with cyclosporiasis and a description of intracellular parasite life-cycle stages. Journal of Infectious Diseases 176(6): 1584–9.

Peter G (Ed.) (1997) Red Book: Report of the Committee on Infectious Diseases. 24th edn. Elk Grove Village, IL: American Academy of Pediatrics.

Petri WA Jr (1996) Recent advances in amebiasis. Critical Reviews of Clinical Laboratory Sciences 33(1): 1–37.

Pothoulakis C (1996) Pathogenesis of Clostridium difficile-associated diarrhoea. European Journal of Gastroenterology and Hepatology 8(11): 1041–7.

Rampal P, Hebuterne X, Fosse T (1989) Infectious diarrhea in the adult. Revista Pratica 39(29): 2583–9.

Settle CD, Wilcox MH (1996) Review article: antibiotic-induced Clostridium difficile infection. Alimentary Pharmacology and Therapeutics 10(6): 835–41.

Shcherbakov IT, Novikova AV, Gracheva NM, Charnyi AM, Partin OS, Avakov AA, Gavrilov AF, Fokin SN, Leont'eva NI, Glokhina TI (1995) Pathomorphology of the large intestinal mucosa in acute infectious colitis. Arkhiv Patologii 57(3): 23–7.

Su C, Brandt LJ (1995) Escherichia coli O157: H7 infection in humans. Annals of Internal Medicine 123(9): 698–714.

Chapter 17
Rectal Prolapse, Volvulus of the Colon and Intussusception

LUKE MELEAGROS MD, FRCS, Consultant Colorectal Surgeon and Honorary Senior Lecturer in Surgery, Homerton Hospital and Medical College of the Royal London and St Bartholomew's Hospital, London, UK

Rectal Prolapse

Definition

Prolapse of the rectum is a distressing, but uncommon, condition. The term implies a partial or circumferential, full-thickness descent of the rectum through the pelvic floor, often to emerge from the anus (Goligher, 1984; Keighley, 1992).

There are three types of rectal prolapse (Andrews and Jones, 1992; Keighley, 1992):

1. incomplete or mucosal prolapse: only a section of the lower rectal mucosa, usually situated anteriorly, prolapses;
2. internal or concealed prolapse: the upper rectum prolapses into the lower rectum but does not emerge through the anus (intranal or recto-rectal intussusception);
3. complete prolapse: the entire rectum, consisting of two layers of gut tube often with an intervening peritoneal sac, is extruded.

Incidence

More than 85% of affected patients are elderly women (Launer et al., 1982; Goligher, 1984), although young children and men can also be affected (Goligher, 1984; Keighley, 1992). The condition is equally common in multiparous and nulliparous women and the incidence increases with age (Goligher, 1984; Duthie and Bartolo, 1991; Andrews and Jones, 1992). In men, the condition occurs at a younger age (Goligher, 1984), and the majority are from tropical countries. Its incidence peaks in the fourth decade, becoming very uncommon in older age-groups (Goligher, 1984; Watts et al., 1985).

Aetiology

The aetiology is debated. Rectal prolapse is characterized by certain anatomical abnormalities (Thomson, 1981; Goligher, 1984; Finlay and Aitchison, 1991; Keighley, 1992):

- deep rectovaginal/rectovesical pouch;
- lack of fixation of the rectum;
- lax pelvic floor and anal sphincter muscles.

Clinical Features

Symptoms

The commonest and often most distressing complaint is of 'something coming down'. At first the patient notices the prolapse only at defecation when it either reduces spontaneously or has to be reduced manually. In more severe cases the rectum may prolapse during minor straining on standing or walking. The prolapse can soil underwear, make walking and sitting uncomfortable and mucous leakage can cause perineal excoriation.

Some patients present with vague symptoms of something obstructing defecation, and there is often overlap with the solitary rectal ulcer syndrome. Patients with a solitary rectal ulcer often respond to behavioural biofeedback. The patient is re-educated by the nurse using biofeedback techniques with emphasis being placed on not straining, and resisting the urge to make frequent trips to the toilet. Mucous discharge is common and may be the only symptom. Patients may describe having to manually evacuate stool. This is distressing and causes great embarrassment and therefore sensitivity is required when taking a thorough history from these patients. Rectal bleeding is uncommon and occurs secondary to traumatic proctitis and ulceration (Thomson, 1981; Goligher, 1984; Andrews and Jones, 1992). When it does occur it is particularly distressing, soils underclothing, causes perineal excoriation and raises in the patient's mind concerns regarding the possibility of cancer.

Faecal incontinence is a very common symptom, affecting more than 70% of patients – mostly elderly multiparous women. Some women experience urgency only, others are incontinent of mucus or flatus, whilst others are incontinent of liquid or solid stool. Owing to the laxity of the musculature, patients are incontinent not only when the rectum is prolapsed but also at other times. Furthermore, impairment of anorectal sensation prevents these patients from experiencing normal call to stool, leading to severe constipation and excessive straining. This state of disorded defecation is a major problem in many patients with rectal prolapse (Thomson, 1981; Goligher, 1984; Keighley, 1992) and requires much sensitivity when discussing the subject as many patients will have coped for many years with the problem without disclosing the fact for fear of the stigma which is perceived to be attached to these problems. It is often the nurse who may be the first person to elicit this information from the patient.

Anorectal examination

On inspection of the perineum the prolapse may be overtly evident (Thomson, 1981; Goligher, 1984; Andrews and Jones, 1992; Keighley 1992). The anal region appears abnormal with a patulous anus and perineal descent at rest or on straining. The prolapse may be visualized if the patient is asked to bear down, best done sittting on a lavatory. There is often associated genital prolapse.

Digital examination may show reduced resting anal tone, which reflects weakness of the internal anal sphincter. When the patient is asked to tighten the anal canal around the examining finger, a diminished squeeze effort will be evident, indicative of impaired external anal sphincter function. There is often loss of the anorectal angle due to a weak puborectalis. Proctosigmoidoscopy allows direct inspection of the mucosa to exclude other lesions. The lumen may contain excessive mucus or there may be evidence of proctitis with bleeding and ulceration. A biopsy may be necessary.

Investigations

Once the diagnosis is established clinically, many patients with rectal prolapse are managed surgically without any detailed preoperative investigations. Some surgeons, however, are in favour of detailed pre-operative assessment such as barium enema, anorectal physiology and proctography (Keighley 1992).

Treatment

The treatment of full-thickness rectal prolapse is surgical, but this must be combined with the medical management of constipation in the hope of reducing the chance of recurrence. At least 17 different opera-tions have been described (Madoff et al., 1992a) but the results of many of these are unsatisfactory and they are no longer employed.

A successful surgical outcome does not depend on the anatomical correction of the prolapse and prevention of recurrence alone. A poor functional result is the source of much patient dissatisfaction. Therefore, the surgeon should aim to correct both the constipation and faecal incontinence which so often accompany the prolapse. The procedures in common use today are classified into perineal and abdominal operations. The potential advantages and possible compli-cations of the various procedures are outlined below; this information will be useful when explaining why a specific operation has been suggested for an individual patient thus assisting patients to make an informed consent to their operation. However, the number of proce-dures which have been used is testament to our lack of complete understanding of this the condition.

Perineal operations

The patient undergoes full bowel preparation and is catheterized prior to operation. The procedures are carried out in the lithotomy position, or in the prone jackknife position. Perineal operations do not involve a laparotomy.

- The operations can be carried out under local or regional, rather than general anaesthesia.
- Therefore, they are better tolerated by elderly frail patients.

Anal Encirclement Procedure (Thiersch Wire)

- This procedure has now been largely superseded. In 1891 Thiersch utilized a subcutaneous stainless steel wire to encircle the anal orifice (Goligher, 1984; Madoff et al., 1992a). Faecal impaction and erosion of the wire were recognized complications.

Delorme's operation

- The mucosa is stripped off the underlying muscle and a series of sutures are inserted into the muscle to plicate the rectum into a doughnut-shaped mass, which is then reduced, and the mucosa sutured circumferentially.
- The reported recurrence rate varies from 4% to 22 % (Monson et al., 1986; Abulafi et al., 1990; Tobin and Scott, 1994; Plusa et al., 1995).
- Incontinence is improved in the majority of patients (Monson et al., 1986; Abulafi et al., 1990).
- Postoperative constipation is not common (Tobin and Scott, 1994; Plusa et al., 1995).

Perineal Rectosigmoidectomy

The prolapse is produced through the anal verge and a circumferential incision is made through the outer rectal wall a few centimetres above the anal canal. The inner tube of rectum and lower sigmoid is fully mobilized, pulled down and excised thus removing all the redundant bowel. The peritoneal sac, anteriorly, is also excised. The two free ends of bowel are anastomosed. Some surgeons carry out concomitant repair of the pelvic floor muscles by suture approximation (Finlay and Aitchison, 1991; Williams et al., 1992; Deen et al., 1994).

- Reported recurrence rates are variable, from 0–1% (Watts et al., 1985; Finlay and Aitchison, 1991) to 10–60% (Goligher, 1984; Madoff et al., 1992a; Williams et al., 1992; Deen et al., 1994).
- In one series 64% of patients regained continence after combined bowel resection and pelvic floor repair, compared with 20% after perineal rectosigmoidectomy alone (Williams et al., 1992). However, in another report, 60% suffered faecal soiling despite total pelvic floor repair (Deen et al., 1994).
- In comparative studies, abdominal rectopexy (see below) has been shown to be superior to perineal rectosigmoidectomy (Watts et al., 1985; Deen et al., 1994). Because the rectal reservoir is excised and anal pressures deteriorate postoperatively, a poor functional outcome with incontinence and increased frequency of defecation is not unknown following perineal rectosigmoidectomy (Deen et al., 1994).

Abdominal Operations

Many different procedures have been described. They can be classified into two broad categories: rectopexy without bowel resection and rectopexy combined with bowel resection. These procedures aim to correct the pathoanatomical features of rectal prolapse with complete mobilization of the rectum down to the pelvic floor and with division of all its attachments. The deep rectovaginal pouch is shortened and the rectum is lifted and attached to the sacrum posteriorly. Preoperatively, all patients undergo mechanical bowel preparation and prophylactic antibiotics are administered. Some surgeons continue antibiotic prophylaxis for 5 days when prosthetic material is employed.

Rectopexy without bowel resection

(i) Sutured rectopexy: In this procedure the posterior mesorectum is simply sutured to the presacral fascia.

(ii) Ripstein procedure (Launer et al., 1982; Goligher, 1984; Madoff et al., 1992a): This is an anterior sling rectopexy, first described in the early 1960s and still popular in the USA, though not in the UK.

- Recurrence of the prolapse can be high after this procedure – 12% in some series (Launer et al., 1982; Madoff et al., 1992a).
- Improvement in continence is only moderate (Launer et al., 1982).
- Its major drawback is faecal impaction resulting from rectal stenosis caused by the sling encircling the rectum (Launer et al., 1982; Madoff et al., 1992a).

(iii) Well's rectopexy: This is the most popular procedure for rectal prolapse in the UK. It employs a rectangular sheet of Ivalon sponge (polyvinyl alcohol) which is secured to the sacrum, wrapped around two-thirds of the circumference of the rectum and sutured to its muscular wall. By leaving the anterior rectal wall free, the problem of rectal stenosis is prevented. It is thought that the sponge induces an intense fibrous reaction thus permanently fixing the rectum to the sacrum.

- There is a 1–4% incidence of infection around the sponge, which necessitates its removal (McCue and Thomson, 1991; Novell et al., 1994).
- Recurrence of prolapse is around 4% (McCue and Thomson, 1991).
- Improvement in continence is variable. Some surgeons report restoration of continence in 30–60% of patients.
- Postoperative constipation, a problem encountered in up to

50% of patients, largely contributes to a poor functional result (Madoff et al., 1992a; Novell et al., 1994). It has been suggested that this is due to kinking at the rectosigmoid junction caused by a floppy redundant sigmoid loop (Watts et al., 1985; Duthie and Bartolo, 1992).

Resection Rectopexy

Bowel resection for the correction of rectal prolapse was first reported by von Eiselsberg at the beginning of the century. In the late 1960s Frykman and Goldberg described the procedure in detail (Frykman and Goldberg, 1969). Since then many surgeons have reported favourable results (Watts et al., 1985; Williams et al., 1991; Duthie and Bartolo, 1992; Madoff et al., 1992b).

After mobilization, the rectum is secured to the presacral fascia with non-absorbable sutures. In addition, a variable length of colon is resected followed by a colorectal anastomosis at the level of the sacral promontory, i.e. at least 12 cm from the anal verge. Most surgeons resect only the sigmoid colon (Frykman and Goldberg, 1969; Duthie and Bartolo, 1992). Some advocate subtotal colectomy with ileorectal anastomosis, in patients with documented evidence of slow-transit constipation (Williams et al., 1991; Madoff et al., 1992b).

The proponents of resection rectopexy emphasize the importance of sigmoid resection in a successful rectopexy. They point out that of all the abnormalities in rectal prolapse, the only factor that can be controlled with certainty is the length of the colon (Frykman and Goldberg, 1969; Watts et al., 1985).

- The main concern with resection and anastomosis is the risk of anastomotic leak. This has not been a major problem in the reported series, because the anastomosis is not low down in the pelvis. A low anterior resection should be avoided for this reason.
- Another disadvantage of an anterior resection is loss of the compliant rectal reservoir with adverse effects on continence.
- Recurrence of prolapse is low, 0–6% (Duthie and Bartolo, 1992).
- Constipation improves in the majority of patients postoperatively (Watts et al., 1985; Williams et al., 1991; Madoff et al., 1992b).
- A significant improvement in continence is noted in 50–70% of patients (Watts et al., 1985; Williams et al., 1991; Madoff et al., 1992b).

Conclusions

In elderly frail patients, perineal procedures under regional anaesthesia may be most appropriate. In the majority of patients, with modern anaesthesia, abdominal procedures are a safe option. The available evidence, outlined above, favours resection rectopexy as the most effective procedure, although this must be offset against the small risk of anastomotic complications as well as damage to the pelvic autonomic nerves.

Volvulus

Volvulus most commonly involves the colon, in which the bowel twists on its mesenteric axis causing partial or complete obstruction of its lumen. The circulation of the bowel is compromised due to venous obstruction, which may lead to venous infarction and gangrene. Occasionally there is interruption of the arterial supply resulting in the rapid development of colonic infarction (Goligher, 1984; Jones, 1992). The sigmoid colon is most commonly affected. Volvulus of the caecum is encountered less frequently whereas the transverse colon is affected rarely.

Volvulus of the Sigmoid Colon

This is a relatively common condition in Eastern Europe, India, Africa and the Middle East where it is responsible for up to 50% of all cases of intestinal obstruction (Sutcliffe, 1968; Wertkin, 1978; Goligher, 1984; Welch and Anderson, 1987; Jones, 1992; Subrahmanyam, 1992). By contrast, in western populations sigmoid volvulus only accounts for 3–5% of all cases of obstruction (Wertkin, 1978; Anderson and Lee, 1981; Welch and Anderson, 1987; Jones, 1992). However, it remains the third commonest cause of large bowel obstruction after carcinoma and diverticular disease (Anderson and Lee, 1981). More importantly, it is the commonest cause of strangulation obstruction, i.e. mechanical obstruction complicated by bowel ischaemia and gangrene, and is therefore associated with a high mortality (Sutcliffe, 1968).

Incidence

The condition affects mainly the elderly with a mean age of over 60 years (Wertkin, 1978; Anderson and Lee, 1981; Jones, 1992). Men and women are affected equally. Long-term inmates of institutions –

psychiatric, geriatric, mentally handicapped – are particularly prone to sigmoid volvulus. Such patients account for 10–26% of all cases in some reports (Sutcliffe, 1968; Wertkin, 1978; Ballantyne et al., 1985; Welch and Anderson, 1987). Many patients also suffer from chronic medical disorders (Wertkin, 1978; Anderson and Lee, 1981; Ballantyne et al., 1985; Jones, 1992). These associated chronic conditions can delay the presentation of the patient, with a consequent higher incidence of gangrene and an increased morbidity and mortality.

Aetiology and Pathology

Important predisposing factors are a long, sigmoid mesentery with a narrow base and a long, redundant colonic loop. In countries where the condition is common, a high-residue diet is thought to contribute to the redundancy of the colon (Sutcliffe, 1968; Welch and Anderson, 1987; Subrahmanyam, 1992). In western practice there is often a history of constipation (Sutcliffe, 1968). This may lead to megacolon which can predispose the sigmoid to rotate around its axis.

Tranquillizers, anticholinergic and antiparkinsonian drugs commonly used in institutionalized patients can also produce megacolon. Volvulus can occur in the postoperative period, presumably precipitated by distension of the sigmoid due to ileus (Sutcliffe, 1968; Anderson and Lee, 1981; Welch and Anderson, 1987), as well as during pregnancy (Sutcliffe, 1968; Ballantyne et al., 1985).

The sigmoid usually rotates through 180°–720° in an anticlockwise direction (Sutcliffe, 1968; Goligher, 1984; Jones, 1992), leading to a closed-loop obstruction. The greater the degree of twist or the longer it persists the higher the risk of strangulation and gangrene.

Clinical Presentation

The presentation is usually acute although the duration of symptoms may range from 6 hours to 21 days. The predominant symptoms are abdominal pain (70% of patients) and marked abdominal distension (90%) (Sutcliffe, 1968; Goligher, 1984; Anderson and Lee, 1981; Welch and Anderson, 1987). The pain is cramp-like in the central or lower abdomen. The distension may be so gross as to affect cardiorespiratory function. Other features include absolute constipation, and later nausea and vomiting. The characteristic feature on examination is abdominal distension (Sutcliffe, 1968; Anderson and Lee, 1981; Welch and Anderson, 1987). Tenderness is common but signs of peritonitis are infrequent (Welch and Anderson, 1987) even in the presence of gangrenous bowel (Anderson and Lee, 1981). Bowel sounds may be tinkling, indicating obstruction (Welch and Anderson, 1987), or absent in cases of gangrene (Anderson and Lee, 1981; Ballantyne et al., 1985).

Sometimes patients, usually from long-term institutions, present late in a moribund state due to arterial occlusion leading to colonic gangrene (Anderson and Lee, 1981; Welch and Anderson, 1987).

A history of previous attacks is not uncommon (Sutcliffe, 1968). Pain and distension resolve after passage of copious amounts of flatus and liquid stool (Goligher, 1984), presumably following spontaneous reduction of the volvulus.

Investigations

Plain abdominal X-ray is diagnostic in more than 80% of cases (Welch and Anderson, 1987). It shows a distended loop of bowel arising from the left iliac fossa and extending to occupy most of the abdomen. The characteristic appearance is said to resemble a 'bent inner tube' or 'ace of spades' (Sutcliffe, 1968; Ballantyne et al., 1985; Welch and Anderson, 1987).

If the diagnosis is in doubt, barium enema examination can be helpful. It produces partial filling of the twisted loop, giving an appearance described as 'bird's beak' or 'snake's head' (Sutcliffe, 1968; Wertkin, 1978; Ballantyne et al., 1985).

As indicated above, it is important to identify patients with gangrene. This is not always possible on clinical grounds. Plain films may show free gas if there is colonic perforation (Anderson and Lee, 1981). A raised white cell count is present in some cases with gangrenous bowel (Anderson and Lee, 1981; Ballantyne et al., 1985).

Management

Sigmoid volvulus can be treated by non-operative means and/or a number of surgical procedures. The appropriateness of each treatment method is assessed according to its success, associated morbidity and mortality and the risk of recurrent volvulus.

Non-operative Management

Sigmoidoscopic reduction is employed when there is no clinical suspicion of gangrene. The technique popularized by Bruusgaard in 1947 is still used today (Sutcliffe, 1968). With the patient in the left lateral position, the sigmoidoscope is inserted up to the site of narrowing, usually at 25 cm (Sutcliffe, 1968; Goligher, 1984). Either the sigmoidoscope or, more usually, a rectal tube is passed through the twist into the bowel. The bowel is untwisted resulting in escape of flatus and liquid stool. The tube is securely taped to the buttock and left *in situ* for at least 48 hours, to allow adequate decompression and prevent early recurrence (Goligher, 1984; Welch and Anderson, 1987). The reported success rate of sigmoidoscopic reduction is high (70–90%) (Wertkin, 1978; Goligher, 1984; Ballantyne et al., 1985; Anderson and Lee 1981; Welch and Anderson 1987). The procedure is well tolerated and has a very low mortality (2–4%) (Sutcliffe, 1968; Wertkin, 1978; Ballantyne et al., 1985; Welch and Anderson, 1987).

Other techniques of non-operative reduction include use of the colonoscope (Starling, 1979) or barium enema (Goligher, 1984; Ballantyne et al., 1985), if sigmoidoscopic reduction fails (10–20% of cases: Anderson and Lee, 1981; Goligher, 1984; Ballantyne et al., 1985). Sigmoidoscopy or colonoscopy allow inspection of the colonic mucosa for signs of ischaemia. If the mucosa is ischaemic or if blood-stained fluid escapes from the bowel, laparotomy should be undertaken (Anderson and Lee, 1981; Welch and Anderson, 1987).

Non-operative reduction is a temporary measure. The recurrence rate can be as high as 90% (Ballantyne et al., 1985) and although sigmoidoscopic reduction can be repeated (Anderson and Lee, 1981; Welch and Anderson, 1987), the mortality from further attacks increases (Goligher, 1984). Therefore, most surgeons recommend surgery soon after non-operative reduction in patients who are medically fit (Wertkin, 1978; Goligher, 1984; Ballantyne et al., 1985; Welch and Anderson, 1987).

Surgical Management

Surgery is indicated if sigmoidoscopic reduction fails, if there is evidence of gangrene, or after successful non-operative reduction. A gangrenous sigmoid is present in 7–12% of cases at presentation (Anderson and Lee, 1981; Ballanytne et al., 1985). In these patients emergency surgery is necessary.

Sigmoid Colon Viable

In an elective procedure, most surgeons perform sigmoid colectomy with anastomosis. A proximal defunctioning stoma is not usually necessary. This policy is successful, associated with a mortality of 0–10% (Wertkin, 1978; Anderson and Lee, 1981; Ballantyne et al., 1985) and without recurrence of the volvulus.

In the emergency situation, the patient is placed in the lithotomy position on the operating table. At laparotomy the volvulus is de-rotated and the colon decompressed via a tube passed per anum. Hartmann's procedure, i.e. sigmoid resection with end colostomy and closure of the distal rectal stump, is performed. This can be associated with a low mortality. Alternative strategies are a Paul-Mikulicz type resection, with a double-barrel colostomy, or resection with primary anastomosis. Such procedures carry higher mortality rates (18–30%) (Welch and Anderson, 1987).

Sigmoid Colon Gangrenous

Postoperative mortality in the presence of gangrene can be as high as 80% (Wertkin, 1978). Hartmann's procedure is probably safest (Anderson and Lee, 1981; Ballantyne et al., 1985). Resection with anastomosis is not recommended in the presence of gangrene.

Volvulus of the Caecum

Caecal volvulus accounts for 25–40% of all cases of colonic volvulus and is responsible for 1% of all cases of intestinal obstruction (O'Mara et al., 1979; Goligher, 1984).

Incidence

It has a reported incidence of 1 per 100 000 population (Ballantyne et al., 1985). The average age of the patients is 50–60 years (Wertkin, 1978; Todd and Forde, 1979; O'Mara et al., 1979; Goligher, 1984; Ballantyne et al., 1985; Neil et al., 1987). In a report from Australia a peak incidence was observed in the 30–40 as well as the 60–80 year age-groups (Neil et al., 1987). Therefore, caecal volvulus tends to occur in a younger age-group compared with sigmoid volvulus. It further differs from sigmoid volvulus in that it is much commoner in women (Wertkin, 1978; O'Mara et al., 1979; Todd and Forde, 1979; Howard and Catto, 1980; Goligher, 1984) and does not occur with increased frequency among institutionalized patients (Wertkin, 1978; O'Mara et al., 1979; Ballantyne et al., 1985).

Aetiology and Pathology

Two types are recognized (O'Mara et al., 1979; Howard and Catto, 1980). In the commoner variety (90% of cases) there is axial twist of the caecum, ascending colon and terminal ileum in a clockwise direction (O'Mara et al., 1979; Howard and Catto, 1980; Jones, 1992). The less common variety is the so-called caecal bascule where the caecum folds upwards to lie in front of the ascending colon.

The primary defect is failure of the peritoneum of the posterior abdominal wall to fuse with the caecum and ascending colon (Howard and Catto, 1980; Weiss, 1982; Jones, 1992). This is a common congenital anomaly, present in 11% of adults. Additional factors thought to precipitate caecal volvulus include the following.

Previous abdominal surgery causes adhesions around which the caecum can rotate. In some series, 25–80% of patients had previous appendectomy, gynaecological procedures or cholecystectomy (O'Mara et al., 1979; Howard and Catto, 1980; Neil et al., 1987). Colonic distension, secondary to chronic constipation or distal colonic obstruction, has been reported in up to 30% of cases (Howard and Catto, 1980; Haskin et al., 1981). Pregnancy, by pushing the caecum out of the pelvis, can cause volvulus (Howard and Catto, 1980; Haskin et al., 1981; Weiss, 1982; Ballantyne et al., 1985). Increased peristalsis, caused by diarrhoea or powerful laxatives, is another precipitating factor (Haskin et al., 1981; Ballantyne et al., 1985).

The incidence of caecal strangulation and gangrene is around 20% (O'Mara et al., 1979; Todd and Forde, 1979; Ballantyne et al., 1985).

Clinical Presentation

Symptoms are non-specific. Abdominal pain is usually felt in the right lower abdomen. Less common symptoms are distension, nausea and vomiting, constipation or diarrhoea (O'Mara et al., 1979; Haskin et al., 1981; Weiss, 1982; Neil et al., 1987).

The common clinical signs are tenderness, usually on the right, and distension (O'Mara et al., 1979; Neil et al., 1987). A compressible abdominal mass may be palpable. The bowel sounds vary and do not correlate well with the presence of ischaemia. Similarly, signs of peritoneal irritation are not reliable in the diagnosis of a gangrenous caecum (O'Mara et al., 1979; Weiss, 1982).

Investigations

Plain abdominal X-rays are abnormal in up to 90% of patients (O'Mara et al., 1979; Weiss, 1982; Neil et al., 1987). They show a greatly dilated caecum, displaced anywhere in the abdomen. The appearance is likened to a 'coffee bean' with its point directed towards the left upper abdomen (Haskin et al., 1981; Ballantyne et al., 1985). Dilated small bowel loops are also present (O'Mara et al., 1979; Haskin et al., 1981). These appearances are frequently not diagnostic. In many series, a preoperative diagnosis was possible in 5–40% of cases (O'Mara et al., 1979; Howard and Catto, 1980; Ballantyne et al., 1985; Neil et al., 1987).

Barium enema is sometimes carried out, provided this will not delay surgery. It is diagnostic in 60–90% of cases, by demonstrating the spiralling folds of the twist (O'Mara et al., 1979; Howard and Catto, 1980; Haskin et al., 1981; Ballantyne et al., 1985).

Management

The management is always surgical. Non-operative reduction by barium enema or colonoscopy have been reported (Wertkin, 1978; Ballantyne et al., 1985) but these forms of treatment are not universally adopted. The type of surgical procedure depends on whether the caecum is viable or gangrenous.

Caecum Viable

The following options are available:

1. tube caecostomy (O'Mara et al., 1979);
2. caecopexy: the caecum and ascending colon are fixed to the abdominal wall, using non-absorbable sutures;
3. detorsion alone: the volvulus is relieved but no fixation of the bowel is undertaken;
4. resection and anastomosis, i.e. right hemicolectomy with ileo-transverse anastomosis.

There is no general agreement on the preferred form of surgery. Operative mortality after resections is below 10% (O'Mara et al., 1979). Therefore, some surgeons recommend resection in every case in order to eliminate the risk of recurrence (Todd and Forde, 1979). However, several series reported very low recurrence rates after non-resectional surgery (Wertkin, 1978; O'Mara et al., 1979; Howard and Catto, 1980; Neil et al., 1987), except with detorsion alone (Neil et al., 1987). Caecostomy can be complicated by sepsis (O'Mara et al., 1979).

Caecum Gangrenous

The only treatment option in the presence of gangrenous bowel is resection, i.e. right hemicolectomy (Wertkin, 1978; O'Mara et al., 1979; Howard and Catto, 1980; Goligher, 1984; Ballantyne et al.,

1985). Primary ileo-transverse anastomosis can be performed in selected patients. However, if there is doubt about bowel viability or fitness of the patient, the bowel ends should be exteriorized and the anastomosis delayed for a second procedure (Ballantyne et al., 1985).

Mortality in these cases is high, ranging between 30% and 40% (O'Mara et al., 1979; Todd and Forde, 1979; Ballantyne et al., 1985).

Intussusception

Definition

Intussusception is defined as the invagination of one portion of the gastrointestinal tract into the adjacent one, which is usually immediately distal to it. The inner portion of bowel, which invaginates, is called the intussusceptum and the outer portion into which it invaginates is called the intussuscepiens.

Intussusception is primarily a disease of young children. Only 5% of cases occur in adults (Weilbaecher et al., 1971).

Intussusception in Infants and Children

Incidence

Epidemiological studies in the UK in the 1950s and 1960s reported an incidence of 1.5–4.3 per 1000 live births (Stringer et al., 1992). Approximately 700 children per year are admitted into hospital with intussusception. Peaks in incidence in the spring/summer and in the winter have been linked to an increased incidence of gastroenteritis and respiratory infections, respectively (Ravitch, 1986).

There is a strong male preponderance with 60–70% of cases occuring in boys (Hutchison et al., 1980; Ravitch, 1986; Stringer et al., 1992). The condition is commonest in the first year of life. More than 50% of infants with intussusception are aged between 3 and 9 months. Only 10–25% of cases occur after 2 years of age (Hutchison et al., 1980; Stringer et al., 1992).

Pathology

Intussusception is the leading cause of intestinal obstruction in infants and young children. The great majority (80–90%) start in the region of the ileocaecal valve and are referred to as ileocolic. The apex of the intussusception is usually in the ascending colon, but can be further distally or even prolapsed through the anus on rare occasions. Other vareties are much rarer: ileoilial, caecocolic, colocolic and jejunojejunal.

The invagination of the bowel results in compression and angulation of the mesenteric blood vessels leading to strangulation. Initially there is only venous obstruction with tissue oedema. Excess mucus is produced and discharged into the bowel lumen. Mucus mixed with blood, seeping from engorged vessels, gives rise to the 'redcurrant jelly' stools characteristic of the condition. If the condition persists, the rising tissue pressure eventually exceeds arterial pressure leading to bowel ischaemia and gangrene. The outer layer of the intussusception is affected first, followed by the inner layer (Ravitch, 1986; Stringer et al., 1992). In some cases the intussusceptum may reduce spontaneously.

Aetiology

Intussusception usually has no identifiable underlying cause. In approximately 10% of cases it is secondary to an underlying abnormality.

In idiopathic intussusception there is frequently hyperplasia of the bowel lymphoid tissue. Enlarged lymph nodes project into the bowel lumen and are propelled distally by peristalsis thus acting as the lead point of the intussusception. Adenoviruses and rotaviruses have been implicated in lymphoid hyperplasia. These viruses cause respiratory tract infections and gastroenteritis, hence the common association between these conditions and intussusception.

Secondary intussusception is commoner in older children and in those with recurrent attacks. Common conditions associated with recurrent attacks include benign polyps, Meckel's diverticulum and duplication cysts. Small bowel lymphoma and lymphosarcoma can present with intussusception (Stringer et al., 1992).

Clinical Presentation

Sudden onset of colicky abdominal pain classically sees the child scream, appear pale and draw up his or her legs. Between episodes the child initially appears well. Vomiting is common and may be the only symptom in infants. Bleeding per rectum, in the form of the characteristic 'redcurrant jelly', may occur in up to 95% of children.

On clinical examination, the child appears listless and apathetic. In the later stages there may be dehydration and collapse. The abdomen is usually soft but becomes distended later. The typical finding is of a tender sausage-shaped mass, palpable in 50–90% of children.

The clinical presentation is often atypical leading to a delay in the diagnosis. In one series there was more than 48 hours delay in 36% of patients (Hutchison et al., 1980). The acute presentation described above is commonly seen in infants and young children. Older children can present with chronic intussusception, with symptoms lasting more than 2 weeks and even up to 93 days (Reijnen et al., 1989). These children present with anorexia, vomiting, weight loss and intermittent abdominal pain. The bowel habit may be normal or there may be diarrhoea.

Investigations

Plain abdominal X-rays show absence of a gas-filled caecum in the right iliac fossa. In late cases, dilated loops of small bowel, consistent with obstruction, will be seen. Ultrasound scan is being increasingly used in diagnosis (Stringer et al., 1992). Barium enema remains the mainstay of radiological diagnosis and is also used extensively in the non-operative treatment of the condition.

Management

Initial treatment consists of resuscitation with intravenous fluids, colloids and/or crystalloids or blood depending on the condition of the child. A nasogastric tube may be required especially in cases of established small bowel obstruction.

The treatment of intussusception used to be surgical. However, in recent years non-operative reduction of ileocolic intussusception has become established as the method of choice in nearly all cases.

Non-operative Reduction

Resuscitation of the child is continued in the X-ray room, attended by both the radiologist and surgeon. A Foley catheter, or soft rubber rectal tube, is inserted in the rectum and the buttocks are strapped together. The catheter is connected to the reservoir of barium which is raised to a maximum height of three and a half feet. The barium is run into the colon and the meniscus of the intussusception is outlined. With continued flow, the hydrostatic pressure of the column of barium effects reduction of the intussusception. A successful reduction is indicated by free flow of barium into the small bowel. This should be accompanied by clinical improvement of the patient, return of faeces or flatus with the barium per rectum and disappearance of the sausage-shaped abdominal mass.

Reduction may be very rapid or can take up to an hour, provided progress is being made. If the intussusception remains static for 10 minutes, non-operative reduction will fail and therefore operation is advised.

Barium enema reduction is successful in up to 80% of patients in whom the technique is employed. The technique has been criticized for its high recurrence rate, incomplete success and the risks of reducing gangrenous bowel, causing perforation and overlooking any underlying pathological lead points. However, published series do not report a higher recurrence rate compared with operative reduction. Pathological lead points in young children are very uncommon, not in themselves dangerous and come to light because of recurrent intussusception which is treated surgically. The risks of perforation or of reducing gangrenous bowel can be prevented by a careful reduction technique and avoidance of high hydrostatic pressures (Ravitch, 1986). Any disadvantages of barium reduction are outweighed by the significantly reduced morbidity and mortality of this method, compared with surgery.

Operative Reduction

Surgery is indicated when hydrostatic reduction has been unsuccessful or if there is uncertainty about complete reduction. It is usually required in cases where the diagnosis has been delayed, where there is established small bowel obstruction (Stringer et al., 1992), in recurrent intussusception, and in chronic intussusception when hydrostatic reduction usually fails (Reijnen et al., 1989). Surgery is always recommended in the presence of peritonitis, perforation or when a pathological lead point is demonstrated radiologically.

At operation, the abdomen is opened via a right transverse incision. The intussusception is reduced by gently compressing its apex and 'milking' it back rather than pulling the intussuceptum, which may result in tearing. Following successful reduction, the bowel is observed carefully in order to ensure its viability. Cases where the intussusception is irreducible or the bowel is gangrenous require bowel resection with anastomosis.

Intussusception in Adults

Compared with infants and children, intussusception in adults is a rare condition. It has an estimated annual incidence of two to three per million population (Carter and Morton, 1989). The condition accounts for 0.1% of all adult hospital admissions (Agha, 1986). Unlike paediatric intussusception, the adult disease is not confined to the ileocaecal region. It affects the small and large bowel with equal frequency (Weilbaecher et al., 1971; Aston and Machleder, 1975; Agha, 1986; Carter and Morton, 1989).

Aetiology

In adults, secondary intussusception is more frequent than primary intussusception, especially in the colon. Benign or malignant neoplasms form the pathological lead point. Benign neoplasms are commoner in the small bowel, whilst in the colon malignant tumours are encountered more frequently. Small bowel lesions commonly associated with intussusception are lipoma, leiomyoma, hamartoma, lymphoma and metastatic melanoma. Colonic lesions include adenocarcinoma, adenoma and lymphoma (Weilbaecher et al., 1971). Meckel's diverticulum is the commonest non-neoplastic lesion causing intussusception (Aston and Machleder, 1975).

Clinical Presentation

Presentation in adults is chronic with non-specific symptoms of intermittent intestinal obstruction which resolve spontaneously but tend to recur over weeks, months or years.

The commonest symptom is colicky abdominal pain. Depending on the type of intussusception other symptoms may be present. Vomiting may be a symptom in small bowel intussusception, constipation or diarrhoea and rectal bleeding in colonic intussusception (Weilbaecher et al., 1971; Carter and Morton, 1989). An abdominal mass was present in 36% of patients in one series (Carter and Morton, 1989).

Investigations

Plain abdominal X-rays will show features of intestinal obstruction during an acute attack, especially when the small bowel is involved.

In colonic cases, barium enema will reveal typical appearances, with the concave meniscus of the intussusception (Weilbaecher et al., 1971). However, because the condition is uncommon in adults, there is often delay in reaching a diagnosis. In one series, the diagnosis was made at laparotomy in 91% of patients (Carter and Morton, 1989).

Management

The usual treatment is surgical resection of the affected segment of bowel. Reduction by hydrostatic pressure is inappropriate because of the high incidence of underlying pathological conditions. Some surgeons recommend resection without prior manual reduction of the intussusception. They maintain that excessive manipulation may lead to tumour dissemination (Weilbaecher et al., 1971). However, prior reduction allows assessment of the causative lesion which may be amenable to local excision (Aston and Machleder, 1975) thus avoiding unnecessary bowel resection. In idiopathic cases, the bowel can be preserved, resection being necessary only in the presence of gangrenous bowel (Carter and Morton, 1989).

References

Abulafi AM, Sherman IW, Fiddian RV, Rothwell-Jackson R (1990) Delorme's operation for rectal prolapse. Annals of the Royal College of Surgeons of England 72: 382–5.

Agha FP (1986) Intussusception in adults. American Journal of Radiology 146: 527–31.

Anderson JR, Lee D (1981) The management of acute sigmoid volvulus. British Journal of Surgery 68: 117–20.

Andrews NJ, Jones DJ (1992) Rectal prolapse and associated conditions. British Medical Journal 305: 243–6.

Aston SJ, Machleder HI (1975) Intussusception in the adult. American Surgeon 41: 576–80.

Ballantyne GH, Brandner MD, Beart RW, Ilstrup DM (1985) Volvulus of the colon. Incidence and mortality. Annals of Surgery 202 (1): 83–92.

Carter CR, Morton AL (1989) Adult intussusception in Glasgow, UK. British Journal of Surgery 76: 727.

Deen KI, Grant E, Billingham C, Keighley MRB (1994) Abdominal resection rectopexy with pelvic floor repair versus perineal rectosigmoidectomy and pelvic floor repair for full-thickness rectal prolapse. British Journal of Surgery 81: 302–4.

Duthie GS, Bartolo DCC (1991) Pathophysiology and management of rectal prolapse. In Taylor I, Johnson CD (Eds) Recent Advances in Surgery 14. Edinburgh: Churchill Livingstone.

Duthie GS, Bartolo DCC (1992) Abdominal rectopexy for rectal prolapse: a comparison of techniques. British Journal of Surgery 79: 107–13.

Finlay IG, Aitchison M (1991) Perineal excision of the rectum for prolapse in the elderly. British Journal of Surgery 78: 687–9.

Frykman HM, Goldberg SM (1969) The surgical treatment of rectal procidentia. Surgery, Gynecology and Obstetrics 129: 1225–30.

Goligher JC (1984) Surgery of the Anus, Rectum and Colon. London: Ballière Tindall.

Haskin PH, Teplick SK, Teplick JG, Haskin ME (1981) Volvulus of the cecum and right colon. Journal of the American Medical Association 245 (23): 2433–5.

Howard ES, Catto J (1980) Cecal volvulus. A case for nonresectional therapy. Archives of Surgery 115: 273–7.

Hutchison IF, Olayiwola B, Young DG (1980) Intussusception in infancy and childhood. British Journal of Surgery 67: 209–12.

Jones DJ (1992) Large bowel volvulus. British Medical Journal 305: 358–9.

Keighley M (1992) Rectal prolapse: clinical features and pathophysiology. In Henry MM, Swash M (Eds) Coloproctology and the Pelvic Floor. 2nd edn. Oxford: Butterworth-Heinemann.

Launer DP, Fazio VW, Weakley FL, Turnhull RB, Jagelman DG, Lavery IG (1982) The Ripstein procedure: a 16-year experience. Diseases of the Colon and Rectum 25(1): 41–5.

McCue JL, Thomson JPS (1991) Clinical and functional results of abdominal rectopexy for complete rectal prolapse. British Journal of Surgery 78: 921–3.

Madoff RD, Watts JD, Rothenberger DA, Goldberg SM (1992a) Rectal prolapse: treatment. In Henry MM, Swash M (Eds) Coloproctology and the Pelvic Floor. 2nd edn. Oxford: Butterworth-Heinemann.

Madoff RD, Williams JG, Wond WD, Rothenberger DA, Golderberg SM (1992b) Long-term functional results of colon resection and rectopexy for overt rectal prolapse. American Journal of Gastroenterology 87(1): 101–4.

Monson JRT, Jones NAG, Vowden P, Brennan TG (1986) Delorme's operation: the first choice in complete rectal prolapse? Annals of the Royal College of Surgeons of England 68: 143–6.

Neil DAH, Reasbeck PG, Reasbeck JC, Effeney DJ (1987) Caecal volvulus: ten year experience in an Australian teaching hospital. Annals of the Royal College of Surgeons of England 69: 283–5.

Novell JR, Osborne MJ, Winslet MC, Lewis AAM (1994) Prospective randomized trial of Ivalon sponge versus sutured rectopexy for full-thickness rectal prolapse. British Journal of Surgery 81: 904–6.

O'Mara CS, Wilson TH, Stonesifer GL, Cameron JL (1979) Cecal volvulus. Annals of Surgery 189 (6): 724–31.

Plusa SM, Charig JA, Balaji V, Watts A, Thompson MR (1995) Physiological changes after Delorme's procedure for full-thickness rectal prolapse. British Journal of Surgery 82: 1475–8.

Ravitch MM (1986) Intussusception. In Welch KJ, Randolph JG, Ravitch MM, O'Neill JA, Rowe MI (Eds) Pediatric Surgery. 4th edn. Chicago: Year Book Medical.

Reijnen JAM, Festen C, Joosten HJM (1989) Chronic intussusception in children. British Journal of Surgery 76: 815–16.

Starling JR (1979). Initial treatment of sigmoid volvulus by colonoscopy. Annals of Surgery 190(1): 36–9.

Stringer MD, Pablot SM, Brereton RJ (1992) Paediatric intussusception. British Journal of Surgery 79: 867–76.

Subrahmanyam M (1992) Mesosigmoplasty as a definitive operation for sigmoid volvulus. British Journal of Surgery 79: 683–4.

Sutcliffe MML (1968) Volvulus of the sigmoid colon. British Journal of Surgery 55: 903–10.

Thomson JPS (1981) Anorectal prolapse. In Hadfield J, Hobsley M (Eds) Current Surgical Practice. Vol. 2. London: Edward Arnold.

Tobin SA, Scott IHK (1994) Delorme's operation for rectal prolapse. British Journal of Surgery 81: 1681–4.

Todd GJ, Forde KA (1979) Volvulus of the cecum: choice of operation. American Journal of Surgery 138: 632–4.

Watts JD, Rothenberger DA, Buls JG, Goldberg SM, Nivatvongs S (1985) The management of procidentia: 30 years' experience. Diseases of the Colon and Rectum 28(2): 96–102.

Weilbaecher D, Bolin JA, Haern D, Ogden W (1971) Intussusception in adults. Review of 160 cases. American Journal of Surgery 121: 531–5.

Weiss BD (1982) Cecal volvulus. A diagnostic and therapeutic challenge. Postgraduate Medicine 72 (2): 189–94.

Welch G H, Anderson J R (1987) Acute volvulus of the sigmoid colon. World Journal of Surgery 11: 258–62.

Wertkin MG (1978) Management of volvulus of the colon. Diseases of the Colon and Rectum 21(1): 40–5.

Williams JG, Rothenberger DA, Madoff RD, Goldberg SM (1992) Treatment of rectal prolapse in the elderly by perineal rectosigmoidectomy. Diseases of the Colon and Rectum 35 (9): 830–4.

Williams JG, Wong WD, Jensen L, Rothenberger DA, Goldberg SM (1991) Incontinence and rectal prolapse: a prospective manometric study. Diseases of the Colon and Rectum 34(3): 209–16.

Chapter 18
Drug Considerations in Coloproctology

STEPHANIE E. GUERRIERO PharmD, Clinical Coordinator, Department of Pharmacy, Cleveland Clinic Hospital, Florida, USA

THOMAS GUERRIERO PharmD, Clinical Coordinator, Department of Pharmacy, North Ridge Medical Center, Florida, USA

Medication is often an integral part of treatment for many patients with diseases of the colon and rectum. In some instances drug therapy can be curative, but more frequently it is an adjunct to other treatment modalities and aimed at control of symptoms. The use of medication to control symptoms can help many patients achieve an acceptable quality of life. Individualization of drug therapy based on specific patient characteristics can minimize side-effects and drug interactions. Familiarity with factors affecting drug therapy and a knowledge base of the individual agents will lead to improved patient outcome. This chapter is aimed at providing an overview of factors affecting drug therapy. A review of commonly used medication in the treatment of diseases of the colon and rectum is also presented.

Factors Affecting Drug Therapy

Effects of Age on Drug Therapy

The Elderly Patient

Significant changes occurring with ageing have clinical implications for drug administration. Several age-related body composition changes may affect the pharmacologic action of drugs. Often a decrease in dosage is needed in order to maximize the therapeutic effects of drug therapy and minimize the toxicity and adverse effects. Age-related changes are gradual over a lifetime rather than abrupt at a specific age. Therefore, care must be taken to assess chronic drug therapy periodically.

Ageing also brings various changes in gastrointestinal tract function. Increased gastric pH, decreased gastric emptying, impaired intestinal motility and reduced splanchnic circulation are most commonly seen. Usually the changes do not alter absorption to the extent that a dosage adjustment is warranted. However, these changes can affect absorption when concomitant conditions such as diarrhoea, achlorhydria or malabsorption, which can be seen in the elderly and in inflammatory bowel disease patients, exist. In this situation a higher dose or an alternative route of drug administration may be needed in order to achieve a desired therapeutic effect. Alternative routes of medication administration include rectal or parenteral administration.

Changes in drug distribution can be due to a decrease in total body water, decrease in lean body mass, increase in body fat, or a decrease in serum albumin. Lean body mass loss is the most significant of these. Losses occur in muscle tissue, visceral compartments and other protein moieties such as connective tissue and collagen, immune bodies, carrier proteins and other protein bodies (Chernoff, 1990). These changes are often accompaniments to ageing, but can also occur with poor nutritional status, congestive heart failure, dehydration, oedema, ascites, hepatic failure and renal failure. Medications that are highly water soluble, fat soluble or highly protein bound may require a reduction in dosage.

Albumin is the most abundant visceral protein in the body. It is the most significant component in protein binding of pharmacological agents. The effect of protein binding on drug distribution is important. Drugs that are protein bound cannot cross biological membranes in the body and are pharmacologically inactive until released from the binding site. Only the unbound portion of a drug is able to exert its therapeutic effect (Zimmerman and Feldman, 1981). In conditions where serum albumin is deficient there are fewer binding sites available to the drug. There is an increase in free drug concentration in blood and tissue. This increase in free drug concentration can have serious consequences of toxicity in the case of potent drugs. Clinically relevant effects occur with agents that are usually at least 90% protein bound (Hansten and Horn, 1986). Examples of highly protein-bound drugs include warfarin, diazepam and furosemide.

Age-related decreases in liver function can cause alterations in drug metabolism. With ageing, blood flow to the liver decreases, as does the

size of the liver and enzymatic activity. Disease states such as congestive heart failure, fever, hepatic failure, malignancy, malnutrition and
viral infection can impair drug metabolism. These factors lead to
decreased drug metabolism and can often result in increased adverse
effects to the patient if dosage adjustments are not made. Long-acting
benzodiazepines, such as diazepam, chlordiazepoxide and
flurazepam, have extended half-lives in the elderly or in individuals
with impaired metabolism. With repeated administration they may
cause daytime sedation and lethargy. These adverse effects may be
more pronounced in the presence of cimetidine, a well known hepatic
microsomal enzyme inhibitor.

Decreased drug excretion occurs due to loss of kidney function,
decreased blood flow to the kidneys and decreased renal tubular function. Age-related decrease in renal function is often clinically significant. Accumulation and toxicity is a concern with renally eliminated
drugs. Renal function decline can be seen in measurements of creati-
nine clearance. An increase in plasma half-life occurs in those drugs
which are renally eliminated. A reduction in the dosage of renally
eliminated drugs such as cimetidine, famotidine, ranitidine,
cyclosporine and certain antibiotics can prevent accumulation and
toxicity.

The Paediatric Patient

Paediatric pharmacotherapy has come to be recognized as a well-
defined specialty. Drug safety and efficacy must be maintained in this
delicate population. Drug response in children is influenced by age,
size and stage of development. Additionally, drugs may have unique
reactions on children. For example, corticosteroid use in children
affects linear growth, whereas in adults this cannot occur (Loeb, 1976).
Other adverse effects seen solely in children include the cartilage toxicity seen with fluoroquinolone antibiotics and the increase in dystonic
reactions to metoclopramide, prochloperazine and other dopamine
agonists (Hooper and Wolfson, 1985; Terrin et al., 1984).

Special problems in drug delivery exist in children. Children
require smaller volumes than adults, limiting the amount of fluid as
well as the maximal rate of intravenous fluids that can be administered. Formulations of drugs available for adults may not be suitable
for or tolerable by children. It is often necessary to prepare special
dosage formulations from commercially available adult products.
Absorption differs in children in that newborns absorb drugs more
slowly, but not necessarily less completely than older children or

adults. The effect of age on absorption is not uniform and cannot be predicted.

Body composition of children differs from adults. Total body water in the newborn is greater than that of the adult and gradually decreases as the newborn reaches childhood. Adipose tissue is doubled during the first year of life and skeletal muscle mass is relatively less than in the adult. Protein binding of drugs in the neonate or infant is decreased (Morselli et al., 1980). Drugs that are highly lipid soluble, water soluble or protein bound must be carefully adjusted to account for these differences.

Age-related differences exist in drug metabolism and elimination in the paediatric patient. Certain types of hepatic metabolism increase from birth and during childhood, occurring at rates that exceed those of adults. Renal clearance increases from birth and at six months of life is equally proportional to adult function when based on body surface area (Aperia et al., 1975).

One must remember that children are not small adults. Drug doses must be individualized and based on the important differences that exist pharmacokinetically and pharmacodynamically between adults and children.

Drug Interactions

Management of drug interactions plays an important role in drug therapy. Interactions can be so severe as to totally negate the therapeutic action of a drug or to enhance its effect to the point of toxicity. A drug–drug interaction occurs when the effects of one drug are modified by the concomitant administration of another. For the sake of this discussion, the 'target drug' will refer to the agent that is being affected and the 'object drug' will refer to the offending agent. Interactions can be classified in two general categories; pharmacokinetic and pharmacodynamic. Pharmacokinetic interactions deal with the object drug's disposition. One may see changes in absorption, distribution, metabolism and excretion. Pharmacodynamic interactions deal with changes in the patient's response to the drug combination without changes in the two agents' pharmacokinetics. Synergism, antagonism and additive effects are examples of pharmacodynamic interactions.

Alterations in the extent of absorption can occur when the target drug has an interacting effect on the absorption of the object drug. These interactions can merely slow absorption or affect the total extent of absorption. Decreases in the amount of drug absorbed can result from formation of large complexes or changes in gastrointestinal pH. These types of reactions can be avoided simply by separating the administration time of the interacting agents.

Absorption rate can be slowed by agents that slow gastric motility, such as anticholinergic drugs. In contrast, agents that increase gastric motility can increase the absorption rate. Metoclopramide is an agent that increases gastric motility. Few clinically important drug–drug interactions fall into this subcategory.

Protein binding may play an important role in the distribution of drug–drug interactions. This is especially true when two agents that are both highly protein bound (greater than 90%) are used. In this situation, one agent (object drug) can displace the other (target drug) from its protein binding and thus potentiate the displaced agent's (target drug) pharmacological action. An example of this is the concomitant use of sulfazalazine and warfarin. A temporary increase in the effect of warfarin is seen due to an increase in its free blood level.

Drug–drug interactions that affect the metabolism of the target drug are clinically important. The metabolic rate may be increased or decreased. These types of reactions are a result of the object drug's effect on the cytochrome P-450 system. This a mixed-function oxidase system responsible for the metabolism of many drugs. Cytochrome P-450 inhibitors include cimetidine, allopurinol and disulfiram. Barbiturates are well-known cytochrome P-450 inducers.

Combination therapy with object drug and target drug is usually not a problem if dosage adjustments are made to keep the target drug's blood levels within therapeutic ranges. Clinically significant interactions can occur when the object drug is discontinued. As the effects of the object drug are no longer present, there is a potential for the target agent's blood levels to fall into the subtherapeutic range or toxic range, depending on the nature of the interaction (induction or inhibition). Since the effects of the object drug can continue for days after it is discontinued, dose adjustments of the target are hard to predict. Close observation of the patient and laboratory values, if pertinent, are prudent .

Changes in glomerular filtration rate, tubular secretion or urine pH may alter the excretion of some drugs. There are few clinically significant drug–drug interactions which fall into this subcategory. An example of historical interest was the co-administration of penicillin and probenecid. Probenecid impairs the secretion of penicillin. This interaction was used so that lower doses of penicillin could be administered when this agent was first developed.

Synergism occurs when the combined effect of two agents is greater than the algebraic sum of their individual effects. Synergistic interactions can be desired or unwanted. An unwanted synergistic effect usually involves potentiation of an adverse effect. An example of a desired synergism is the use of gentamicin with a beta-lactam antibiotic to enhance antibacterial activity.

Antagonism occurs when there is opposition between two medicines. In this situation, the antagonistic agent can be though of as an antidote. Examples of this type of interaction are the administration of vitamin K to reverse the effects of warfarin or the administration of romazicon to reverse the sedative effects of benzodiazepines.

In contrast to synergistic interactions, additive interactions occur when the effect of combination therapy is equal to the algebraic sum of the agents' individual effects. These types of interactions are usually unwanted. Additive interactions are usually expressed as pronounced side-effects. An example would be the sedative effects of an elderly patient receiving long-acting benzodiazepines and narcotic analgesics. Excessive sedation in this patient population can lead to altered mental status.

Compliance with the Medication Regimen

When drug therapy is prescribed the patient must be educated and motivated in order to assume active responsibility for the management of their medication regimen. Compliance with a medication regimen averages 50%, and ranges between 30% and 80% (Sackett, 1976). Morbidity and mortality associated with medication use costs the US health care system billions of dollars each year and results in approximately 10% of all hospital admissions (Manasse, 1995). Patient involvement in medication management results in increased compliance. Nurses and other health care workers can be involved with identifying, resolving and preventing potential and actual drug-related problems by counselling patients about medication information, management and compliance. Information given to the patient should include written and verbal instruction. It should include the name, dosage, route, and duration of the medicine, as well as any special precautions, drug interactions, self-monitoring techniques, and instructions of what to do in the event of a missed dose.

Drug Therapy

Drugs Used in Inflammatory Bowel Disease (see Table 18.1)

Sulfasalazine

Sulfasalazine combines sulfapyridine with 5-aminosalicylate by means of a chemical bond. This bond must be cleaved by colonic bacteria in

Table 18.1: Common drug interactions of medication used in IBD.

Target drug	Object drug		Description
corticosteroids	salycilates, isoniazid	↓	decreased serum levels of object drug
hydantoins, barbiturates, ephedrine	corticosteroids	↓	decreased effect of corticosteroid may be observed
oral contraceptives, macrolide antibiotics, estrogens, ketoconazole	corticosteroids	↑	clearance of corticosteroids may be decreased
corticosteroids	cyclosporine, digoxin	↑	increased risk of toxicity of object drug
sulfasalazine	digoxin, folic acid	↓	decreased absorption of object drug when coadministered
sulfasalazine	oral anticoagulants, methotrexate, oral hypoglycemic agents	↓	decreased effect of object drug
methotrexate	phenytoin	↓	decreased phenytoin effectiveness
non-steroidal anti-inflammatory drugs	methotrexate	↑	increased risk of methotrexate toxicity
6-mercaptopurine	trimethoprim-sulfamethoxazole	↑	increased risk of bone marrow suppression
azathioprine	anticoagulants, cyclosporine	↓	decreased action of object drugs
allopurinol, methotrexate	azathioprine	↑	increased risk of azathioprine toxicity
ACE inhibitors	azathioprine	↑	concurrent use may induce severe neutropenia
anticonvulsants, rifampin	cyclosporine	↑	increased cyclosporine metabolism
diltiazem, erythromycin, fluconazole, ketoconazole ranitidine, vancomycin, cimetidine, quinolones	cyclosporine	↑	increased risk of nephrotoxicity
cyclosporine	digoxin	↑	elevated digoxin levels

order for the drug to be activated. Sulfasalazine exerts its beneficial effects in ulcerative colitis due to the local effects of the 5-aminosalicylic acid, not the sulfapyridine (Klotz et al., 1980). Its exact mechanism of action is unknown. Once the 5-aminosalicylic acid reaches the diseased colonic mucosa it acts locally to suppress inflammation. Up to 21% of patients taking sulfasalazine experience adverse effects (Dukes and Duncan, 1992). Adverse reactions to sulfasalazine can be dose related or idiosyncratic. The majority of sulfazalazine's adverse effects are dose related, tend to occur early in therapy, and are increased when doses reach or exceed 4 g per day. Dose-related reactions include nausea, vomiting, anorexia, headache, fever and arthralgias. Haematological side-effects such as anaemias can also occur. Dose-related side-effects can be minimized by initiating therapy with low doses of 0.5 g/day and increasing in gradual increments as tolerated by the patient. The drug should be temporarily discontinued until dose-related side-effects resolve, and then reinstituted at a lower dose if tolerated by the patient. Enteric-coated sulfasalazine is available, with the advantage of decreasing gastrointestinal irritation. Idiosyncratic reactions to sulfasalazine are infrequent, but more severe. Such reactions include agranulocytosis, skin rashes, topical epidermal necrolysis, exfoliative dermatitis, pulmonary complications, hepatotoxicity, pancreatitis, Lupus-like syndrome, nephrotic syndrome and worsening of colitis. Withdrawal of sulfasalazine at the first indication of such a reaction will help minimize the sequelae. Patients should be informed that sulfasalazine will cause yellow-orange discoloration of the urine and photosensitivity. Folic acid supplementation may be necessary in patients taking sulfasalazine. Impaired folate absorption can occur and result in macrocytic anaemia. Folic acid 1 mg/day reduces the incidence of folate depletion.

5-Aminosalicylic Acid Derivatives

Dosage formulations of 5-aminosalicylic acid derivatives have been developed to deliver the active moiety of sulfasalazine and avoid the side-effects of sulfapyridine. These formulations are generally better tolerated than sulfasalazine and deliver higher doses of active drug to specific sites within the intestine. Both oral and rectal formulations are available by the name of mesalamine in the USA and mesalazine in Europe. Mesalamine is available in the USA as a retention enema, rectal suppository and controlled-release oral system. Rectal administration requires local contact to exert its effect (Kruis et al., 1982). This therapy is therefore limited to patients with distal colon involvement. The most common side-effects are anal irritation and pruritus (McPhee et al., 1987). Oral formulations of controlled release mesalamine and osalazine were developed to increase the area of exposure of 5-aminosalicylic acid and eliminate the sulfapyridine. Osalazine is associated with profuse watery diarrhoea, which appears to be dose related.

Corticosteroids

Corticosteroids are used in the treatment of both ulcerative colitis and Crohn's disease. It is thought that their mechanism of action in inflammatory bowel disease is through non-specific anti-inflammatory properties and that they probably do not alter the underlying disease process (Hawthorne et al., 1989). Parenteral steroids are reserved for severe or exacerbated disease. Extensive disease requires the use of oral steroids, while active ulcerative proctitis, distal ulcerative colitis and distal Crohn's disease respond to treatment with hydrocortisone enemas or foam. Up to 50% of patients treated with high-dose prednisone therapy experience side-effects and almost 33% experience side-effects at prophylactic doses (Singleton et al., 1979). Frequent adverse effects include facial mooning, acne and skin rash. Peptic ulcer disease, hypertension, severe emotional disturbance, immunosuppression and diabetes may also occur. Of importance to patients with inflammatory bowel disease, corticosteroids can mimic, mask or intensify the symptoms or complications of this disease. Cutaneous atrophy caused by corticosteroids can increase the predisposition of intestinal wall perforation in the patient with ulcerative colitis (Colomb, 1971). Decreased wound healing caused by cutaneous atrophy can also increase surgical morbidity and mortality (Knudsen et al., 1976). Patients requiring long-term steroids may benefit from alternate-day dosing or the addition of an immune modifier to reduce steroid requirements and minimize side-effects (Linn and Peppercorn, 1992a). Additional doses of steroids may be necessary in patients receiving chronic corticosteroid therapy when undergoing surgery or other stressful events. During physiological stress the adrenal glands can secrete between 200 and 500 mg of hydrocortisone per day. Patients receiving chronic exogenous glucocorticoid therapy may be unable to increase endogenous cortisol production in response to stress-related events. This is due to suppression of the hypothalmic-pituitary-adrenocorticoid (HPA) axis via chronic feedback inhibition of adrenocorticotropin. When circulating levels of cortisol are low during an acute stress event, hypotension, hypoglycaemia and cardiovascular collapse can result. The amount of suppression is related to steroid

dose, schedule, route of administration and duration of therapy
(Melby, 1974). Doses of prednisone (or its equivilent) greater that 7.5
mg per day are associated with slower recovery of HPA axis respon-
siveness after stopping therapy than in patients receiving lower doses.
Recommendations are aimed at corticosteroid supplementation to
those patients undergoing surgery who have used steroids in the past
year or are currently receiving steroids. The most frequently used agent
for steroid supplementation is intravenous or intramuscular hydrocortisone either as the hemisuccinate or phosphate salt. For major surgical
procedures doses equivalent to the known maximal endogenous hydrocortisone production have been recommended (Roizen, 1986; Atkinson
et al., 1987). Hydrocortisone should be administered every 6 hours
intravenously or intramuscularly starting immediately prior to surgery
and rapidly tapered over 2 to 3 days, based on the patient's clinical
status (Symerng et al., 1981; Roizen, 1986).

Immune Modifiers

The immunosuppressive agents azothioprine and its metabolite 6-
mercaptopurine (6-MP) have become accepted therapy for refractory
cases of inflammatory bowel disease. They are used more commonly
in Crohn's disease than ulcerative colitis, where surgery is more often
used for refractory cases. Immune modifiers have been used to treat
enteric and perianal fistulae (Present, 1989). These drugs have also
been shown to be useful in maintaining remission and reducing steroid
doses in patients with Crohn's disease. One study found that steroid
doses were able to be reduced or discontinued in 75% of patients
receiving 6-MP as compared with 36% receiving placebo. 6-MP was
more efficacious in fistula healing as compared with placebo (Present
et al., 1980). The onset of action can take up to 3 months. Doses are
lower than those used in transplant patients and range from 1 to 2
mg/kg/day. Toxicity can be severe and occurs in 7.6% of patients.
Bone marrow suppression, pancreatitis, allergic reactions and nausea
are among the side-effects (Present et al., 1989).

Cyclosporine has been investigated for its use in inflammatory
bowel disease. Its use is well established in preventing organ rejection
in transplant patients. Continuous infusion cyclosporine was studied in
severe ulcerative colitis refractory to steroids, in a randomized, double-
blind, controlled trial. Some 82% of cylcosporine-treated patients
showed improvement compared with none in the placebo group. The
study was terminated prematurely because of these positive results and
five of the placebo group patients were then treated with cyclosporine.

Each of these patients responded to cyclosporine treatment (Lichtiger et al., 1994). Oral cyclosporine has been shown to have some benefit in short-term management of Crohn's disease when corticosteroids fail (Peppercorn, 1990). However, once cyclosporine therapy is discontinued, disease relapse occurs. Cyclosporine has numerous significant drug interactions as well as serious side-effects. Nephrotoxicity and neurotoxicity are associated with long-term use.

Metronidazole

Antibiotics have been used in the treatment of inflammatory bowel disease based on the theory that infection may have a role in the disease process. Only metronidazole has been shown to have a clear role in the treatment of Crohn's disease (Linn and Peppercorn, 1992b). In perianal Crohn's disease, metronidazole has been shown to be safe and effective in a 3-year follow-up study (Brandt et al., 1982). Side-effects of metronidazole are nausea, anorexia, fatigue, metallic taste and coated tongue. Long-term therapy is associated with dose-related, persistent paraesthesias.

Methotrexate

The use of methotrexate in the treatment of inflammatory diseases such as rheumatoid arthritis, asthma and psoriasis has led to the investigation of its use in persistent inflammatory bowel disease. Doses of 25 mg of methotrexate administered by intramuscular injection weekly to patients with chronically active ulcerative colitis and Crohn's disease have demonstrated clinical benefit as well as steroid reduction. Methotrexate can cause gastrointestinal distress, hepatic enzyme elevation and leucopenia.

Nicotine

Nicotine cessation has been associated with the development of ulcerative colitis, although its exact role is unclear. The use of nicotine has been tested in the treatment of ulcerative colitis in recent years. Studies using both nicotine transdermal patches and nicotine gum have been conducted (Lashner et al., 1990; Pullan et al., 1994; Thomas et al., 1995). Adverse effects of dizziness, sleep disturbances, headache and tremor led to patient withdrawal. Results of these studies show mixed results, leading to the conclusion that the role of nicotine in ulcerative colitis remains in question.

Cromolyn

Cromolyn sodium, which inhibits the release of inflammatory substances from sensitized mast cells, has been theorized to have a role in ulcerative colitis. Initial trials demonstrated prevention of acute attacks and improvement of rectal biopsy tissue. Relapse rate was unaffected (Heatley et al., 1975; Della Calla et al., 1976; Mani et al., 1976). More recent studies show no benefit of cromolyn over placebo and less efficacy of cromolyn over sulfasalazine (Babb, 1980; Binder et al., 1981; Dronfield and Langman, 1978).

Antidiarrhoeal Agents

The frequency of a patient's stool is highly variable. Diarrhoea is defined as an abnormal frequency and liquidity of faecal discharge compared with the patient's norm. In some instances, this condition is the body's defence mechanism against harmful substances or pathogens as in infectious colitis, and stopping the diarrhoea at any cost is not warranted. However, if symptomatic relief is desired, the clinician can choose an agent from the following categories: antimotility, absorbents, antisecretory compounds and intestinal microflora.

Antimotility agents include diphenoxylate, difenoxin, loperamide, paragoric and tincture of opium. Opiates and opioid derivatives are the most common drugs used to treat diarrhoea. Their mechanism of action is slowing intestinal motility which results in increased gastrointestinal contact and absorption. Diphenoxylate and difenoxin are combined with atropine in order to discourage deliberate over-use. Tincture of opium is reserved for cases that do not respond to the other agents or for intractable diarrhoea. The most common side-effects are nausea, vomiting, dry mouth and headache. Reduction of intestinal motility may be deleterious in diarrhoea resulting from certain bacteria as well as from pseudomembranous enterocolitis associated with broad-spectrum antibiotic use. The use of opiates can predispose patients with inflammatory bowel disease to toxic megacolon and is therefore not recommended.

Kaolin-pectin mixture and attapulgite comprise the adsorbent category. Their exact mechanism of action is unknown. It is thought that these agents adsorb toxins, drugs and digestive juices. Since they have the potential to interfere with the absorption of other pharmacological agents, their administration should be 2 hours apart from other agents.

Bismuth subsalicylate is a trivalent bismuth compound. Its exact mechanism of action is not known. It may be due to both antimicrobial and antisecretory properties (Gorbach, 1990; Lambert, 1991). Each molecule contains 42% salicylate and 58% bismuth. Salicylate has the potential to displace warfarin from protein binding and thus increase its anticoagulant effect. Patients should be informed that stools may temporarily appear grey-black. Salicylate toxicity is a risk when recommended doses are exceeded.

Lactobacillus preparations are used in diarrhoea in the hope of replacing the colonic microflora. These preparations have been tried in diarrhoea secondary to antibiotic therapy. Their use is controversial owing to the lack of clinical studies.

Octreotide has been effective in the treatment of secretory diarrhoea. Octreotide is an analogue of naturally occurring somatostatin. Doses of 50 to 200 µg subcutaneously two to three times daily have been used for control of diarrhoea. This agent has also been used to decrease high stoma output. Octreotide can cause glucose intolerance in some non-diabetic individuals and conversely may reduce insulin requirements in insulin-dependent diabetics.

Laxatives

Treatment of underlying disease and correction of any predisposing factors that may be causing constipation should be undertaken whenever possible when considering laxative use. Drugs such as narcotics, aluminium hydroxide antacids, anticholinergics, iron supplements and some antihypertensive agents can induce constipation. Often a change in diet and an increase in fluid intake will alleviate constipation. Laxatives can be used in conjunction with dietary modification to facilitate bowel evacuation.

Fibre is often beneficial in patients with chronic constipation. It increases the mass and moisture content of the stool. Fibre can be added by increasing dietary sources or by using bulk-forming agents. Several fibre supplements are available in tablet and wafer forms.

Emollient laxatives are surface-active wetting and dispersing agents that work by softening the stool and allowing water and fat to penetrate the faecal mass. Emollient laxatives are available as various salts of docusate. The amount of sodium, calcium or potassium in the formulations is considered clinically insignificant. Concurrent use of docusate and mineral oil is contraindicated because of the increased risk of toxicity from the mineral oil. Liquid formulations of docusate should be mixed with milk or fruit juice to mask the bitter taste.

Bulk-forming agents adsorb water in the intestine to increase the mass of the stool which promotes peristalsis and reduces transit time.

The most common preparations are psyllium derivatives. These are available as powders, granules and wafers which must be mixed in water or juice before drinking. Bulk-forming agents must not be used in patients with faecal impaction or gastrointestinal obstruction. Patients with insufficient fluid intake may be predisposed to faecal impaction or intestinal obstruction. The effects of digoxin, warfarin, salicylates, potassium-sparing diuretics, tetracyclines and nitrofurantoin are decreased with concurrent administration. Products containing aspartame as a sweetener are contraindicated in patients with phenylketonuria. Patients should be advised that the full effect of psyllium can take up to two to three days.

Stimulant cathartics include castor oil, bisacodyl, senna and cascara. These agents have a direct action on the intestinal mucosa resulting in an increased rate of colonic motility and a change in fluid and electrolyte secretion. All stimulant laxatives produce some degree of intestinal discomfort, nausea and mild cramps. Stimulant laxatives can be habit forming and result in a loss of normal bowel function with long-term use. Castor oil acts primarily in the large intestine and produces bowel evacuation within two to six hours. Chilling the liquid or taking it with juice or carbonated beverages improves the palatability. Castor oil can increase the risk of toxic megacolon in patients with inflammatory bowel disease. Bisacodyl is available as either oral tablets or rectal suppositories. Tablets have an onset of six to 10 hours and suppositories exert their effect within 15 minutes to an hour. Bisacodyl can decrease the effect of warfarin. Patients should be informed not to crush or chew the tablets. Antraquinone cathartics such as extract of cascara and extract of senna have an onset of action of between six and 10 hours. Liquid and tablet formulations are available. Pink to red or brown discoloration of the urine can occur.

Saline laxatives attract and retain water on the intestinal lumen resulting in an increase in intraluminal pressure. Therapeutic doses usually produce semi-fluid or watery stool in three to six hours or less. Milk of magnesia, magnesium citrate solution, lactulose and lavage solutions of sodium phosphates or polyethylene glycol are considered saline laxatives. Caution should be taken when magnesium-containing laxatives are used in renal impairment, as hypermagnesaemia can occur due to decreased renal excretion of magnesium.

A polyethylene glycol-electrolyte solution is often used for mechanical bowel preparation when necessary. The solution, administered orally, induces diarrhoea within 30 to 60 minutes and results in a rapid cleansing of the bowel, usually within four hours. The electrolyte concentration of the non-absorbable solution results in a lack of absorption or secretion of ions. Large volumes of this solution can be administered without a significant change in water or electrolyte balance.

The solution is administered to the patient in a fasting state of three to four hours. The adult dosage is four litres of solution. The patient should be instructed to drink 240 ml every 10 minutes until 4 litres are consumed or the rectal effluent is clear. The solution may be given via a nasogastric tube, at a rate of 20 to 30 ml per minute, to those patients unable or unwilling to drink the solution. The solution must be reconstituted with a volume of 4 litres of water. Tap water can be used. Chilling the solution prior to administration improves the palatability. The most common adverse reactions are nausea, abdominal fullness and bloating. Abdominal cramps, anal irritation and vomiting occur less frequently. Adverse reactions are considered transient and rapidly subside.

Sodium phosphate solution is also used for mechanical bowel evacuation. The solution exerts its osmotic effect by drawing water into the lumen of the gut, producing distension and promoting peristalsis and evacuation of the bowel. The onset of action is within three to six hours. Adverse effects include electrolyte imbalances, nausea and vomiting. Cautious use is recommended for patients with renal failure, congestive heart failure or cirrhosis. Patient tolerability to sodium phosphate solution was shown to be better when compared with polyethylene glycol solution. Patients were better able to tolerate the smaller volume of solution, and had less abdominal pain, bloating and fatigue (Oliveira et al., 1997).

Antiflatulents

Simethicone disperses and prevents the formation of gas pockets in the gastrointestinal tract. It decreases the surface tension of gas bubbles enabling them to coalesce. Gas is eliminated by belching or passing flatus. It is effectively used as an adjunct in many conditions producing gas retention. Simethicone is available in a variety of dosage forms including capsules, tablets, chewable tablets and drops. The drug is safe for use in infants. Simethicone can cause a false negative gastric guaiac result as a result of test interference.

Charcoal is an adsorbent, detoxicant and soothing agent that reduces the volume of gastrointestinal gas and relieves the discomfort this causes. Diarrhoea is a common side-effect. A major disadvantage of the use of charcoal is the adsorption of other drugs when taken concurrently. Charcoal can also remove drugs from the systemic circulation. It is recommended that charcoal be taken 2 hours before or 1 hour after other medication. Patients should be informed that charcoal can cause the stools to turn black.

Anorectal Preparations

Ointments, suppositories and foams can be effective for relief of symptoms associated with haemorrhoids and perianal itching. The available preparations contain various ingredients. Hydrocortisone is added to reduce inflammation, itching and swelling. Local anaesthetics provide temporary relief of pain, itching and irritation. Burning and itching are the most frequently encountered adverse effects of the local anaesthetics. Vasoconstrictors reduce the swelling and congestion of the anorectal tissues. Astringents such as witch hazel and zinc oxide coagulate the cell protein in the skin, protecting the underlying tissue and decreasing the cell volume thereby reducing inflammation and irritation. Emollients and protective agents include glycerine, lanolin, mineral oil, petrolatum, zinc oxide, shark liver oil, cocoa butter and bismuth salts. These agents form a protective barrier on the skin surface. Camphor may be used as a counter-irritant to distract the perception of pain and itching by producing a cool, tingling or warm sensation. Keratolytics such as resorcinol cause sloughing of the epidermal layer and may help expose underlying tissue to therapeutic agents. Resorcinol should not be used on open wounds. Wound-healing agents are claimed to promote tissue repair. This claim has not been conclusively demonstrated.

Antimicrobial Surgical Prophylaxis

Antimicrobial prophylaxis is of benefit in surgical procedures associated with a high incidence of infection. Surgical procedures that enter the gastrointestinal tract benefit from the use of antibiotics administered prophylactically. The most common complication following colorectal surgery is wound infection. Specifically, the goal of antimicrobial prophylaxis for elective colorectal surgery is to minimize the risk of bacterial contamination to the operative wound. The concentration of resident bacteria must be reduced in order to achieve a decreased risk of infection. Infection rates as high as 40% have been associated with the lack of reduction of resident bacteria (Polk and Lopez-Meyer, 1969; Burton, 1973). Risk factors associated with an increased risk of postoperative infection include impaired immunity, age greater than 60 years, hypoalbuminaemia, poor preoperative bowel preparation, and bacterial contamination of the surgical wound.

The timing of antimicrobial administration is crucial in preventing postoperative infection. Administration of the antibiotic within 30 minutes of surgical incision and persisting in adequate tissue concentrations throughout the operative procedure ensures efficacy (Classen et al., 1992). Antimicrobial administration after bacterial contamination markedly diminishes efficacy. When a short-acting antimicrobial is administered, it should be repeated if the operation exceeds 3 to 4 hours. The use of an agent with a longer half-life and duration of action is appropriate when an operation is expected to last 6 to 8 hours.

Various drug regimens have been studied for prophylaxis for colorectal surgery including oral and parenteral agents. The choice of prophylactic regimen should include activity against Gram-positive and Gram-negative aerobes and anaerobic bacteria (Page et al., 1993). Oral regimens may include neomycin in combination with erythromycin, metronidazole or clindamycin in doses high enough to reduce resident colonic flora (Anonymous, 1992). Preoperative oral antimicrobials are not used in infants and young children as the safety and efficacy of such regimens have not been documented. Several different regimens of intravenous antimicrobials have been used with successful results. Intravenous antibiotic choice often includes, either singly or in combination, a cephalosporin, an aminoglycoside, metronidazole, or erythromycin. Often a combination of oral and intravenous antibiotics is used in an attempt to further decrease the rate of postoperative infection in adults. The results of such studies remain inconsistent. Postoperative wound infection rates have declined from 30–60% to less than 10% in clean-contaminated procedures when antimicrobial agents are combined with mechanical bowel preparation.

References

Anonymous – ASHP Commission on Therapeutics (1992) ASHP therapeutic guidelines on antimicrobial prophylaxis in surgery. Clinical Pharmacy 11: 483–513.

Aperia A, Bromberg O, Thodenius K, Zelterstrom R (1975) Development of renal control of salt and fluid homeostasis during the first year of life. Acta Paediatrica Scandinavica 64: 393.

Atkinson RS, Rushman GB, Lee JA (Eds) (1987) A Synopsis of Anaesthesia, 10th edn. Bristol: Bath Press, pp 423–4.

Babb RR (1980) Cromolyn sodium in the treatment of ulcerative colitis. Journal of Clinical Gastroenterology 2: 229–31.

Binder V, Elsborg L, Greibe, Henderiksen C, Hoj L, Jensen KB, Kristensen E, Madsen JR, Marner B, Riis P, Willumsen L (1981) Disodium cromoglycate in the treatment of ulcerative colitis and Crohn's disease. Gut 22: 55–60.

Brandt LJ, Bernstein LH, Boley SJ, Frank MS (1982) Metronidazole therapy for perianal Crohn's disease: a follow-up study. Gastroenterology 83: 383–7.

Burton RC (1973) Postoperative wound infection in colon and rectal surgery. British Journal of Surgery 60: 363–8.

Chernoff R (1990) Physiologic aging and nutritional status. Nutrition in Clinical Practice 5: 8–13.

Classen DC, Evans RS, Pestotnik SL, Horn SD, Menlove RL, Burke JP (1992) The timing of prophylactic administration of antibiotics and the risk of surgical-wound infection. New England Journal of Medicine 326: 281–6.

Colomb D (1971) Cutaneous manifestations in long term general corticotherapy. Study of 100 cases. Presse Medicale 79: 1011.

Della Calla G, Garibaldi LR, Durand P (1976) Ulcerative colitis and disodium cromoglycate. Lancet 1: 1129.

Dronfield MW Langman MJ (1978) Comparative trial of sulphasalazine and oral sodium cromoglycate and sulfasalazine in the maintenance of remission in ulcerative colitis. Lancet 1: 119.

Dukes GE, Duncan BS (1992) Inflammatory bowel disease. In Young LY and Koda-Kimble MA (Eds) Applied Therapeutics: The Clinical Use of Drugs. Vancouver: Applied Therapeutics.

Gorbach SL (1990) Bismuth therapy in gastrointestinal diseases. Gastroenterology 99: 863–75.

Hansten PD, Horn JR (1986) Mechanisms of drug interactions: protein binding displacement. Drug Interactions Newsletter 6: 9–12.

Hawthorne AB, Hawkey CJ et al. (1989) Immunosuppressive drugs in inflammatory bowel disease. A review of their mechanisms and place in therapy. Drugs 38: 267–88.

Heatley RV, Calcraft BJ, Rhodes J, Owen E, Evans BK (1975) Disodium cromoglycate in the treatment of chronic proctitis. Gut 16: 559–63.

Hooper DC, Wolfson JS (1985) The fluoroquinolones: pharmacology, clinical uses, and toxicities in humans. Antimicrobial Agents and Chemotherapy 28: 716.

Klotz U, Maier K, Fischer C, Henkel K et al. (1980) Therapeutic efficacy of sulfasalazine and its metabolites in patients with ulcerative colitis and Crohn's disease. New England Journal of Medicine 303: 1499–502.

Knudsen L, Christiansen L, Jarnum S (1976) Early complications in patients previously treated with corticosteroids. Scandinavian Journal of Gastroenterology 11(Suppl 3): 123–8.

Kruis W, Bull U, Eiseberg J, Paumgartner G (1982) Retrograde colonic spread of sulfasalazine enemas. Scandinavian Journal of Gastroenterology 17: 933.

Lambert JR (1991) Pharmacology of bismuth-containing compounds. Review of Infectious Diseases 13(Suppl 8): 691–5.

Lashner BA, Hanauer SB, Silverserstin MD (1990) Testing nicotine gum for ulcerative colitis patients. Digestive Diseases and Sciences 35: 827–32.

Lichtiger S, Present DH, Kornbluth A, Gelernt I, Bauer J, Galler G, Michelassi F, Hanauer S (1994) Cyclosporine in severe ulcerative colitis refractory to steroid therapy. New England Journal of Medicine 330: 1841–5.

Linn FV, Peppercorn MA (1992a) Drug therapy for inflammatory bowel disease: Part I. American Journal of Surgery 164: 85–9.

Linn FV, Peppercorn MA (1992b) Drug therapy in inflammatory bowel disease: Part II. American Journal of Surgery 164: 178–85.

Loeb JN (1976) Corticosteroids and growth. New England Journal of Medicine 295: 547.

McPhee MS Swan JT, Biddle WL, Greenberger NJ (1987) Proctocolitis unresponsive to conventional therapy. Response to 5-aminosalicylic acid enemas. Digestive Diseases and Sciences 32(Suppl 12): 76S–81S.

Manasse HR (1995) Toward defining and applying a higher standard of medication use in the United States. American Journal of Health System Pharmacy 52: 374–7.

Mani V, Lloyd G, Green FH, Fox H, Turnberg LA (1976) Treatment of ulcerative colitis with oral disodium cromolglycate – a double-blind trial. Lancet 1: 439–41.

Melby JC (1974) Systemic corticosteroid therapy: pharmacology and endocrinologic considerations. Annals of Internal Medicine 81: 505–12.

Morselli PL, Franco-Morselli R, Bossi L (1980) Clinical phamacokinetics in newborns and neonates. Clinical Pharmacokinetics 5: 485.

Oliveira L, Wexner SD, Daniel N, DeMarta D, Weiss EG, Nogueras JJ, Bernstein (1997) Mechanical bowel preparation for elective colorectal surgery. A prospective, randomized, surgeon-blinded trial comparing sodium phosphate and polyethylene glycol-based oral lavage solutions. Diseases of the Colon and Rectum 40(5): 585–91.

Page CP, Bohnen JM, Fletcher JR, McManus AT, Solomkin JS, Wittmann DH (1993) Antimicrobial prophylaxis for surgical wounds: guidelines for clinical care. Archives of Surgery 128: 79–88.

Peppercorn MA (1990) Advances in drug therapy for inflammatory bowel disease. Annals of Internal Medicine 112: 50–60.

Polk H, Lopez-Meyer J (1969) Postoperative wound infection: a prospective study of determinant factors and prevention. Surgery 66: 97–103

Present DH (1989) 6-mercaptopurine and other immunosuppresive agents in the treatment of Crohn's disease and ulcerative colitis. Gastroenterological Clinics of North America 18(1): 57–71.

Present DH, Korelitz BI, Wisch N, Glass JL, Sachar DB, Pasternack BS (1980) Treatment of Crohn's disease with 6-mercaptopurine. New England Journal of Medicine 302(18): 981–7.

Present DH, Meltzer SJ, Krumholtz MP, Wolke A, Koreelitz BI (1989) 6-mercaptopurine in the management of inflammatory bowel disease: short- and long-term toxicity. Annals of Internal Medicine 111: 641–9.

Pullan RD, Rhodes J, Ganesh S, Mani V, Morris JS, Williams GT, Newcombe RG, Russell MA, Feyerabend C, Thomas GA (1994) Transdermal nicotine for active ulcerative colitis. New England Journal of Medicine 330: 811–15.

Roizen MF (1986) Anesthetic implications of concurrent diseases. In Miller RD (Ed.) Anesthesis. Vol 1, 2nd edn. New York: Churchill Livingstone, pp 265–8.

Sackett DL (1976) The magnitude of compliance and noncompliance. In Sackett DL, Haynes RB (Eds) Compliance with Therapeutic Regimens. Baltimore, MD: Johns Hopkins University Press.

Singleton JW, Law DH, Kelley ML, Mekhjian HS, Sturdevant RA (1979) National

Cooperative Crohn's Disease Study: adverse reactions to study drugs. Gastroenterology 77: 870–2.

Symerng T, Karlberg BE, Kagedal B, Schildt B (1981) Physiological cortisol substitution of long-term steroid-treated patients undergoing major surgery. British Journal of Anaesthesia 53: 949–54.

Terrin BN, McWillians NB, Maurer HM (1984) The effects of metoclopramide as an antiemetic in childhood cancer therapy. Journal of Pediatrics 104: 138.

Thomas GA, Rhodes J, Mani V, Williams GT, Newcombe RG, Russell MA, Feyerabend C (1995) Transdermal nicotine as maintenance therapy for ulcerative colitis. New England Journal of Medicine 332: 988–92.

Zimmerman JJ, Feldman S (1981) Physical-chemical properties and biological activity. In Foye WO (Ed.) Principles of Medicinal Chemistry. 2nd edn. Philadelphia: Lea & Febiger.

Index

References to figures and tables occurring separately from their corresponding page ranges are indicated in *italic* and **bold** respectively.

abdomen, examination *see also* physical examination 55, 200
abdominal bloating 55, 71, 224, 230
abdominal pain
  and abdominal examination 55
  colorectal cancer 99
  diverticular disease 190–191, 199
  and endoscopy 71
  intussusception 394, 397
  key symptom 52
  types 54, 99
abdominoperineal excision of rectum (APER) 39, 309
abdominoperineal resection, laparoscopic 266–267
abscess
  and anal fistula 87
  diverticular 194
  drainage 64, 93, 196
  hidradenitis suppurativa 86, 92
  ischiorectal 87, 92–93
  pelvic 188
  perianal 87, 92–93
  perirectal 56
  pilonidal 84, 92
absorbent antidiarrhoeal agents 412
ACE *see* antegrade colonic irrigation
acupuncture 137, 249–250

acute anorectal sepsis 92–94
  microbiology 93, 94
  surgical management 93–94
adenoma-to-carcinoma sequence 97, 147, 150, 154
adenomatous polyps 97
adhesions
  and constipation 212
  laparoscopic lysis 268–269
  and volvulus 391
adjuvant therapy 106–107, 152–153
Aeromonas 358–360
age effects
  body composition 402, 404
  drug therapy 401–406
  drug toxicity 403
  gastrointestinal function 402
  liver function 402–403
albumin, protein binding 402, 404, 405
altered mental states, and rectal sensation 23
alverine citrate (Spasmonal, Relaxyl) 233, 236
5-aminosalicylic acid derivatives 132, 133, 135, 408–409
amoebicide treatment, *Entamoeba histolytica* 325
anaemia 99, 100, 113, 135
anal *see also* anorectal; rectoanal
anal canal
  anatomy 27–28, *79*
  epithelium 27–28
  innervation 39–40

anal conditions
  common 76–78
  presenting as emergencies 92–95
anal encirclement procedure (Thiersch
      wire) 382
anal fissure 82–83
  and constipation 82
  and Crohn's disease 83
  examination 56, 57
  management 83
  symptoms 53–54
anal fistula
  associated conditions 84, 87
  classification 88
  clinical examination 88
  incidence 87
  surgical management 88–92
  wound management 90–91
anal irritation 139
anal plug 299
anal seepage, skin irritation 76–77
anal sensation 23–26, 40
anal sinuses 27
anal sphincterotomy 218
anal sphincters
  anatomy 29–30
  and faecal incontinence 293
  function testing see anorectal
      manometry
  inappropriate contraction 212–213
  muscle tone 24–25, 56–57, 77, 381
  role in defecation 207–208
  voluntary control 208, 295
anal ulcers 323, 326
anal verge 28
anismus 212–213, 215, 218
anogenital warts 321
anoplasty 335, 342
anorectal angle 25–26, 295, 381
anorectal examination 55–57, 58, 381
anorectal herpes 320
anorectal malformations
  classification 333–334
  and faecal incontinence 348–350
  female babies 339–342
  incidence 333
  male babies 336–339
  nursing care 332, 334, 336
  surgical treatment 332, 342–348

anorectal manometry 64–65, 141, 215,
      226, 297
anorectal myectomy 218
anorectal pain 52, 53
anorectal physiology 40, 64–66
anorectal preparations 416
anorectal region, muscles 29–31
anorectal ring 31
anorectal sensation
  loss 381
  testing 297
anorectal ultrasonography 66, 102, 106,
      297–298
anorectovaginal fistula 87
antegrade colonic irrigation (ACE)
      see also irrigation 309–310
anterior levatorplasty, pelvic floor repair
      301–302
anthelmintics 376
antibiotic treatment
  Aeromonas 360
  Campylobacter 361
  Chlamydia spp. 320
  Clostridium difficile 362
  gonorrhoea 319
  hidradenitis 86
  and irritable bowel syndrome 226
  Mycobacterium avium-intracellulare 324
  overuse 361
  preoperative 274, 416–417
  Salmonella, infection 364
  Shigella 326, 365
  syphilis 319
  Yersinia spp. 367
anticancer drugs 110
anticholinergics 234
anticoagulants 69
antidepressants 235
antidiarrhoeal agents 232–233, 235,
      351, 355, 412–413
  viral infections 369, 370
antiflatulents 415–416
antimotility agents 372, 412
antiparasitic treatment
  Cryptosporidium 372
  Isospora belli 325
antispasmodics 226, 228, 233–234
antiviral treatment
  cytomegalovirus 323

herpes simplex virus 321
anus
    digital examination 214
    dilation 81, 83, 342, 346–347
anxiety
    about investigations 67–68
    preoperative 72, 82
APC gene 97, 102, 146, 155–156
APER *see* abdominoperineal excision of
        the rectum
apocrine glands, circumanal 86
appendectomy, laparoscopic 264–265
appendices epiploicae 21, 22, 263
appendix (vermiform) 23
aromatherapy 248–249
Aromatherapy Organisations Council
        249, 255
artificial bowel sphincter (ABS)
        313–314
ascending colon, anatomy 21, 23
aspirin, preventive effects 110
aspirin-containing products, avoidance
        69, 71
Association to Aid the Sexual and
        Personal Relationships of People
        with a Disability (SPOD) 132, 145
astringents 416
astroviruses 367–368
attapulgite 412
azathioprine 132, 135, 410–411

bacillary dysentery 365
bacterial colitis 358–367
bacterial metabolism and fermentation,
        colonic 28
barium enema
    colorectal cancer 100
    constipation 214
    contraindications 63
    diverticular disease 191
    intussusception 394, 397
    irritable bowel syndrome 226
    procedures 63–64
    and volvulus 388, 389, 391
barium meal
    inflammatory bowel disease 126
    irritable bowel syndrome 226
benzodiazepines 235, 403
bichloroacetic acid 322

bile, carcinogenic effect 109, 150
biofeedback therapy
    constipation 217
    faecal incontinence 299
    irritable bowel syndrome 231–232,
        244–245
    rectal ulcer 380
biopsy
    colonoscopic 71
    endoscopic 214
    sigmoidoscopic 59
bismuth salicylate 412–413
blood supply, large intestine 33–37, 103
blood tests 62–63
Blumer's shelf 57
body composition, age effects 402, 404
body image
    colorectal surgery 114
    inflammatory bowel disease 128
    stoma patients 72, 73, 139, 176–177
books and videos *see* patient education
bowel cancer *see* colorectal cancer
bowel cleansing *see* bowel preparation
bowel evacuation, mechanical 415
bowel habit
    medical history 213
    privacy and dignity 210, 219, 220
    re-education 78, 80
bowel habit change
    and abdominal examination 55
    colorectal cancer 99, 113, 212
    diverticular disease 190–191, 199
    irritable bowel syndrome 231
    key symptom 52–53
Bowel Management Program 350–357
bowel obstruction *see* intestinal
        obstruction
bowel preparation
    for colonoscopy 214
    Fleet's enema 59, 61
    laparoscopy 274
    paediatric patients 344–345
    preoperative 274, 300
    procedures 71
    solutions 61, 414–415
    timing 69
bowel sounds 55, 200, 388
Bowenoid papulosis 322

bran *see also* dietary fibre 109, 215–216,
        231, 237
British Acupuncture Council 250, 255
British Colostomy Association 145
British Digestive Foundation 145
British Homeopathy Association 247,
        255
Brooke ileostomy 155
bulking agents 216, 226, 228, 231, 232,
        234–235, 299, 413–414
Buschke–Lowenstein tumours 322

caecum
    anatomy 21, 22–23
    volvulus 390–393
caliciviruses 368–369
call to stool, deferral 22, 381
camphor 416
Campylobacter infection 360–361
cancer, colorectal 97–116
cancer *see also* tumours
cancer registry, role 156–162
Candida albicans, and irritable bowel
        syndrome 240–241
carcinoembryonic antigen (CEA) 63,
        237
cascara 414
castor oil 414
chancre 319
chancroid 326
charcoal 230, 415–416
chemotherapy, desmoid tumours
        152–153
chemotherapy *see* adjuvant therapy
children *see* paediatric patients
Chlamydia spp. 319–320
cholera 366
cinedefecography 66, 72
Citrucel 202
Cleveland Clinic continence score 296,
        297
Cleveland Clinic Foundation familial
        adenomatous polyposis (FAP)
        Registry 147, 151, 157
Clostridium difficile 124, 361–362
coccydynia 53–54
codeine 298
colectomy
    with ileorectal anastomosis 139

segmental 103, 193
subtotal 162
total 138
colitis
    infectious 358–377
    parasitic 324–325
Collaborative Group of the Americas on
        Inherited Colorectal Cancer 162
coloenteric fistula 197
colovaginal fistula 197
colon
    anatomy 21–24
    blood supply 103
    contractile activity 41–22
    diverticular disease 188–204
    emptying into rectum 22
    metabolic function 26–28
    microflora 28
    water absorption 22, 120, 207, 209,
        211, 212
colonic *see also* colorectal
colonic cancer, treatment 103
colonic conduit 310–313, **314**
colonic constipation 211–213
colonic irrigation 350–355
colonic reservoir 106
colonic transit time 41, 209, 210, 211
    gender differences 41
    studies 65–66, 214–215
colonoscopy
    colorectal cancer 100–101
    constipation 214
    indications 61
    inflammatory bowel disease 124–126
    instrument *61*
    nurse's role 71
    procedure 61–62
    risks 62, 101
    sedation 71
    and sigmoidoscopy 80
    volvulus reduction 389
colorectal cancer
    abdominal pain 99
    adjuvant therapy 106–107
    aetiology 97
    associated findings 100
    associated with intussusception 397
    barium enema 100
    bowel habit change 99, 212

colonoscopy 100–101
diagnostic studies 99–101
dietary aspects 108–111
Dukes' staging 106
family history 100
gender differences 98
genetic factors 97, 102, 110–111
health education 108–111
high-risk patients 61, 102, 111, 120
imaging studies 100, 102
incidence and prevalence 97, 98
laparoscopic surgery 269–271
left- and right-sided 98–99, 103, 113
liver involvement 100–102
nurse–patient relationship 113–115
nursing care 108
physical examination 99–101
presentation 113
prognosis and outcome 106
psychological aspects 114
rectal bleeding 98–99, 113
screening and early detection 98,
    108, 111–113
signs and symptoms 98–99
staging 37, 64, 66, 101–102
support 113–115
surveillance and follow-up 107–108
systemic effects 53, 99
treatment options 103–106, 114
colorectal patients
body image 114
nursing aspects 14–15, 67–68
paediatric 332–357
patient education 300
postoperative care 300–301
sexual concerns 114
symptoms 52–54
voluntary/self-help groups 115
colorectal surgery
laparoscopic 256–285
nurse specialists 115–116
colostomy
closure 347–348
descending 193, *194*
output 170, 171
paediatric 335, 342–344
permanent 168–169, 355
procedures 168–171

temporary 169–171
transverse loop 198
colouretericfistula 197
colovaginal fistula 195
colovesical fistula 191, 195, 197
complementary therapies
inflammatory bowel disease 137
irritable bowel syndrome 245–251
compliance, drug regime 80, **82**, 406
condyloma
examination 56
and human papilloma virus 321
and perianal mass 54
condyloma acuminata 54
condyloma latum 319
congenital malformations, anorectal
    293, 332–357
constipating agents *see also*
    antidiarrhoeal agents 298
constipation
and adhesions and strictures 212
and anal fissure 82
biofeedback therapy 217
causes 208–213
colonic 211–213
and colorectal cancer 53, 99
colostomy patients 180
definition 206–207
and diabetes 210
dietary aspects 208–209
and diverticular disease 211
as drug side-effect 210, 220
extracolonic 208–211
gender differences 210
hospital patients 210
and hypothyroidism 210
imaging studies 214
investigations 213–215
and irritable bowel syndrome 211,
    231–232
and laxative use 217
and menstrual cycle 210
misperceived 80
and neurological disorders 211
nursing management 218–220
patient education 217
and pregnancy 210–211
and psychiatric disorders 210
surgical treatment 217–218

symptoms 206–207
    treatment 215–218
constipation *see also* bowel habit
contrast studies *see also* barium enema
    63
corticosteroids 403, 409–410
cosmesis, improved 258, 267, 272
counselling 137, 176, 231–232, 327
Crohn's disease
    and anal fissures 83
    and anal fistula 87, 90
    associated conditions **124**
    azathioprine and 6-mercaptopurine
        410–411
    corticosteroid treatment 409–410
    disease pattern 120–124, *125*
    perianal 56
    signs and symptoms **124**
    surgery 143
Crohn's disease *see also* inflammatory
    bowel disease
cromolyn 412
cryoablation, rectal cancer 106
cryptoglandular infection 87, 93
Cryptosporidium spp. 324, 370, 371–372
CT scanning
    colorectal patients 64, 102
    diverticular disease 191
    fistula 87–88, 195
cultural aspects, stoma patients
    181–182
Cyclospora, HIV/AIDS patients 370
Cyclosporiasis infection 372–372
cyclosporin 134, 410–411
cytomegalovirus 322–323, 326

defecation
    adequate cleaning 79, **82**, 86
    deferred *see also* call to stool 26, 208,
        231
    frequency and ease 80
    mechanisms 40
    nervous control 207–208
    normal process 22, 26, *27*, 207–208
    position 217, 231, 244
    straining 26, 78, 80
defecation reflex 207–208, 215
defecatory proctography 215, 226, 298
Delorme's operation 383

dentate line 27, 83, 106
descending colon, anatomy 21, 24
desmoid tumours 147, 151, 152–153
diabetes 54, 210, 294
diarrhoea
    colorectal cancer 99
    colostomy patients 180
    and faecal incontinence 294–295
    and irritable bowel syndrome
        232–233
diarrhoea *see also* bowel habit
dicyclomine (Merbentyl) 233
diet, changing 80, 215
dietary aspects
    colorectal cancer 108–111
    constipation 208–209
    diverticular disease 189–190,
        201–202
    faecal incontinence 298
    inflammatory bowel disease 136–137
    irritable bowel syndrome 230, 233,
        237–238
    paediatric 342, 348, 355
    pruritus ani 86
    stoma care 180
    volvulus 387
dietary fibre 109, **203**, 208–209, 215,
    232, 237, 413
    and diverticular disease 201–202
    food content **200**
    increasing 231
    supplementary 80
difenoxin 412
digital examination 56–57, 62, 77–78,
    93, 100, 214, 381
digitation (manual evacuation) 206,
    212, 380
diphenoxylate (Lomotil) 298, 412
direct sphincter repair 302
disease states, and drug metabolism 403
diverticular disease
    abdominal pain 199
    abscess 194
    aetiology 190
    bowel habit change 199
    chronic 64
    clinical features 190–191, 199
    colon 188–204
    complications 192–198

and constipation 211
diagnosis and investigation 191
dietary aspects 189–190, 201–202
epidemiology 188–189, 190, 201
Hinchey staging 196
laparoscopic approach 198
medical history 199
nursing aspects 198–201
and obstruction 195–196, 197–198
pathophysiology 189–190
patient assessment 199
patient education 199, 202
sigmoidoscopy 195
surgical treatment 192
diverticular disease *see also* diverticulitis;
    diverticulosis
diverticulitis
    acute 192–194
    definition 188
    and fistula 195
    inpatient therapy 196–198
    outpatient therapy 196
    surgical treatment 193–194
diverticulosis
    definition 188
    endoscopy *189*
double-barrelled colostomy 171
Down's syndrome 339
Drapolene 299
drug excretion, kidney 403, 405
drug interactions 404–406, **407**
drug therapy
    age aspects 401–406
    compliance 80, **82**, 406
    faecal incontinence 298
    paediatric patients 403–404
drug toxicity, age effects 403
drug-induced megacolon 387
Dukes' staging, colorectal cancer 101,
    106
duodenoscopy, side-viewing 150, 154
duplication cysts, and intussusception
    394

elderly patient, drug therapy 401–403
electromyography 65
electrophysiology 65, 298
electrosurgery 277

elimination diets 239–240
embarrassment for patient
    enema 216
    faecal incontinence 68
    history taking 68, 380, 381
    inflammatory bowel disease 127,
        129, 130
    investigations 68, 296–297
    pilonidal disease 84
    pruritus ani 85
emergencies
    anal conditions 92–95
    perforation 197
emergency procedures
    laparoscopic appendectomy
        264–265
    laparotomy 323
    stoma formation 175
    volvulus reduction 390
emollient laxatives 413
emollients and protective agents 416
encopresis (overflow incontinence) 43,
    350
end (permanent) ileostomy 173
endocrine adenoma 148
endoscopy
    and abdominal pain 71
    diverticular disease *189*, 191
    inflammatory bowel disease 124–126
    irritable bowel syndrome 226
enema, embarrassing for patient 216
enema administration 69, 351
Entamoeba histolytica infections 323, 325,
    373–374
enterostomal therapist *see* stoma care
    nursing
enteroviruses (non-polio) 369–370
epidermoid cysts 148
episiotomy 54, 293
Escherichia coli infections 362–363
Eurofap 161
examination *see also* physical
    examination
examination under anaesthetic 77–78,
    93, 94, 327
external anal sphincter *see* anal
    sphincters
extrasphincteric fistula 87

faecal continence
  normal mechanism 40–46, 295,
    350–351
  postoperative 348–350
  prognosis 349
  psychological aspects 293
  and sensory innervation 40
faecal continence *see also* faecal
    incontinence
faecal diversion 262
faecal impaction 23, 54, 293, 298, 320,
    414
faecal incontinence
  and anal sphincter damage 293
  anorectal malformation patients
    348–350
  appliances 292, 299
  assessment 296
  biofeedback therapy 299
  causes 54, 293–295
  and diarrhoea 294–295
  dietary aspects 298
  drug therapy 298
  embarrassing for patient 68
  examination 57
  investigations 296–298
  key symptoms 52
  multidisciplinary management
    295–196
  odour 299
  physiotherapy 299
  postoperative 23, 31, 81–82, 83, 92,
    294
  prevalence 292
  and rectal prolapse 381
  school problems 292, 350, 356
  sexual problems 292
  social support 299–300
  surgical management 300–314
faecal matter, volume 22, 207
faeces *see* stool
familial adenomatous polyposis (FAP)
  epidemiology 149–150
  extracolonic manifestations 147–154
  Gardner's syndrome 147
  high-risk patients 102
  historical aspects 146–147
  incidence 146
  patient education 110–111, 160–161

registries 156–162
screening 154
surgical options 154–155
familial polyposis coli *see* familial
    adenomatous polyposis
family history, colorectal cancer 100
fat intolerance 299
fertility, and inflammatory bowel disease
    132
fibre *see* dietary fibre
fistula
  CT scan 195
  and diverticulitis 195
  formation 188
  and hysterectomy 195, 197
  incidence, gender differences 87
fistula *see also* individual fistulae
flatus
  distinguishing from faeces 24, 26,
    142, 295
  in irritable bowel syndrome 224,
    225, 230
Fleet's enema 59, 61, 274, 351
fluid intake 80, 109, 202, 209, 215, 216,
    231, 234
fluid replacement *see* rehydration
5-fluorouracil 107
foam dressings 84, 85
folinic acid 107
folliculitis 92–93
food hygiene *see* infectious colitis
food intolerance, and irritable bowel
    syndrome 226, 233, 237, 239–241
fulguration, rectal lesions 59, 106
Fybogel *see* bulking agents

gangrene 388, 389, 390, 392–393
Gardner's syndrome 147
garlic (*Allium stratum*) 110, 241
gastric and duodenal polyps 149–150
gastrocolic reflex 217
gastroenteritis
  Aeromonas 358–360
  and irritable bowel syndrome 242
gastrointestinal infections, HIV/AIDS
    370
gastrointestinal tract defects 335
gastrointestinal tract function, age effects
    402

gelatine 298
gender differences
    anal canal anatomy 27
    anal fistula incidence 87
    caecal volvulus 390
    colonic transit time 41
    colorectal cancer 87, 98
    cryptoglandular sepsis 93
    desmoid tumours 153
    hidradenitis suppurativa 86
    inflammatory bowel disease 119,
        129–130
    intussusception 393
    irritable bowel syndrome 222
    lymphatic drainage 37
    postoperative sexual complications 39
    rectal anatomy 25
genetic factors, colorectal cancer 97,
    102, 110–111
Giardia lamblia infection 325, 374–375
glycerine trinitrate ointment 83
gonorrhoea 318–319
gracilis neosphincter 303–308, **309**
gut flora 28, 239–240

haemorrhagic colitis 362
haemorrhoidal disease
    and anal seepage 76
    anorectal preparations 416
    causes 78
    classification 79
    investigations 77
    nursing management 80, 81
    prolapsing 54, 68
    strangulated haemorrhoids 94
    surgical treatment 81–82
    thrombosed external haemorrhoids
        95
    treatment 80–84
Hartmann procedure 171, 193, 197,
    198, 390
Hasson technique 262
health food products 230
heat, external application 232
Helicobacter 124
helminth infections 376
hemicolectomy 21, 103, *104*
herbal medicines 110, 250–251
hereditary nonpolyposis colorectal

cancer (HNPCC) 102, 111, 156,
    157
herpes simplex virus 320–321, 323
hidradenitis suppurativa 86–87, 92
high-risk patients, colorectal cancer 61,
    102, 111
Hinchey staging, diverticular disease
    194, 196
Hirschsprung's disease 169, 212, 215,
    218
history taking, embarrassing for patient
    68, 380, 381
HIV/AIDS patients
    anal ulcerations 326
    Cryptosporidium infection 370
    Cyclospora infection 370
    cytomegalus infection 322–323
    gastrointestinal infections 370
    infectious protocolitis 324–325
    Isospora infection 370
    Microsporidium infection 370
    Mycobacterium avium-intercellulare
        infection 324
HNPCC *see* hereditary nonpolyposis
    colorectal cancer (HNPCC)
homeopathy 246–247
hormonal therapy, desmoid tumours
    153
hospital patients
    constipation 210
    easy access to toilet 128, 135
human papilloma virus (HPV) infection
    54, 321–322
hydrocortisone 416
hygiene *see* infectious colitis
hyoscine hydrobromide (Buscopan) 234
hypertrophic retinal pigmentation
    (CHRPE) 148, 156
hypnotherapy 137, 247–248
hypothyroidism, and constipation 210
hysterectomy, and fistula 195, 197

IBS Network 229, 233, 236, 251–252,
    253, 255
ileoanal pouch 141, 155, 218
ileocaecal sphincter 22–23
ileocolitis 322
ileorectal anastomosis (IRA) 155
ileostomy

end (permanent) 139, 173
inflammatory bowel disease 171
loop (temporary) 138, 142, 155,
        172–173, 193
output 142, 173
Ileostomy and Internal Pouch Support
        Group 145
imaging studies
    colorectal cancer 100
    constipation 214
    inflammatory bowel disease 126, 136
imaging studies *see also* radiological
        studies, CT scanning;
        ultrasonography 63–64
immune modifiers 410–411
imperforate anus, without fistula
        338–339, 341
imperforate anus *see also* anorectal
        malformation
incontinence appliances 292, 299
infectious colitis 358–377
inflammatory bowel disease
    acute exacerbation 135
    aetiology 119–120
    body image 128
    and colorectal cancer 111
    complementary therapy 137
    diagnosis 124–126
    dietary aspects 136–137
    disease pattern 119
    drug therapy 406–412
    embarrassing for patient 129, 130
    endoscopy 124–126
    epidemiology 119
    and fertility 132
    and growth retardation 128
    ileostomy 171
    imaging studies 126, 136
    medical treatment 133–137
    nursing care 119–144
    odour 129, 130, 132
    patient education 126–127
    psychological effects 126–128, 129
    rectal bleeding 53
    rehydration 135
    school problems 129
    sexual problems 129–131
    and smoking 119
    social implications 132–133

surgical treatment 137–143
symptoms 53
inflammatory bowel disease *see also*
        Crohn's disease; ulcerative colitis
inspection, in abdominal examination 55
internal anal sphincter *see* anal
        sphincters
International Collaborative Group for
        the Study of Familial
        Adenomatous Polyposis 162
intestinal obstruction
    and diverticular disease 188,
        195–196, 197–198
    and fluid intake 414
    and intussusception 393
    laparoscopy 268–269
    volvulus 386–390
intussusception
    in adults 396–398
    associated conditions 394, 397
    definition 393
    diagnosis 66
    gender difference 393
    and intestinal obstruction 393
    paediatric 393–396
    and viral infections 394
irrigation 178–180, 302, 309–310
irritable bowel syndrome
    aetiology 222–223
    and antibiotics 226
    attitudes towards 223–224
    and biofeedback therapy 244–245
    and bloating 224
    and bowel habit change 231
    and *Candida albicans* 240–241
    and complementary therapies
        245–251
    and constipation 211, 231–232
    definition 222–223
    diagnosis 224, 225–228
    and diarrhoea 232–233
    dietary aspects 230, 233, 237–238
    diurnal variation 232
    effect on life 236–237
    epidemiology 222
    and flatus 224, 225
    and food intolerance 226, 233, 237,
        239–241
    gender differences 222

investigations 226–227
and laxative use 226
long-term treatment 235–236
medical treatment 233–236
and menstrual cycle 224
nursing care 228–229
patient education 228, 229
and physical exercise 245–246
presentation 223–225
professional associations 255
and psychiatric problems 242
self-help/support groups 225, 228,
    229–233, 251–253, 255
and stress 226, 237, 242
symptoms 224–225
ischiorectal abscess 87, 92–93
Isospora belli infection 324–325, 370,
    375–376
itching and soreness, perianal see also
    pruritus ani 78–79

jackknife position 56, 68, 69–70
jejunostomy 173
juvenile polyposis 156, 157

K-ras 97, 102, 150
kaolin–pectin 412
keratolytics 416
kidney function, drug excretion 403,
    405
knee–chest position 56
knee–elbow position see jackknife
    position
kock pouch 140
Koenig bag 167

lactobacillus preparations 413
lactose intolerance 226–227, 237, 239
lactulose (Duphalac) 234, 414
lambliasis see Giardia lamblia
laparoscopic surgery
    abdominoperineal resection
        266–267
    advantages 257–259, 272
    appendectomy 264–265
    bowel preparation 274
    clinical trials 198, 258, 270–271
    colorectal 256–285
    colorectal malignancy 269–271

controversial issues 271–272
disadvantages 259–262
diverticular disease 198
equipment 274–279, **280–281**
historical aspects 256–257
intestinal obstruction 268–269
nursing care 272–274, 284–285
patient education 273–274
patient preparation and positioning
    279–282
perioperative evaluation 272–274
postoperative management 282–284
preoperative procedures 274
rectopexy for rectal prolapse 271
right hemicolectomy 267–268
sigmoid colectomy 265–266
stoma formation 262–264
total abdominal colectomy 267
laparotomy, obtaining consent 274
large bowel see large intestine
large intestine
    anatomy and physiology 21–28
    blood supply 33–36
    innervation 37–40
    lymphatic drainage 37
    venous drainage 36
lavatory see toilet
laxative use
    and constipation **209**, 210, 217
    and faecal incontinence 293
    and irritable bowel syndrome 226
    short-term treatment 216
laxatives, types 216, 413–415
Leeds Castle Polyposis Registry 161
left colon
    anatomy 21
    innervation 38–39
    splenic flexure 21, 24
left lateral (Sims') position 56, 70, 76, 77
levamisole 107
levator ani muscles see pelvic floor
    muscles
levator spasm 53–54
LGV 326
lifestyle
    changes 80, 213
    and constipation 208–209
linseed 232, 241
liquorice 232

liver function, age effects 402–403
liver involvement, colorectal cancer
    100–102
local anaesthetics, anorectal
    preparations 416
loop colostomy 170
loop ileostomy, temporary 155,
    172–173, 193
loperamide see also antidiarrhoeal agents
    133, 142, 235, 298, 412
lymph nodes 269–270
lymphatic drainage, large intestine 37
lymphosarcoma, and intussusception
    394

magnesium citrate 414
magnetic resonance imaging (MRI) 64,
    87–88
manual evacuation (digitation) 206,
    212, 380
marijuana, contaminated 364
mass movements, colonic 41–22
massage 137, 232, 248–249
masses, examination 57
mebeverine hydrochloride (Colofac)
    233, 236
Meckel's diverticulum, and
    intussusception 394, 397
medical history 52–54, 76, 199, 213,
    273
megabowel, idiopathic 218
megacolon 213, 214, 326, 361, 387, 414
megarectum 213
megasigmoid 354, 355
menstrual cycle
    and constipation 210
    and irritable bowel syndrome 224
6-mercaptopurine 410–411
mesalazine (mesalamine; Asacol,
    Pentasol) 133, 135, 408
mesoappendix 23
mesocaecum 22
mesorectum 26
methotrexate 411
metronidazole 411
Microsporidium infection 370
Miles procedure (abdominoperineal
    resection) 103, 105
milk of magnesia 414

milk products, intolerance 237–238
missile injuries see trauma
mucous discharge 79, 99
muscle tone, sphincter muscles 24–25,
    56–57, 77, 381
Mycobacterium avium-intracellulare infection
    324
Mycobacterium tuberculosis infection 326

National Association for Crohn's and
    Colitis 128, 145
Neisseria gonorrhoeae infection 318
neoplasms see cancer; tumours
neorectal pouch 23
nervous control, defecation 207–208
neurological disorders, and constipation
    211
neurological injuries 54
newborn, physical examination 334
nicotine 411
NSAID therapy, desmoid tumours 153
nurse specialists, colorectal surgery
    115–116
nurse–patient relationship 68, 72, 113,
    199
nursing care
    after haemorroidectomy 82
    anorectal malformations 332, 334,
       336
    bowel habit re-education 78
    colorectal patient 67–68, 108
    constipation 218–220
    diverticular disease 198–201
    during endoscopy 62, 70–71
    during laparoscopy 284–285
    during screening 112–113
    haemorrhoidal disease 81
    inflammatory bowel disease 126–127
    irritable bowel syndrome 228–229
    laparoscopic colorectal surgery
       272–274
    paediatric patients 332, 336, 344
    preoperative preparation 72–73
nursing care see also stoma care nursing
nursing profession
    UK perspective 1–11
    US perspective 11–18
nutritional assessment, inflammatory
    bowel disease 136–137

obstetric problems 66, 293, 297
obstruction *see* intestinal obstruction
octreotide 413
odour
   faecal incontinence 299
   irritable bowel disease 129, 130, 132
   stoma patients 177, 178
olasalazine (Dipentum) 133
onion (*Allium cepa*) 110
opiates 210, 412
osteoma 148
ostomies *see* stoma
ostomy patients *see* stoma patients
overflow incontinence (encopresis) 43,
   350

paediatric patients
   colorectal problems 332–357
   dietary aspects 348, 355
   drug therapy 403–404
   nursing care 344
pain management, postoperative 301,
   346
palpable masses, key symptom 52
palpation 55, 77–78, 93, 200, 201
pan-protocolectomy 139
para-anal spaces 31–33
paradoxical contraction 212–213
pararectal spaces 31–33
parasitic infections 371–376
paregoric 412
passiflora 235
patient education
   bowel surgery 300
   colorectal cancer 108–111
   constipation 217
   diverticular disease 199, 202
   familial adenomatous polyposis (FAP)
     110–111, 160–161
   inflammatory bowel disease 126–127
   irritable bowel syndrome 228, 229
   laparoscopic surgery 273–274
   stoma care 72–73, 142, 174–175,
     177–180, 273
   toilet use 78, 217, 231, 380
patient support groups *see* self-
   help/support groups
pectinate line *see* dentate line
pelvic abscess 188

pelvic floor muscles
   anatomy 29, *30*, 31
   evaluation by cinedefacography 66
   and faecal continence 295
   inappropriate contraction 212–213
   repair (anterior levatorplasty)
     301–302
pelvic floor neuropathy 293–294
pelvic outlet obstruction 212
peppermint 230, 250
peppermint oil 234, 236
percussion 55, 200
perforation, surgical emergency 197
periampullary carcinoma 151, 153–154
perianal abscess 87, 92–93
perianal area
   anorectal preparations 416
   examination 56–57
   hygiene 142, 299
   skin problems 56, 78–79, 86–86,
     320, 416
   trauma 54
perianal itching *see* pruritus ani
perianal mass, and condyloma 54
perianal pain 320
perianal surgery, wound infection 301
perineal fistula 335, 336–338, 339, *340*
perineal surgery
   advantages 386
   procedures 382–386
   rectosigmoidectomy 383
perineum
   inspection 76
   skin problems 76–77, 346, 348
perirectal abscess, examination 56
peristomal area, skin care 139, 142, 167
peritoneal reflection 26
peritonitis 188, 195, 197
persistent cloaca 341–342, 343
Peuts-Jager's syndrome 156, 157
phlegmon 188, 193, 194
physical examination
   abdomen 55, 200
   anal fistula 88
   auscultation 200
   colorectal cancer 99–101
   importance 54–55
   newborn 334
   position 76

safety precautions 69–72
visual inspection 200
physical exercise 208–209, 216, 232,
    241
    and irritable bowel syndrome 244,
        245–246
physiology, anorectal 40
physiotherapy, faecal incontinence 299
piles
    prolapse 76
    strangulated 79
piles see also haemorrhoidal disease
pilonidal disease 83–85, 92
plague (Black Death) 367
podophyllin 322
polyethylene glycol 61, 414, 415
polyps
    adenomatous 97
    and intussusception 394
    gastric and duodenal 149–150
    snare removal 59, 62, 71
postanal repair 301–302
posterior sagittal anorectoplasty
        (PSARP)
    for anorectal malformations 332,
        339, 341
    postoperative care 346–348
    preoperative care 344–345
    surgical procedure 345–346
posterior sagittal
        anorectovaginalurethroplasty
        (PSARVUP) 342
postoperative care
    colorectal patients 300–301
    laparoscopic surgery 282–284
    posterior sagittal anorectoplasty
        (PSARP) 346–348
    stoma patients 175–180
postoperative faecal continence
        348–350
postoperative problems
    faecal incontinence 23, 31, 81–82,
        83, 92, 294
    sexual dysfunction 39, 73, 139, 175
    urinary dysfunction 39
postoperative sexual activity 131–132,
    301
pouch of Douglas 77
pouchitis 143

pre-investigation preparation 68–69
prednisolone 134, 135
prednisone see also corticosteroids
        409–410
pregnancy
    and constipation 210–211
    and volvulus 391
preoperative preparation
    laparoscopic surgery 274
    nursing care 72–73
    posterior sagittal anorectoplasty
        (PSARP) 344–345
    stoma patients 174–175
privacy and dignity, importance for
        bowel habit 210, 220
proctectomy, total 154–155
proctitis, gonorrhoeal 318
proctocolectomy 162
    restorative 141–143, 155
proctocolitis, infectious 324–326
proctoscopy
    acute anal sepsis 93
    colorectal cancer 100
    haemorrhoidal disease 78
    procedure 57–59
proctosigmoidoscopy 381
professional associations, irritable bowel
        syndrome 255
prolapse
    inspection 77
    piles 76
prone position 56
propantheline bromide (Pro-Banthine)
    234
prostate gland 56, 77
protein binding 402, 404, 405
pruritus ani 85–86, 322, 408–409
pseudomembranous colitis 361
psychiatric conditions
    and constipation 210
    and irritable bowel syndrome 242
psychiatric conditions see also altered
        mental states
psychological aspects
    colorectal cancer 114
    faecal continence 293
    inflammatory bowel disease 129
psychological problems, stoma patients
        174, 175–176, 302

psyllium derivatives 414
puborectalis muscles, and anorectal
    angle 25–26
pudendal neuropathy 81, 294, 298, 301
pyoderma gangrenosum *123*, **123**

RADAR 133, 145
radiological studies
    anorectal malformations 336
    colorectal patients 63–64
    constipation 214
radiotherapy
    desmoid tumours 152
    rectal cancer 106
randomized clinical trials, laparoscopic
    colorectal surgery 198, 258,
    270–271
rectal *see also* colorectal
rectal atresia and stenosis 339, 341
rectal bleeding
    blood tests 62–63
    causes 53
    colorectal cancer 98–99, 113
    haemorrhoidal disease 78
    and HPV infection 322
    inflammatory bowel disease 53
    key symptom 52, 76
    quality and quantity 53, 78
rectal cancer
    adjuvant therapy 107
    local therapy 106
    surgical treatment 103–106
rectal capacity and compliance 22–23
rectal columns 28
rectal myectomy 218
rectal prolapse 54, 66, 68, 271, 379–386
rectal sensation 23
rectal ulcer, biofeedback therapy 380
rectal washouts 299
rectoanal inhibitory reflex 23–26,
    207–208
rectobladder neck fistula 338
rectocele 212, 214, 218
rectopexy 271, 384–385
rectosacral fascia 26
rectosigmoid junction 22, 24, 25
rectourethral fistula 338
rectourinary fistula 338
rectum

anatomy 24–26
    fascial relationships 26–27
    innervation 38–39
'redcurrant jelly' stools 394
reflexology 137, 251
rehydration
    infectious disease 360, 361, 363, 365,
        366, 368, 369, 370, 371, 372
    inflammatory bowel disease 135, 142
relaxation 241, 242–244
repair genes 102
resection rectopexy 385
restorative proctocolectomy 141–143,
    154, 155
retinal pigmentation, hypertrophic 148,
    156
retrograde movements, colonic 41–22
right colon
    anatomy 21
    hepatic flexure 21, 23
    innervation 37
right hemicolectomy, laparoscopic
    267–268
Ripstein procedure 384
road traffic accidents *see* trauma
rotavirus 370–371
roughage *see* dietary fibre

safety precautions, physical examination
    69–72
St Mark's Hospital 87, 147, 151, 155,
    156
St Mark's Hospital Operation Sheet 88,
    89
salicylate 413
saline enemas 351
saline laxatives 414
Salmonella spp. infections 363–364
school problems
    faecal incontinence 292, 350, 356
    irritable bowel disease 129
The Scope of Professional Practice 7–11
screening
    colorectal cancer 111–113
    familial adenomatous polyposis (FAP)
        154
    nursing care 112–113
    sigmoidoscopy 61
sedation 57, 71

segmentation, colonic 41
self-help/support groups
    irritable bowel syndrome 225, 228,
        229–233, 251–253, 255
    stoma patients 73, 143, 166
senna (Senokot) 234–235, 414
sexual activity
    postoperative 131–132, 301, 313
    traumatic 132, 294
sexual function, nervous regulation 39
sexual history, importance 54
sexual problems
    colorectal surgery 114
    and faecal incontinence 292
    inflammatory bowel disease 129–131
    postoperative 39, 73, 139, 175
sexually transmitted diseases 54,
    319–327
Shigella spp. 325–326, 362, 363, 365
shigellosis 365
sigmoid colectomy 103, *105*, 389
    laparoscopic 265–266
sigmoid colon
    anatomy 21, 24
    volvulus 386–390
sigmoidoscopy
    acute anal sepsis 93
    and colonoscopy 80
    colorectal cancer 100
    constipation 214
    diverticular disease 195
    instruments *60*, 69, *70*
    procedure 59–61
    rigid 78
    risk of perforation 59
    screening 61
    volvulus reduction 388–389
simethicone 415
skin problems
    and anal seepage 76–77
    perianal area 56, 78–79, 320, 416
    perineal 76–77, 346, 348
    peristomal area 139, 142, 167
    stoma 167
skin tags 54, 56, 79, 82–83
small bowel lymphoma, and
    intussusception 394
smoking
    and inflammatory bowel disease 119

and irritable bowel syndrome 241
and ulcerative colitis 411
social implications, inflammatory bowel
    disease 132–133
sodium phosphates 414, 415
soiling, causes 76
specimen bags 260, *261*, *265*
sphincter-preserving surgery 105–106,
    141
sphincters *see* anal sphincters
SPOD (Association to Aid the Sexual
    and Personal Relationships of
    People with a Disability) 132, 145
staging, colorectal cancer 37, 66,
    101–102, 106
steroid treatment, inflammatory bowel
    disease 128, 134, 409–410
stimulant laxatives 414
stoma
    classification 165
    granulomas 186
    herniation 185–186
    necrosis 183–184
    problems 139, 182–186
    prolapse 182–183
    retraction 184
    sites 73, *168*, 175, 262
    stenosis 185
    temporary (reversible) 142, 167
stoma *see also* colostomy; ileostomy;
    jejunostomy
stoma care
    appliances 139, 167, 344
    dietary aspects 180
    paediatric 344
    patient education 273
    self-help/support groups 166
stoma care nursing
    history 166–167
    patient education 72–73
    referral 114
    sexual advice 131, 132
    UK perspective 1–11
    US perspective 11–18
stoma formation
    emergency procedure 175
    for faecal incontinence 302–303
    incidence 167
    laparoscopic 262–264

reversal 142, 167
stoma formation *see also* colostomy;
    ileostomy; jejunostomy
stoma patients
    body image 72, 73, 139, 176–177
    cultural aspects 181–182
    follow-up and community care
        180–181
    odour 177, 178
    patient education 142, 174–175,
        177–180
    postoperative care 175–180
    preoperative care 174–175
    psychiatric problems 302
    psychological 174, 175–176
    self-help/support groups 73, 143,
        166
    skin problems 139, 142, 167
stool, gross or occult blood *see also* rectal
    bleeding 57
stool quality 57, 77–78
    colorectal cancer 99
    loop colostomy 170
    permanent colostomy 169
straining at stool 80, 94, 220
stress, and irritable bowel syndrome
    226, 237, 242
strictures 57, 391
Strongyloides infections 376
subtotal colectomy 162
sulfasalazine (Salazopyrin) 133,
    406–408
sulindac 153
suppositories 216
sutured rectopexy 384
syphilis 319, 326

TAC *see* total abdominal colectomy
taeniae coli 21–22, 23
tenesmus 99, 318, 320, 325, 360
Thiersch wire (anal encirclement
    procedure) 382
thrombosed external haemorrhoids 94,
    95
TME *see* total mesorectal excision
toilet
    ease of access 128, 132, 133, 225,
        232, 233, 252, 292
    hospital patients 128, 135

optimum use 217, 231, 380
    prolonged sitting 78, 80
toilet training 349, 350
total abdominal colectomy (TAC) 155
    laparoscopic 267
total colectomy 138, 155, 267
total mesorectal excision (TME) 106
total proctocolectomy with ileostomy
    154–155
toxinogenic diarrhoea 366
TPC *see* total proctocolectomy
transanal endoscopic surgery 106
transanal excision, rectal cancer 106
transanal ultrasound *see* anorectal
    ultrasonography
transverse colon, anatomy 21, 24
transverse loop colostomy 198
trauma, anorectal 54, 66, 87, 298, 313
traveller's diarrhoea 227, 360, 375
Treponema pallidum 319
tuberculosis, and anal fissure 87, 90
tumours
    and constipation 212
    recurrence (wound implantation)
        270
tumours *see also* cancer
Turcot syndrome 147
typhoid fever 363–364
ulcerative colitis
    associated conditions **123**
    corticosteroid treatment 409–410
    disease pattern 119, *120, 122*
    signs and symptoms **123**
    and smoking 411
    surgical treatment 138–143
ulcerative colitis *see also* inflammatory
    bowel disease
ulcers, idiopathic 326
ultrasonic scalpel 260, *261,* 267, 268,
    277
ultrasonography
    abdominal 335
    anorectal 66, 102, 106, 297–298
    equipment *67*
    fistula 87–88
ureters, vulnerability 24, 271
urinary dysfunction 190–191, 296
    postoperative 39
urinary tract defects 335, 343, 344

vaginal fistula 335, 341
valves of Houston 59
vasoconstrictors 416
venous drainage, large intestine 36
Veress technique 262
vestibular fistula 335, 339–341
Vibrio spp. infections 366
viral infections 367–371
    and intussusception 394
vitamin B12 143, 173
vitamins
    antioxidant effects 110
    deficiency 210
volvulus
    caecum 390–393
    definition 386
    sigmoid colon 386–390

wasting syndrome 323
water absorption, colon 22, 120, 207,
    209, 211, 212
Well's rectopexy 384–385
wheat intolerance 237–238
worms *see* helminth infections
wound dressings, types 91
wound implantation (tumour
    recurrence) 270
wound infection, perianal surgery 301
wound management 84–85, 86, 90–91,
    106, 160

Yersinia spp. infections 367
yoga 244